PSYCHONEPHROLOGY 2

*Psychological Problems in
Kidney Failure and Their Treatment*

PSYCHONEPHROLOGY 2

Psychological Problems in Kidney Failure and Their Treatment

EDITED BY

NORMAN B. LEVY, M.D.

Professor of Psychiatry, Medicine and Surgery
New York Medical College
Valhalla, New York

ASSISTANT EDITORS

WILLIAM MATTERN, M.D.

Associate Professor of Medicine
University of North Carolina
Chapel Hill, North Carolina

AND

ALFRED M. FREEDMAN, M.D.

Professor and Chairman
Department of Psychiatry and Behavioral Science
New York Medical College
Valhalla, New York

SPRINGER SCIENCE+BUSINESS MEDIA, LLC

Library of Congress Cataloging in Publication Data

International Conference on Psychonephrology (2nd: 1981: New York, N.Y.)
  Psychonephrology 2.

  Bibliography: p.
  Includes index.
  1. Hemodialysis—Psychological aspects—Congresses. 2. Renal insufficiency—
Psychological aspects—Congresses. 3. Kidneys—Transplantation—Psychological
aspects—Congresses. I. Levy, Norman B. II. Mattern, William. III. Freedman, Alfred
M. [DNLM: 1. Hemodialysis—Psychology—Congresses. 2. Kidney failure, Acute—
Therapy—Congresses. 3. Kidney failure, Acute—Psychology—Congresses. 4. Kid-
ney failure, Chronic—Therapy—Congresses. 5. Kidney failure, Chronic—Psychology
—Congresses. WL PS748F v.2/WJ 342 P974 1981]
  RC901.7.H45I58 1981   616.6′14′0019   83-8015

  ISBN 978-1-4899-6671-1   ISBN 978-1-4899-6669-8 (eBook)
  DOI 10.1007/978-1-4899-6669-8

To Eli A. Friedman, M.D.
distinguished nephrologist, inspiring teacher, and friend

Contributors

STEPHEN ARMSTRONG, PH.D. • Associate Clinical Professor, Tufts University School of Medicine; Pediatric Psychology, Baystate Medical Center, Springfield, Massachusetts

BERND ARONOW, M.A. • Psychologist, Psychosomatic Research Unit, University of Hamburg, German Federal Republic

FRIEDRICH B. BALCK, PH.D. • Dipl. Psych., Psychosomatic Research Unit, University of Hamburg, German Federal Republic

JUNE BURLEY, A.I.M.S.W. • Social Worker, University Hospital, London, Ontario, Canada

HOWARD J. BURTON, M.S.W., M. SC. (Hig.) • Assistant Professor, Faculty of Nursing, University of Western Ontario, London, Ontario, Canada

VITO M. CAMPESE, M.D. • Associate Professor of Medicine, University of Southern California School of Medicine, Los Angeles, California

LINO CANZONA, B.S.W., M.S.W., D.S.W. • Associate Professor, Social Work Department, King's College, University of Western Ontario, London, Ontario, Canada

JOHN A. CONLEY, B.P.E., PH.D. • Health Promotion Directorate, Department of Health and Welfare, Ottawa, Canada

KATHLEEN DEGEN, M.D. • Assistant Clinical Professor of Psychiatry, Columbia University College of Physicians and Surgeons; Assistant Attending Psychiatrist, Consultation–Liaison Service, St. Luke's-Roosevelt Hospital Center, St. Luke's Site, New York, New York

ATARA KAPLAN DE-NOUR, M.D. • Chairman and Professor, Department of Psychiatry, Hebrew University and Hadassah Medical Center, Jerusalem, Israel

DENNIS DROTAR, PH. D. • Division of Pediatric Psychology, Associate Professor in Psychiatry and Pediatrics, Case Western Reserve University, School of Medicine, Cleveland, Ohio

MARITA DVOŘÁK, M.A. • Psychologist, Psychosomatic Research Unit, University of Hamburg, German Federal Republic

RICHARD A. FAMULARO, M.D. • Clinical Instructor of Child Psychiatry, Harvard Medical School, Boston, Massachusetts

ANNETTE C. FRAUMAN, R.N., M.S.N. • Assistant Professor, College of Nursing, University of Florida, Gainesville, Florida

HELLMUTH FREYBERGER, M.D. • Professor of Psychosomatics and Chairman, Center of Psychological Medicine, Department of Psychosomatics, Hannover Medical School, Hannover, German Federal Republic

ROBERT JOEL FRIEDLANDER, JR., M.D. • Former Fourth-Year Medical Student, Cornell University Medical College, New York, New York. Present affiliation: Resident Physician in Medicine, New York Hospital, Cornell Medical Center, New York, New York

ELI A. FRIEDMAN, M.D. • Professor of Medicine, Director of Renal Division, Downstate Medical Center, Brooklyn, New York

MARY ANN GANOFSKY, A.C.S.W. • Pediatric Social Service, Rainbow Babies and Children's Hospital, Cleveland, Ohio

DAVID A. GOLDSTEIN, M.D. • Associate Professor of Medicine, University of Southern California School of Medicine, Los Angeles, California

WILLIAM A. GREENE, M.D. • Professor of Medicine and Psychiatry, University of Rochester Medical Center, Rochester, New York

ROBERT W. HAMILTON, M.D. • Associate Professor of Medicine, Department of Medicine; Medical Director, Artificial Kidney Clinic, Bowman Gray School of Medicine, Winston-Salem, North Carolina

RONALD R. HOLDEN, M.A., PH.D. • Researcher, Health Care Research Unit, University of Western Ontario, London, Ontario, Canada

CHASE P. KIMBALL, M.D. • Professor of Psychiatry and Medicine, Division of Biological Sciences, and Professor in the College, University of Chicago, Chicago, Illinois

OSCAR A. KLETZKY, M.D. • Associate Professor of Obstetrics and Gynecology, University of Southern California School of Medicine, Los Angeles, California

NORMAN B. LEVY, M.D.• Professor of Psychiatry, Medicine and Surgery, New York Medical College; Director, Liaison Psychiatry Division, Westchester County Medical Center, Valhalla, New York

ROBERT M. LINDSAY, M.D., F.R.C.P.(C.), M.R.C.P. (EDIN.) • Director of Renal Unit, Victoria Hospital, Faculty of Medicine, University of Western Ontario, London, Ontario, Canada

SUDESH MAKKER, M.D. • Associate Professor, Case Western Reserve University, School of Medicine, Division of Pediatric Nephrology, Rainbow Babies and Children's Hospital, Cleveland, Ohio

SHAUL G. MASSRY, M.D.• Professor of Medicine, University of Southern California School of Medicine, Los Angeles, California

JOHN P. MERRILL, M.D. • Professor of Medicine, Harvard Medical School, Director, Renal Division, Peter Bent Brigham Hospital, Boston, Massachusetts

JOHN NEWMANN, PH. D., M.P.H. • President, National Association of Patients on Hemodialysis and Transplantation, Brookline, Massachusetts

WARREN R. PROCCI, M.D. • Director, Residency Education in Psychiatry, Harbor-UCLA Medical Center, Torrance, California; Visiting Professor of Psychiatry and the Biobehavioral Sciences, University of California at Los Angeles School of Medicine, Los Angeles, California.

JAMES C. ROMEIS, PH. D. • Assistant Professor of Sociology, Department of Family and Community Medicine, Bowman Gray School of Medicine, Winston-Salem, North Carolina

ROGER J. SHERWOOD, D.S.W., A.C.S.W. • Assistant Professor, Hunter College Graduate School of Social Work, City University of New York, New York, New York.

ROBERTA G. SIMMONS, PH. D. • Professor of Sociology and Psychiatry, University of Minnesota, Minneapolis, Minnesota

SUE E. SLEVIN, R.N., M.S. • Psychiatry Nurse–Clinician, Maimonides Medical Center, Brooklyn, New York

CELIA A. SNAVELY, A.C.S.W. • Instructor (Social Work), Department of Medicine, and Social Worker, Artificial Kidney Clinic, Bowman Gray School of Medicine, Winston-Salem, North Carolina

HUBERT SPEIDEL, M.D., PH. D. • Professor and Director, Psychosomatic Department, University of Hamburg, German Federal Republic

JAMES J. STRAIN, M.D. • Professor of Clinical Psychiatry, Director, Psychiatry Consultation–Liaison Service, Mt. Sinai School of Medicine, City University of New York, New York

JON STRELTZER, M.D. • Associate Professor of Psychiatry, University of Hawaii at Manoa, John A. Burns School of Medicine, Honolulu, Hawaii

MILTON VIEDERMAN, M.D. • Professor of Clinical Psychiatry, Cornell University Medical College; Director, Consultation–Liaison Division, Department of Psychiatry, New York Hospital, New York, New York

LOKKY WAI, M.A., PH.D. • Staff, Health Care Research Unit, University of Western Ontario, London, Ontario, Canada

ROSALYN JONES WATTS, ED.D, R.N., • Associate Professor, University of Pennsylvania School of Nursing, Philadelphia, Pennsylvania

ANNE WOODS, M.S.W. • Nephrology Social Worker, Baystate Medical Center, Springfield, Massachusetts

BARNETT ZUMOFF, M.D. • Chief, Division of Endocrinology and Metabolism, Department of Medicine, Beth Israel Medical Center, New York, New York

Preface

This book is the product of the research of its 44 contributors whose work was presented at the Second International Conference on Psychonephrology. Therefore, a knowledge of the background of the Conference is essential to understanding this book.

In 1978 its predecessor, the First International Conference on Psychological Factors in Hemodialysis and Transplantation, was held at the Downstate Medical Center. It fulfilled the need of those working in this area who in the past had to rely upon meetings of specialty organizations to hear presentations by the major contributors in this field. The latter forum is typically restricted in the time devoted to this subject and restricted in its appeal to professional people outside the host specialty group. Therfore, the success of the First Conference was attributed to its interdisciplinary setting and its exclusive devotion to psychological factors surrounding patients with renal failure.

The Second International Conference on Psychonephrology, held on October 3–5, 1981, attracted over 500 registrants from 45 states, six Canadian Provinces, and six other countries. This Conference could not have been held without the generosity of the American Kidney Fund; its National Executive Director, Kay Hatch; her staff; its Community Service Grant; its help in distributing brochures; and its fellowship support of travel for expenses for many registrants. The contract for this book has been drawn up so that all editorial royalties are sent directly to the American Kidney Fund as my personal expression of gratitude to this organization.

I am indebted to the Conference's Program Committee for its hard work and guidance. Its members were Elizabeth Cameron, Elisabeth Enright, Susan Molumphy, and Virgil Smirnow.

The Conference was cosponsored by the Council of Nephrology Social Workers of the National Kidney Foundation; International College of Psychosomatic Medicine, of which Dr. Adam J. Krakowski served as President and Prof. Cairns Aitken as Chairman of its Education Committee; New York Medical College; and New York State Kidney Disease Institute.

Concerning the use of the term *psychonephrology*, Dr. Atara Kaplan De-Nour and I pondered a single word encompassing the scope of the work that we do. We rejected *nephropsychiatry* because it implies only the activity of physicians. The term was inverted to *psychonephrology* and selected because it is interdisciplinary.

This book contains all but two of the papers presented at that Conference, elaborated upon from their time-restricted presentations and updated to the time of manuscript submission to the editors. As in the case of its two predecessors, *Living or Dying: Adaptation to Hemodialysis* (Charles C. Thomas, Publisher, 1974) and *Psychonephrology I: Psychological Factors in Hemodialysis and Transplantation* (Plenum Press, 1981), the purpose of this book is not to review all the literature in the area. All feasible sources were not tapped in creating it. Nevertheless, I believe it gives the reader a good overview of the subject and an excellent update of recent developments by the major workers in this area.

I wish to also thank the Chairman of the Department of Psychiatry and Behavioral Sciences of New York Medical College, Dr. Alfred M. Freedman, for his support of the Conference; Dr. Susan Molumphy, for editing two of the manuscripts, and her secretary Mrs. Nancy Calvert; my family for putting up with me during the strenuous days immediately before and during the Conference; and the book's many contributors. Last but not least my secretary, Mrs. Camille Damiano, deserves much credit for her patience and hard work in helping organize the Conference, for doing the many small and big things necessary to make it a success, and for her work on the manuscripts which constitute this book.

NORMAN B. LEVY, M.D.

Valhalla, N.Y.

Contents

II. Dialysis and Renal Transplantation

III. Renal Transplantation

I
Dialysis

An Overview of Psychological Problems in Hemodialysis Patients

ATARA KAPLAN DE-NOUR

INTRODUCTION

Psychiatry has been involved in chronic hemodialysis from its early stages as a clinical modality of treatment of terminal renal failure. The first psychiatric reports were published in the mid-sixties by Shea et al.,[1] Wright et al.,[2] Cramond et al.,[3] and of course, by Abram.[4,5] Since then many hundreds of papers have been published about psychological aspects of chronic dialysis, yet it is quite impossible to present an overview of the psychological problems associated with dialysis. We find ourselves in the strange position that although the psychiatric research has been going on for more than 15 years, we still lack sufficient knowledge about many of the psychological problems associated with dialysis, and the available information about some of the problems is often contradictory. One can find many reasons for this poor state of affairs. For example, many of the studies are based on clinical observations. While some of these studies supplied fascinating information, they covered only small samples. Comparison of results, replication, and assessment of change have been nearly impossible. Another factor that greatly hampered the psychiatric research in dialysis is the fact that many professionals from the behavioral sciences started to work in dialysis units, too many of them transferring within a short time to less stressful (if not greener) fields.

The aim of this report, therefore, is neither to summarize nor to provide information but to highlight some of the main issues and especially the dire need for systematic, integrated, large-scale, and long-term research.

When speaking about the psychological problems associated with dialysis it should be remembered that we are dealing with three partners. One, of course, is the patient, but over the years it became quite

ATARA KAPLAN DE-NOUR, M.D. • Chairman and Professor, Department of Psychiatry, Hebrew University and Hadassah Medical Center, Jerusalem, Israel.

clear that the family and the medical staff are also partners of great importance. Thus, an integrated study should devise methods to study all three partners. So far this has not been done. Furthermore, an integrated study should try to eludicate (1) the sources of stress for each of the partners, (2) the methods used for handling the stresses, and (3) the reactions of each of the partners to the stresses. The reactions to the stresses are certainly influenced, if not determined, by the methods of handling the stresses. The reactions, therefore, might be regarded as end results and are the observable behavior of patients, families, and staff. These reactions may be adjustive or maladjustive and they may also increase the stressfulness of the situation for one or another of the partners. Thus an integrated study should concentrate on the sources of stress, on the methods for handling stress, and on the reactions of the patients, families, and staff. Such studies have not yet been carried out.

Sources of Stress

Let us have a brief look at what we know or do not know about the sources of stress. As for the patients, very many sources of stress have been described, as briefly summarized in Table 1. However, so far we have actually only inferred that these are indeed major sources of stress. In only one study[6] a small group of patients was asked to rank ten items describing various concerns of dialysis patients: Fear of death was ranked lowest while dependency and loss of mastering were ranked as most stressful. Thus we still do not know the relative importance of the various stresses, nor have we been able to measure them. The list in Table 1 includes the stresses believed to be inherent in the dialysis situation. In recent years it also became evident that interaction with the other two partners may be stressful (Table 2).

Change of roles within the family have been described clinically only.[7,8] It has been possible, however, to measure double-bind commu-

TABLE 1
Sources of Stress—Patients

Loss or threat of loss of external objects
Restrictions
Dietary
Freedom of planning
Loss of body function (body image problems)
Urination
Sexual activity
Increased dependency
Increased aggression
Threat of death

TABLE 2
Sources of Stress—Patients

Change of roles within the family
Double-bind communication from staff
Rejection from staff

TABLE 3
Sources of Stress—Families

Financial and vague general insecurity[a]
Worry over patient; change in patient behavior[b]
Increase in aggression
Change in roles[c]
Patient control + minimal overt communication + withdrawal from social life[d]
Staff attitudes

[a]Holcomb et al.[12]
[b]Shulman et al.[13]
[c]Stewart et al.[14]
[d]Maurin et al.[8]

nication[9,10] and rejection by staff[11] and both attitudes were found to hamper patients' adjustment. Thus it seems quite clear that some of the patients' stresses might be inherent in the chronic dialysis situation. Other stresses, however, are linked to the reactions of the other two partners or to the patients' interaction with them.

Much less is known about the sources of stress for the other two partners. As to families, many stresses were described in a few studies of small groups (Table 3).[8,12–14] Usually no differentiation was made between the stressfulness for the families of well- and poorly adjusted patients.

As to sources of stress for the staff, very many stresses have been described which can be summarized into four categories (Table 4). One could say that the fourth stress—increased aggression—which I believe is extremely important, is already a reaction to the situation and one that indeed increases very much the stressfulness of the situation.

In the present report one cannot go into details about the second question, that is, how patients, families, and staff handle the stresses.

TABLE 4
Sources of Stress—Medical Staff

Patient's interpersonal behavior (uncooperative, hostile, etc.)
Frustration of expectations (chronic patients often psychologically ill)
Doubts about "rightness" of treatment/modality of treatment
Increased aggression (caused by first and second sources listed above)

Yet, before going on to the questions of reactions and adjustment, one has to mention one method for handling the stress, that is, denial. Denial as a major method has been repeatedly described.[15,16] Patients' denial has been measured on the MAPI[17,18] and staff denial was also measured, though by different methods.[19] On a number of psychological tests, patients came out as normal, which was understood to be caused by denial. Furthermore, patients, families, and maybe also staff too often use suppression. Because of that combination of denial and suppression, many people, including myself, avoided for many years any method but clinical observations. Patients, staff, and families do use denial and are inclined to suppress. Yet it seems to be possible to gather meaningful information also by questionnaires. In the following part of the report on adjustment, more attention will be paid to results of such studies, not because these are better studies but because of the wish to demonstrate that large-scale studies are not only necessary, but also possible.

Patients' Reactions/Adjustment

Only a number of aspects will be brought up. *Compliance with the diet* is one aspect of adjustment about which information is badly lacking (Table 5).[20,21] There is little information about patients' compliance or noncompliance, although it is easily measured. Surprisingly we do know something about the personality factors[21] and the staff attitudes that influence compliance.[10]

The problem of *vocational rehabilitation* has received quite a lot of attention. Different studies, however, report very different rates of rehabilitation. Table 6 presents only those center dialysis patients medically fit to work. As can be seen, the study from Australia[22] reported full rehabilitation in half of the patients, while other studies reported much lower rates.[21,23] Some of these differences may be due to variances in definition and criteria. There is no doubt, however, that many factors in addition to the patients' personality and medical condition influence rehabilitation, for example, staff attitudes or social welfare policy.

TABLE 5
Compliance with the Diet

Friedman et al.[20]	Gross abuse 25%
Kaplan De-Nour et al.[21]	Abuse 39%
	Fair compliance 38%
	Good compliance 23%

TABLE 6
Vocational Rehabilitation

Study	No. of patients	Complete	Partial	None
Disney et al.[22]	300	51%	31.5%	17.5%
Strauch et al.[23]	178	29%	—	71%
EDTA statistics		37%	31%	32%
Kaplan De-Nour et al.[21]	95	28%	37%	35%

TABLE 7
Vocational Rehabilitation—Patients

	Patients' rating			
Physician's rating	Complete	Partial	None	
Complete	16	7	8	31 (28.4%)
Partial	2	12	7	21 (19.3%)
None	0	1	56	57 (52.3%)
	18	20	71	109
	(16.5)	(18.4)	(65.1)	
		$\chi^2 = 79.457$		

It should be added that patients do not deny or suppress vocational rehabilitation problems. The group presented in Table 7 is not composed only of patients medically fit to work, a factor which accounts, in part, for the poor rehabilitation. In this group—which dialysed in a number of centers—a high agreement was found between the patients' and the physicians' rating of rehabilitation, with the patients reporting somewhat poorer rehabilitation than the physicians.

As to the patients' *social activities*, there has been only limited and contradictory information (Table 8). It has also been pointed out that passive social activities decrease less than active ones.[23] Altogether, this seems to be another area in which the patients do not deny or repress. Or rather, even if they do, what they report is very bad indeed. The Derogatis psychosocial adjustment to physical illness scale[24] was administered to patients in a number of units. The patients reported sepa-

TABLE 8
Social Activities—Patients

	Friedman et al.[20]	Shulman et al.[13]
No change	55%	22%
Decrease	25%	60%
Marked decrease	20%	18%

TABLE 9
Social Rehabilitation—Interest (118 Patients)

	Unchanged	Slightly reduced	Significantly reduced	None
Individual leisure activities	69	15	17	17
Family leisure activities	43	24	21	30
Social leisure activities	36	28	20	34

$$\chi^2 = 22.53$$
$$p = 0.01$$

TABLE 10
Social Rehabilitation—Participation (118 Patients)

	Unchanged	Slightly reduced	Significantly reduced	None
Individual leisure activities	39	27	34	18
Family leisure activities	39	8	60	11
Social leisure activities	28	21	34	35

$$\chi^2 = 37.23$$
$$p = 0.01$$

rately on interest (Table 9) and actual participation (Table 10) in three fields of social activity. The patients reported severe and differential drops in interest, and an even greater drop in actual participation. An especially high number of patients reported that family leisure activities were significantly reduced. The next analysis (Table 11) combined the patients' reports on interest and participation and highlights once more

TABLE 11
Social Rehabilitation—Comparison of Interest and Participation (%)

	Unchanged	Slightly reduced	Significantly reduced	None
Individual				
Interest	59	13	14	14
Participation	33	23	29	15
$\chi^2 = 17.5$			$p = 0.006$	
Family				
Interest	36	20	18	26
Participation	33	7	51	9
$\chi^2 = 35.77$			$p = 0.001$	
Social				
Interest	30	24	17	29
Participation	24	18	29	29
$\chi^2 = 5.6$			$p = $ n.s.	

TABLE 12
Sexual Relationship (66 Male Patients)

	No decrease	Slight decrease	Marked decrease	Sexual activities have stopped
Frequency of sexual activity	21%	20%	32%	27%
	None	Slight	Constant	Complete
Sexual dysfunction	29%	31%	11%	29%
	No loss	Slight loss	Marked loss	
Sexual interest	35%	23%	21%	21%
	No loss	Slight loss	Marked loss	
Pleasure or satisfaction	41%	21%	15%	23%

the severe drop in interest and in participation, especially in social activities, while in individual activities participation dropped much more than interest. As to patients' sexual problems, it seems that patients do not deny or suppress information. The picture that emerges on the Derogatis scale is grim indeed (Table 12). The 66 male patients were all on hospital hemodialysis. They reported many problems, especially in frequency and somewhat less in interest and satisfaction. Altogether about half of them reported severe problems and a quarter reported no interest, satisfaction, or function at all. One could, of course, argue that the patients are denying and that the magnitude of the problem is even bigger. There is indeed little doubt that the patients are denying the impact of their condition on their wives. Nearly 70% of the patients claimed that the sexual problems do not cause any problems with their wives and only 7% were ready to admit that it caused frequent or constant problems. As to the female patients, compared to the male population, no significant differences were found in the frequencies of the various dysfunctions. More than a quarter of them, however, reported that the sexual problems led to frequent or constant arguments and problems. This statistically significant difference can be understood as indicating that female patients can use less denial or that female spouses are more tolerant than male spouses.

The last, but not least area of psychological problems that should be mentioned is that of *psychological symptoms*. One would imagine that by now there would be a lot of information about frequency of psychiatric symptoms as well as their severity and optimal treatment. That is not the case. Recent British publications found that the psychiatric morbidity on the General Health Questionnaire is only 22% and thus similar to

TABLE 13
Depression—Clinical Assessments

Shea et al.[1]	60% severely depressed
Cramond et al.[3]	About a quarter of patients
Forester et al.[27]	Nearly half of patients
Kaplan De-Nour et al.[21]	33% moderately depressed
	20% severely depressed
Lowry[28]	22% depressed
Farmer et al.[26]	13% depressed

general practice patients.[25] In another study, involving a standardized semistructured interview, it was found to be 31%.[26] Other studies reported different results. Let us take as an example depression, which by no doubt is the most common psychiatric problem (Table 13).[1,3,21,26-28] All the samples were small, the largest including 100 patients. It is difficult to hazard an opinion whether the differences are due to differences in patient population, in units, or in the psychiatrists. Psychological tests which aimed at measuring depression, added information but not clarity (Table 14).[2,12,17,18,29,30] Of course, the fact that different tests have been used does not help. Furthermore, a major question is which tests are suitable to measure depression in dialysis patients. For example, one should hesitate to use any test questionnaire that includes the somatic manifestations or equivalents of depression.

This raises the question of whether the patients themselves can be asked about their psychological condition or whether they will deny or suppress difficulties. Table 15 includes the answers of 120 patients on the psychological distress section of Derogatis' questionnaire. On the whole, the patients do not feel guilty, but only a third of them negated any feeling of depression. A high frequency of feelings of self-devaluation and even of hostility was reported. One can suggest, therefore, that such a questionnaire seems adequate for large-scale studies. In such a way we could learn about the differences between modalities of

TABLE 14
Depression—Psychological Tests

Beck Depression Inventory[a]	70% of patients depressed
Heimler Scale[b]	40% of patients depressed
MMPI[c-f]	Elevated depression scores
KDS-1[d]	Elevated scores

[a]Daly.[29]
[b]Holcomb and Macdonald.[12]
[c]Wright et al.[2]
[d]Fishman and Schneider.[30]
[e]Pierce et al.[18]
[f]Mlott and Mason.[17]

TABLE 15
Psychological Distress (PAIS) in % (120 Patients)

	None	Some	Quite a Lot	Extreme
Guilt	71.0	18.0	8.0	30.0
Hostility	46.0	37.5	9.0	7.5
Depression	33.0	42.0	17.5	7.5
Anxiety	31.0	42.0	18.0	9.0
Body image distortion	44.0	32.0	11.0	13.0
Self-devaluation	38.0	38.0	11.5	12.5
Worry	23.0	35.0	23.0	19.0

treatment over time and even about the effectiveness of our therapeutic interventions.

Families' Reactions/Adjustment

Much less is known about families' reactions or adjustment. One could say that for years the attitude towards the spouses was as that directed to assistants and not to people in distress. The spouse was supposed to be supportive and help the patient to adjust. The advance of home dialysis increased the burden of and our expectations from the spouses.

As the information is limited, it can be briefly summarized. Table 16 presents a summary of the information about symptoms of psychological distress.[12,13,31-34] Reviewing such results is, of course, a problem—again the same story of small samples and a great variety of methods. One is inclined, however, to suggest that anxiety and/or depression are fairly frequent problems. In any case, the information highlights the need to carry out large-scale studies of families, the need to look for correlations between the patients' condition and the family members' relationship with the patient, and to find out the effectiveness

TABLE 16
Psychological Distress—Spouses

Steele et al.[31] (hospital)	No depression (KDS-1 questionnaire)
Shulman et al.[13] (home)	Depression or anxiety in 20%
Shambaugh et al.[32] (hospital and home)	Depression (moderate–severe) in a third
Holcomb and Macdonald[12] (home)	65% at times extremely depressed (Heimler Scale)
Mock and Kopel.[33] (home and hospital)	Higher scores on depression, anxiety, and hostility than before dialysis (MAACL)
Brown et al.[34] (home)	42% often anxious, 48% sometimes anxious

TABLE 17
Psychological Distress—Spouses

Giessen Test[a]	Less attractive, less popular, and more socially incompetent
MMPI[b]	Doing less well at work, in marriage, and in recreation
Sentence Completion Test[c]	Differed significantly compared to matched controls, e.g.:
	Lower goals and aims
	Lower active coping
	Lower self-image
	Less energy in instrumental activities

[a]Spiedel et al.[35]
[b]Mock and Kopel.[33]
[c]Soskolni, unpublished.

of therapeutic interventions. Such studies are badly needed, especially in view of recent studies which indicate that the spouses are in distress even when they do not develop signs of psychopathology (Table 17). The first two studies mentioned in this table[33,35] report the spouses' feeling of doing less well in many areas compared to before commencement of dialysis. The last study (unpublished) to some extent explains that feeling by measuring the severe psychological damage that has occurred in the spouses.

The present report will not include the reactions of the third partner, that is, the staff, as this subject will be dealt with separately.

SUMMARY

During the last 15 years great progress has been made in the technical and medical aspects of chronic hemodialysis. Yet the adjustment of the quality of life of the patients did not improve, nor did the distress of staff and families decrease. It seems that the behavioral sciences have failed to keep pace with the technical and medical progress. One can say that we still do not have sufficient information and knowledge about the psychological problems associated with dialysis and therefore have not been able to devise the optimal methods to decrease the distress. Yet the tools for the necessary research are available. The aim of this so-called overview has been to convey the feeling that further research is badly needed and can indeed be carried out.

REFERENCES

1. SHEA, E. J., BOGDAN, D. F., FREEMAN, R. B., and SCHREINER, G.E. Hemodialysis for chronic renal failure. IV. Psychological considerations. *Annals of Internal Medicine*, 1965, *62*, 558–564.

2. WRIGHT, R. G., SAND, P., and LIVINGSTON, G. Psychological stress during hemodialysis for chronic renal failure. *Annals of Internal Medicine*, 1966, *64*, 611–621.
3. CRAMOND, W. A., KNIGHT, P. R., and LAWRENCE, J. R. The psychiatric contribution to a renal unit undertaking chronic haemodialysis and renal homotransplantation. *British Journal of Psychiatry*, 1967, *113*, 1201–1212.
4. ABRAM, H. S., and WADLINGTON, W. Selection of patients for artificial and transplated organs. *Annals of Internal Medicine*, 1968, *69*, 615–620.
5. ABRAM, H. S. The psychiatrist, the treatment of chronic renal failure, and the prolongation of life. I. *American Journal of Psychiatry*, 1968, *124*, 1351–1358.
6. NORTON, C. E. Attitudes toward living and dying in patients on chronic hemodialysis. *Annals of the New York Academy of Science*, 1969, *164*, 720–732.
7. KAPLAN DE-NOUR, A., FISHER, G., MASS, M., and CZACZKES, J. W. Diagnosis and therapy of families of patients on chronic hemodialysis. *Mental Health and Society*, 1974, *1*, 251–256.
8. MAURIN, J., and SCHENKEL, J. A study of the family unit's response to hemodialysis. *Journal of Psychosomatic Research*, 1976, *20*, 163–168.
9. ALEXANDER, L. The double-bind theory and hemodialysis. *Archives of General Psychiatry*, 1976, *33*, 1353.
10. KAPLAN DE-NOUR, A. The influence of physicians' behavior and teams' attitudes on adjustment of chronic patients. In F. Antonelli (Ed.), *Therapy in psychosomatic medicine*. Rome: Edizioni Luigi Pozzi, 1977.
11. KAPLAN DE-NOUR, A., and CZACZKES, J. W. Nurses' rejection and acceptance of patients. *Mental Health and Society*, 1977, *4*, 85–94.
12. HOLCOMB, J. L., and MACDONALD, R. W. Social functioning of artificial kidney patients. *Society of Science and Medicine*, 1973, *7*, 109–119.
13. SHULMAN, R., PACEY, I., and DIEWOLD, P. The quality of life on home haemodialysis. Presented at the *European Conference on Psychosomatic Research*, Edinborough, 1974.
14. STEWART, S., and JOHANSEN, R. A family system approach to home dialysis. *Psychotherapy and Psychosomatics*, 1976/1977, *27*, 86–92.
15. ABRAM, H. S. Psychiatric reflections on adaptation to repetitive dialysis. *Kidney International*, 1974, *6*, 67–72.
16. SHORT, M. J., and WILSON, W. P. Roles of denial in chronic hemodialysis. *Archives of General Psychiatry*, 1969, *20*, 433–437.
17. MLOTT, S. R., and MASON, R. L. The practicability of using an abbreviated form of the MMPI with chronic renal dialysis patients. *Journal of Clinical Psychology*, 1975, *31*, 65–68.
18. PIERCE, D. M., FREEMAN, R., LAWTON, R., and FEARING, M. Psychological correlates of chronic hemodialysis estimated by MMPI scores. *Psychology*, 1973, *10*, 53–57.
19. KAPLAN DE-NOUR, A., and CZACZKES, J. W. Bias in assessment of patients on chronic dialysis. *Journal of Psychosomatic Research*, 1974, *18*, 217–221.
20. FRIEDMAN, E. A., GOODWIN, N. J., and CHAUDHRY, L. Psychosocial adjustment to maintenance hemodialysis: I. *New York State Journal of Medicine*, 1970, *70*, 629–637.
21. KAPLAN DE-NOUR, A., and CZACZKES, J. W. Influence of patients' personality on adjustment to chronic dialysis. *Journal of Nervous and Mental Disease*, 1976, *162*, 323–333.
22. DISNEY, A. P. S., ROW, P. G. Australian maintenance dialysis survey. *Medical Journal of Australia*, 1974, *2*, 651–656.
23. STRAUCH, M., HUBER, W., RAHAUSER, G., WERNER, J., WALZER, P., and HAFNER, H. Rehabilitation in patients undergoing maintenance haemodialysis: Results of a questionnaire in 15 dialysis centres. In J. S. Cameron (Ed.), *Proceedings, European Dialysis and Transplant Association*. Great Britain: Pitman Medical, 1971.

24. MORROW, G. R. CHIARELO, R. J., and DEROGATIS, L. R. A new scale for assessing patients' psychosocial adjustment to medical illness. *Psychological Medicine*, 1978, *8*, 605–610.
25. LIVESLEY, W. J. Psychiatric disturbance and chronic haemodialysis. *British Medical Journal*, 1979, *2*, 306–308.
26. FARMER, C. J., SNOWDEN, S. A., and PARSONS, U. The prevalence of psychiatric illness among patients on home haemodialysis. *Psychological Medicine*, 1979, *9*, 509–514.
27. FOSTER, F. G., and MCKEGNY, F. P. Small group dynamics and survival on chronic hemodialysis. *International Journal of Psychiatry in Medicine*, 1977/78, *8*, 105–115.
28. LOWRY, M. R. Frequency of depressive disorder in patients entering home hemodialysis. *Journal of Nervous and Mental Disease*, 1979, *167*, 199–204.
29. DALY, R. J. Psychiatric aspects of maintenance haemodialysis. In *Proceedings, 4th International Congress of Nephrology*, Vol. 3. Basel/Munchen/New York: Karger, 1970.
30. FISHMAN, D. B., and SCHNEIDER, C. J. Predicting emotional adjustment in home dialysis patients and their relatives. *Journal of Chronic Disease*, 1972, *25*, 99–109.
31. STEELE, T. E., FINKELSTEIN, S. H., and FINKELSTEIN, F. O. Hemodialysis patients and spouses. *Journal of Nervous and Mental Disease*, 1976, *162*, 225–237.
32. SHAMBAUGH, P. W., HAMPERS, C. L., BAILEY, G. L., SNYDER, D., and MERRILL, J. P. Hemodialysis in the home—Emotional impact on the spouse. *Transactions, American Society for Artificial Internal Organs*, 1967, *13*, 41–45.
33. MOCK, L. A. T., and KOPEL, K. Psychosocial aspects of home and in-center dialysis. *Dialysis and Transplantation*, 1977, *6*, 36–43.
34. BROWN, T. M., FEINS, A., PARKE, R. C., and PAULUS, D. A. Living with long-term home dialysis. *Annals of Internal Medicine*, 1974, *81*, 165–170.
35. SPEIDEL, H., KOCH, W., BALCK, F., and KNIESS, J. Problems in interaction between patients undergoing long-term hemodialysis and their partners. Presented at the *4th Congress of the International College of Psychosomatic Medicine*, Japan, 1977.

2

Staff's Problems and Staff's Affective Reactions to Dialysis Patients' Problems

FRIEDRICH B. BALCK, MARITA DVOŘÁK, HUBERT SPEIDEL, AND BERND ARONOW

INTRODUCTION

Attending to and working with patients suffering from chronic renal disease in clinical dialysis is a difficult and psychologically stressful task for the staff.[1,2] According to Czaczkes and Kaplan De-Nour[3] the stress has three main sources: tension between staff and patients, emotional and physical setbacks, and doubts about the effectiveness of dialysis for improving quality of life for the chronically ill patient. The first two stress sources are assumed to lead to an increase of aggression, while the doubts are often handled by reaction formation and overcompensation which in turn lead to high expectation for the patient's medical and psychological adjustment.

The staff's cognitive, affective, and behavioral reactions to the patient with chronic renal failure can be described by the coping strategies and defense mechanisms chosen by the staff members. According to Lipowski[4] coping strategies imply cognitive and motor activities which are selected in an active struggle with the stressful situation and which serve the function of restoring or preserving psychological integrity.

Abram[5] lists three different staff reactions:

1. Exaggerated and excessive concern as well as identification with the patient's problems

FRIEDRICH B. BALCK, PH.D. • Dipl. Psych., Psychosomatic Department, University of Hamburg, German Federal Republic.   MARITA DVOŘÁK, M.A. • Psychologist, Psychosomatic Research Unit, University of Hamburg, German Federal Republic.   HUBERT SPEIDEL, M.D., PH.D. • Professor and Director, Psychosomatic Department, University of Hamburg,   German Federal Republic.   BERND ARONOW, M.A. • Psychologist, Psychosomatic Research Unit, University of Hamburg,   German Federal Republic.

2. Irritation and rejection of the patient who does not cooperate well with the team
3. Indifference as a defense against one's own helplessness and hopelessness

The main defense mechanisms used by the staff according to Czaczkes and Kaplan De-Nour[3] are: regression, denial, and displacement. Defense mechanisms are defined as processes of the ego which do not (in contrast to the coping strategies) imply an active confrontation with the anxiety-producing situation, but represent attempts to reject reality or its significance for the individual.[6]

This paper describes the results of a survey in which 53 dialysis staff members in Hamburg, Germany, participated. The survey was an attempt to investigate the emotional reactions and the resulting behavior of a medical team to its work situation and to the patient with chronic renal failure. First, the stressful elements and the amount of stress the team is confronted with are described. Second, dialysis team members were asked by what means they try to reduce the stress and these results are described.

The patient's most crucial problem is his dependence on the dialysis machine. In clinical dialysis this dependence is transmitted to the medical team. The questions arising from this situation are: To what extent do nurses and physicians recognize the patient's feelings of dependence, and how does the staff react to them?

Czaczkes and Kaplan De-Nour[3] emphasized the significance of the team attitude towards certain characteristics of the dialysis treatment, for instance, restriction of fluid intake, diet, and range of weight gain. We tried to find out how much importance the staff attached to these aspects of the dialysis treatment and in what way they are related to measures by which the patient's activity can be increased.

It is a common view that patients use a lot of denial to handle their problems. In this respect we were interested in the staff's assessment of the patient's willingness to communicate. We also wanted to know whether nurses and physicians wish to establish a close personal relationship with the dialysis patients and in what way they respond to the patients' offer to talk about personal problems.

The results presented are part of a more extensive study carried through in various dialysis units in the Hamburg area (Federal Republic of Germany) by a research team in a special research department of the Hamburg University. The staff of eight dialysis units was interviewed by means of a questionnaire. Most of the items had to be answered on a 6- or 7-point scale, a few were open questions.

Of the 165 questionnaires distributed only 32% were sent back to us. This relatively low return rate calls for two comments:

1. The sample will show a selection effect. It is impossible to judge the degree and direction of selection. At any rate it will make the interpretation of our results difficult.
2. The low return rate allows an inference about the stressful psychological team situation. It can be assumed that those members of the staff who responded are more ready to communicate, more open-minded, and possibly more stressed and dissatisfied. A selection effect of this kind can be expected to affect the coping mechanisms used by them.

DESCRIPTION OF THE SAMPLE ACCORDING TO SOCIODEMOGRAPHIC DATA

Of 53 persons investigated, 15 are male and 38 female. The mean age is 30 years for the nurses and 32.9 years for the physicians. The mean experience in a dialysis unit is 42 months for the nurses and 48 months for the physicians. This rather long work experience does not support the high fluctuation rate for dialysis teams found by other authors (Table 1).[3]

Outside of the dialysis unit the members of the eight medical teams have a very diversified work experience. Their experience ranges from wards of internal medicine, psychiatry, and pediatry to wards more related to dialysis, such as intensive care units (Table 2).

STRESSES IN THE DIALYSIS TEAM AND MODES OF COPING

The stressful work in a dialysis unit has often been described. The close contact with the patient (sometimes over many years), the confrontation with his personal problems, and the helplessness induced by his chronic disease can cause intense feelings of tension and stress. When

TABLE 1
Sociodemographic Data of the 35 Nurses
and 18 Physicians

	Nurses	Physicians
Sex		
Male	5	10
Female	30	8
Age	$\bar{x}$: 30 years	$\bar{x}$: 32.9 years
Average vocational experience in a dialysis unit	$\bar{x}$: 42 months	$\bar{x}$: 48 months

TABLE 2
Previous Occupation of the Nurses and Physicians

	Nurses		Physicians	
	n	%	n	%
Infection	16	19.2	25	50
Surgery	19	22.8	10	20
Gynecology	6	7.2	4	8
Intensive Care	13	15.6	7	14
Psychiatry	10	12	1	2
Pediatrics	5	6		
Ear, nose, + throat	2	2.4		
Orthopedics	1	1.2		
Outside the hospital	8	9.6		
Other departments	3	3.6		
Radiology			1	2
Dermatology			2	4
Number of responses	83		50	

TABLE 3
Rank Order of Stressful Situations in the Dialysis Unit

	Nurses	Physicians
Intrateam tensions	1	2
Death of a patient	2	1
Deterioration of health	3	3
Time pressure	4	4
Problem talks with patients	5	7
Drop of blood pressure during dialysis	6	5
Noncompliance	7	6
Machine alarm	8	8

asked for the main factors that create tension on a dialysis ward, nurses and physicians mention the death of a fellow patient and slow deterioration of a patient's health condition (Table 3). A source of stress equally important as the stress originating from the patient is tension within the team. Tension in nurses is often the result of being involved in team as well as patient stresses. A fourth source of stress is time pressure. Time pressure constitutes a link between the patient-originated and team-originated stressors because it results from dealing with acute and critical dialysis situations within the typical constraints of understaffed facilities.

On the basis of the relatively intense work pressure on a dialysis ward it is not surprising that 47% of the nurses and 50% of the physicians, when asked to compare the stress on a dialysis unit to that in

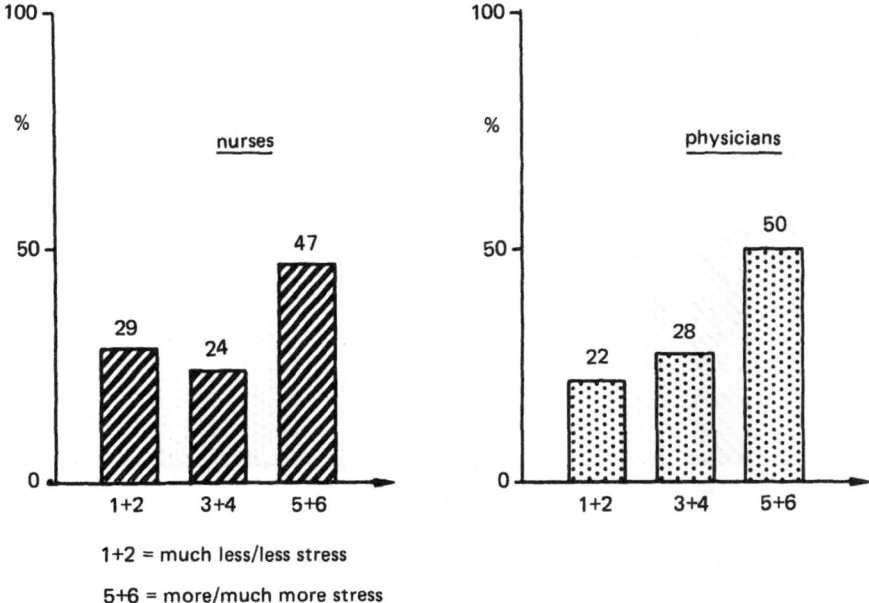

1+2 = much less/less stress

5+6 = more/much more stress

FIG. 1a. Amount of stress experienced on the dialysis ward as compared to other wards.

other departments of the clinic, answer that dialysis confronts them with more stress. On the other hand, 25% of the staff judge the stress as equal to other departments and 29% of the nurses and 22% of the physicians judge the stress as even less than that in other departments (Figure 1a).

Working on a dialysis ward can be viewed as a reduction of stress as illustrated by one nurse's remark. Previously she worked on the surgical ward and had very little contact with the patients. She commented that changing to the dialysis ward made it possible for her to enjoy the rewarding experience of a more direct and prolonged contact with the patients.

Another factor which may be viewed as reducing stress in a dialysis unit is the high level of competence and self-esteem nurses can acquire as compared with the physicians because of the relatively high proportion of routine work.

The experience of high stress mentioned by the majority of the staff is also reflected in the daily experience of exhaustion after work. Fifty-one percent of the nurses and thirty-four percent of the physicians report that they very often or quite often feel exhausted after work (Figure 1b).

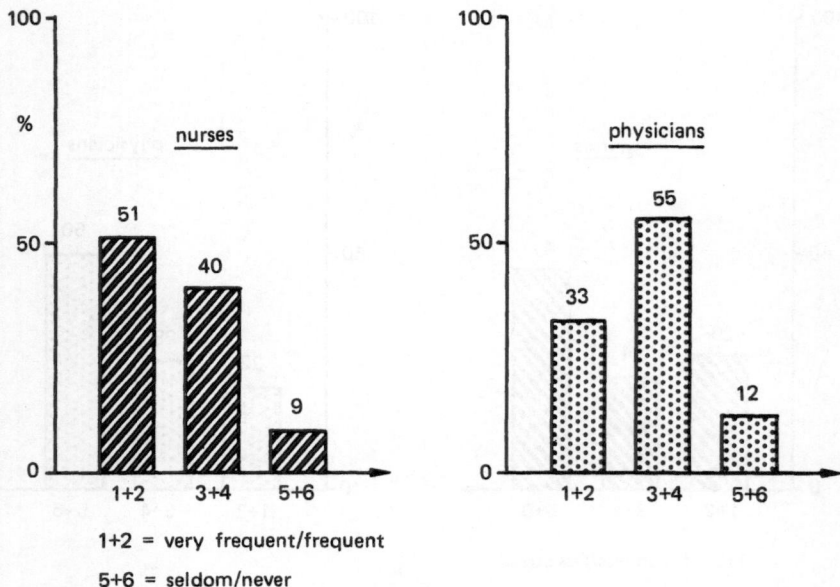

1+2 = very frequent/frequent

5+6 = seldom/never

FIG. 1b. Frequency of daily experience of exhaustion after work in a dialysis unit.

In what way do the members of the dialysis staff cope with stress? One way which is judged as most stress reducing and helpful is to talk with colleagues. But the tension created on the dialysis ward seems to be so serious that 59% of the nurses and 78% of the physicians desire additional stress-reducing conversations with their partners after work (Table 4). The higher percentage for the physicians may be due to the fact that talking to colleagues does not give them as much relief or that they generally integrate their work more into their private life than the nurses do. (On the other hand, perhaps the physicians' role expectations prevent them from conversing about their stress with colleagues or partners—Editor's note.)

TABLE 4
Attempts at Coping with Stress in the Dialysis Unit

Modes of coping with stress	Rank order	
	Nurses	Physicians
Talk it over with somebody	1	1
Recover at home	2	2
Meet other people	3	2
Go out	4	3
Sleep	4	3

Both nurses and physicians indicated recovering at home is the second most stress-reducing coping strategy. These recovering activities seem to be related to the daily experience of exhaustion. Rather than serving as a strategy of coping with the general psychological stress it will function more as a necessary buffer between the work sphere and the private sphere.

The choice of communication with colleagues and partners for reducing stress places some doubt on the often-stated assumption that nurses and physicians have the tendency to deny the problems of the patients as well as their own problems. On the other hand, in interpreting our results we have to consider the bias caused by the low return rate. It could be possible that those nurses and physicians who answered the questionnaire are more highly motivated and open for communication and problems on the dialysis ward, or that our sample does not include that part of the staff which uses defense mechanisms like denial and regression for relief of tension and anxiety.

To the question, "How often are problems occurring with patients talked over in the team?", 74% of the nurses compared to only 44% of the physicians responded with the categories "often" and "very often" (Figure 2a). The nurses obviously make more use of a conversation

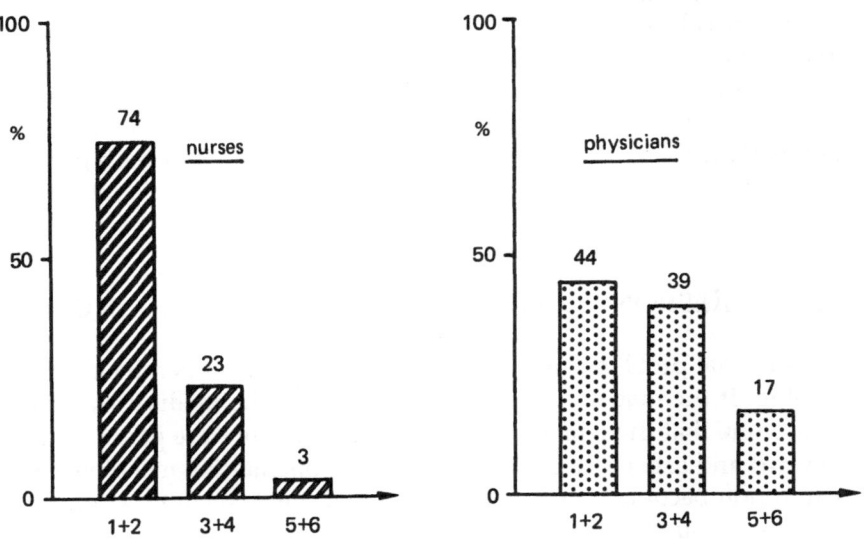

1+2 = very frequent/frequent

5+6 = seldom/never

FIG. 2a.   Frequency of talks about patient problems with team members.

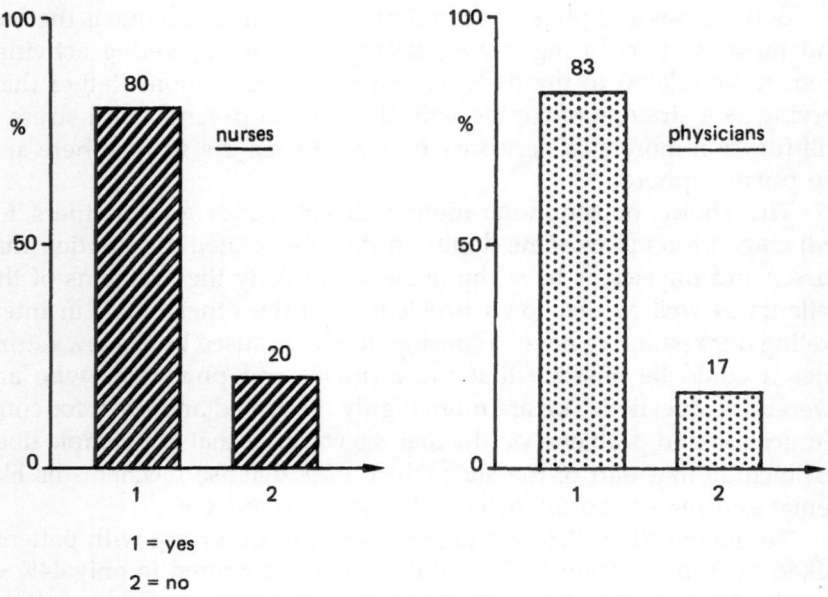

1 = yes

2 = no

FIG. 2b.   Desire for more frequent talks about patient problems with team members.

within the team than do the physicians. This may be due to the greater number of colleagues to be found by the nurses, whereas physicians have fewer colleagues with whom they interact. Beyond the actual rate of conversation 80% of the nurses and 83% of the physicians wish that problems with patients would be talked over in the team more frequently (Figure 2b). Based on the given interpretation, this high percentage is expected for the physicians, while for the nurses it is rather surprising.

STAFF'S RESPONSES TO THE PATIENT'S DEPENDENCE

A crucial problem for the dialysis patient is his dependence on the machine. If the machine is considered a part of the medical ward, one can assume that the patient's feelings of dependence are generalized to the ward and especially to the persons who operate the machines. This assumption becomes even more plausible if one takes into account the patient's constant attempts to master the machine, which means to either integrate the machine into his own body or to dissociate himself from it. In this process the staff as the operator of the machine is viewed as a factor that can be manipulated only to a very small degree. The results are feelings of dependence and aggression.

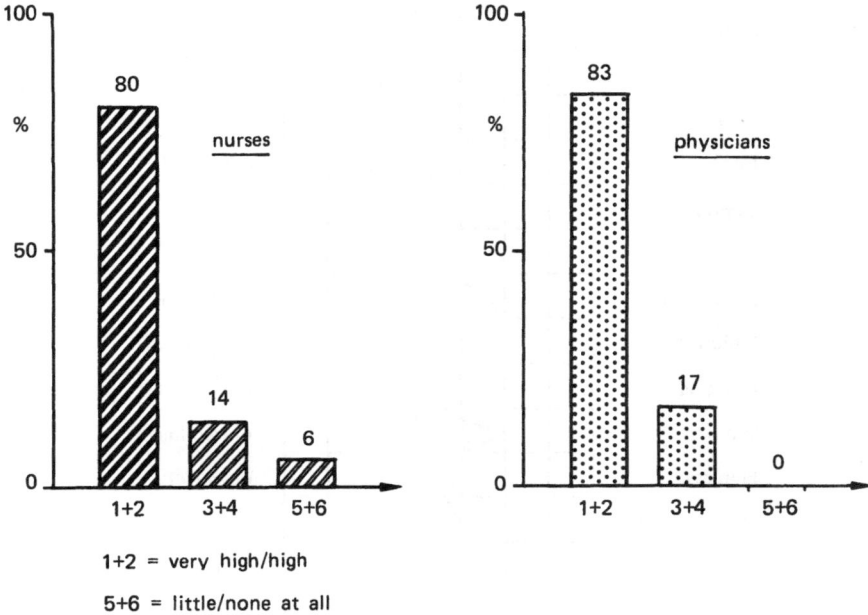

FIG. 3. Amount of consent to the statement of patients' dependence on the dialysis staff.

When asked the extent to which staff members observe dependence on the part of the patients, 80% of the nurses and 83% of the physicians indicated either "to a very high extent" or "to a high extent" (Figure 3).

The nurses' and physicians' emotional reactions to the patient's dependence are presented in Figure 4 in the form of profiles of the mean scores for the two groups. Common to both groups are feelings of tension, concern, and care as well as feelings of confidence and openness. Additionally, the nurses indicate responding with more reactions like compassion, warmth, affection, familiarity, and friendliness than do the physicians.

In general, the patient's dependence is not primarily responded to with rejection, retreat, or aggression. The emotional reactions, especially those of the nurses, rather fit the image of a protective and concerned mother. This behavior, with its constituents of compassion, concern, and caring, when used as an element of therapeutic action is considered by some to further adaptation.[7] Others, however,[3] view it as increasing the patient's dependence and regression and of preventing the expression of aggression.

In an open question we asked the team members to list their emotional responses and resulting behavior towards the patient's depend-

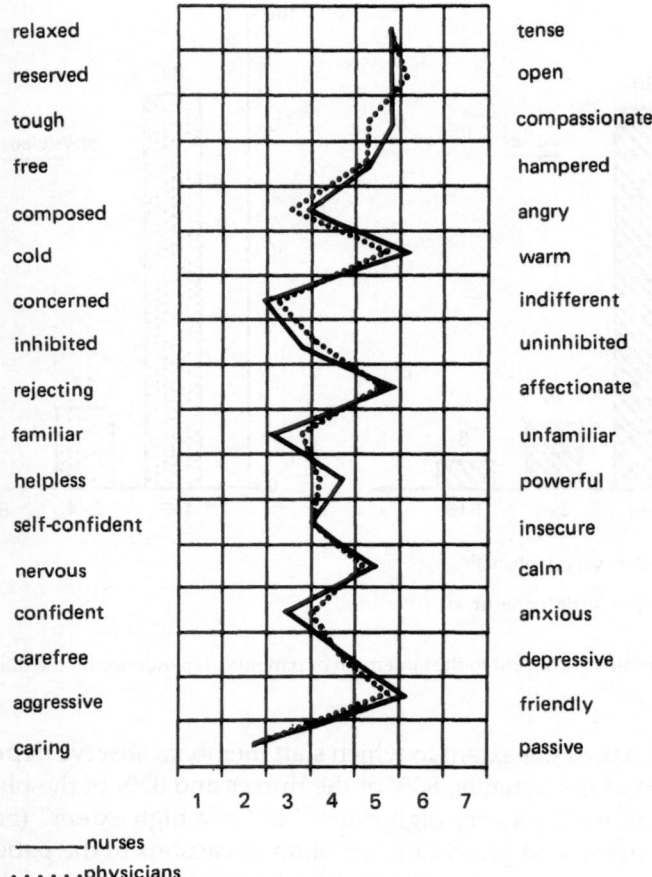

	relaxed									tense
	reserved									open
	tough									compassionate
	free									hampered
	composed									angry
	cold									warm
	concerned									indifferent
	inhibited									uninhibited
	rejecting									affectionate
	familiar									unfamiliar
	helpless									powerful
	self-confident									insecure
	nervous									calm
	confident									anxious
	carefree									depressive
	aggressive									friendly
	caring									passive

1   2   3   4   5   6   7

————— nurses
· · · · · · physicians

FIG. 4. Feelings caused by the experience of patients' dependence.

ence (Table 5). The response frequency shows 21% of the nurses and 20% of the physicians respond with an attitude of rejection, irritability, reserve, or helplessness. Irritability in the sense of open aggression covers only a very small percentage of the answers. Seventeen percent of the nurses and 15% of the physicians show a kind and accepting behavior, and a protective–motherly attitude characterizes 20% of the nurses and only 10% of the physicians. On the basis of the very low aggression rate, some authors (for example, Czaczkes and Kaplan De-Nour[3]) interpret the kind–accepting and the protective–motherly behaviors as reaction formation. One-third of the staff responded that they attempt to reduce patient dependence by encouraging discussion about the dependence and by actively engaging the patients in anxiety-reducing activities.

TABLE 5
Staff Reactions to the Dialysis Patients' Dependence

Staff's response	Nurses	Physicians
Personal reactions		
Rejection		
Wait-and-see attitude		
Helplessness	21%	20%
Irritability		
Anxiety		
Kindness/acceptance	17%	15%
Protective behavior	20%	10%
Attempts to reduce dependence		
Try to get the patient to talk		
Talk about dependence		
Activate the patient	34%	35%
Take away the anxiety of the patient		
Evasive responses	8%	20%

IMPORTANT CHARACTERISTICS OF A "GOOD" DIALYSIS

The relationship between longevity and successful adaptation to dialysis treatment has been investigated. The results show that patients with a high degree of self-control and autonomy and a strong drive to integrate and control the dialysis machine by operating it have a greater chance to survive.[8] Although this behavior is shaped by the patient's premorbid personality structure, it is to a great extent also influenced by the reactions of the staff. Depending on the degree to which it contradicts the team standards, it is either extinguished or reinforced.[3]

In our research we asked the nurses and physicians to rate the importance of some features of the dialysis treatment with respect to the patient's adaptation (Table 6). The correlation between the rank order of the nurses and that of the physicians amounts to 0.68, showing that the degree of similarity is not very high.

Most important for the nurses is the fact that the patient is active and keeps the dialysis times necessary for him. The avoidance of a sudden decrease of blood pressure and the strict adherence to the rules of hygiene are other important criteria for the nurses. This list of criteria reflects two approaches which I should like to call "patient oriented" and "task oriented". The patient-oriented approach, which is reflected in emphasizing the patient's activity, shows the nurses' attempt to support his striving for adaptive behavior. On the other hand the nurses try to achieve a smooth flow of their ward routine. To reach this task-oriented goal, the patient's compliance and the avoidance of complications are necessary.

TABLE 6
Factors Judged as Important for Adjustment to Dialysis

	Nurses[a]	Physicians[a]
Patient's activity	1	1
Adherence to the dialysis time	2	5
Avoidance of blood pressure decrease	2	4
Strong adherence to hygiene instructions	3	3
Restriction of fluid intake	4	6
Patient's assistance during dialysis	4	5
Offering entertainment for the patients (e.g., television, radio, newspaper, games)	5	4
Keeping weight constant	6	8
Social contact between patients	6	2
Quiet atmosphere on the dialysis ward	6	6
Meeting the patient's family members	7	7
Adherence to dietary restrictions	7	9

[a]Nurses and pysicians were asked to rank-order the factors important for 2 patient's adjustment to dialysis

The physicians emphasize the patient-oriented criteria for a good dialysis by rating the patient's activity level and the social contact between the patients as most important. Next to this they list adherence to hygienic rules and to measures, factors which make the stay on the ward more comfortable for the patients. Adherence to the dietary regimen and the necessity of keeping weight within constant limits are considered less important by both groups. As far as restriction of fluid intake is concerned, the physicians consider it a less important factor than do nurses.

The explanation for the greater task orientation observed with the nurses can be their attempt to lessen their work stress by implementing a more rigid control on some part of the work routine. Examples are their time regulations and measures to prevent a drop in patient blood pressure.

INTERACTIONAL BEHAVIOR BETWEEN THE TEAM AND THE PATIENTS

In a dialysis unit the staff has a greater opportunity than in other departments to establish a personal relationship with the patient. However, considering the patient's psychological situation, it can be assumed that his attitude is ambivalent because an intense personal contact implies the danger of breaking down defenses mitigating personal problems caused by his chronic illness.

We asked the nurses and physicians whether the patients are more open and outspoken or more reserved with respect to their social and psychological problems. They had to mark their answer on a 7-point scale with the extremes of "more open" and "more reserved". The nurses' assessment of the patient's readiness to communicate does not differ from the physicians' assessment. The responses of both groups are in the middle range of the scale.

This result can be explained in different ways. It could mean that dialysis patients do not show a unified behavior with respect to their willingness to talk about their social and psychological problems, but instead cover the whole range of possible behaviors. The reason for such a high deviation could be the patient's above-mentioned ambivalence. The result could, on the other hand, also be an assessment effect caused by the staff. It is possible that the staff scores show a regression toward the mean for the variables of proneness towards stress or protective–motherly versus activating behavior towards the patients.

We were also interested in knowing to what extent the team members actually establish an intense personal relationship with the patients. Figure 5 shows the response frequencies to this question. Seventeen percent of the nurses and physicians tend to prefer avoiding personal contact. Three times as many nurses as physicians took a neutral position, and 78% of the physicians versus 66% of the nurses are ready to get involved in a close personal relationship.

What happens if the dialysis patient accepts this offer by talking about his personal and family problems? Do the nurses and physicians

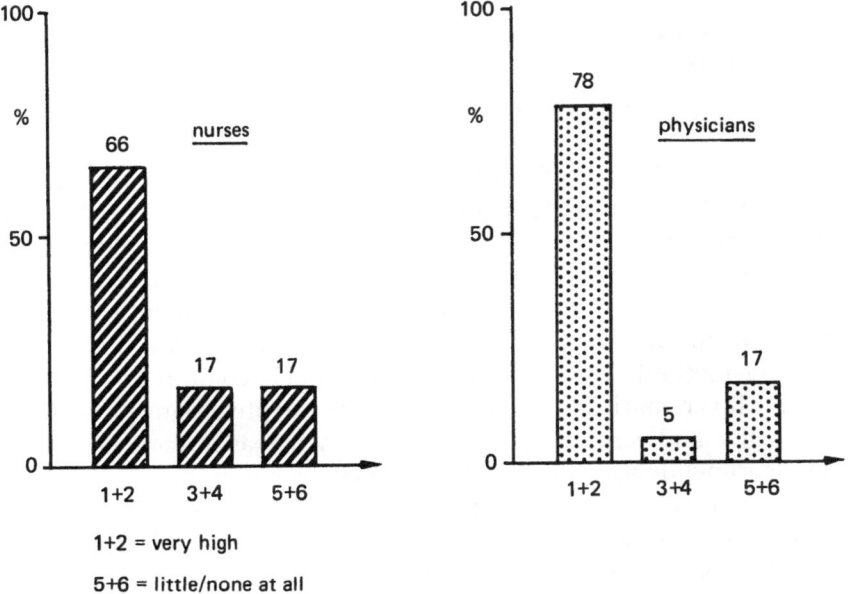

FIG. 5. Tendency to establish an intense personal relationship with the patient.

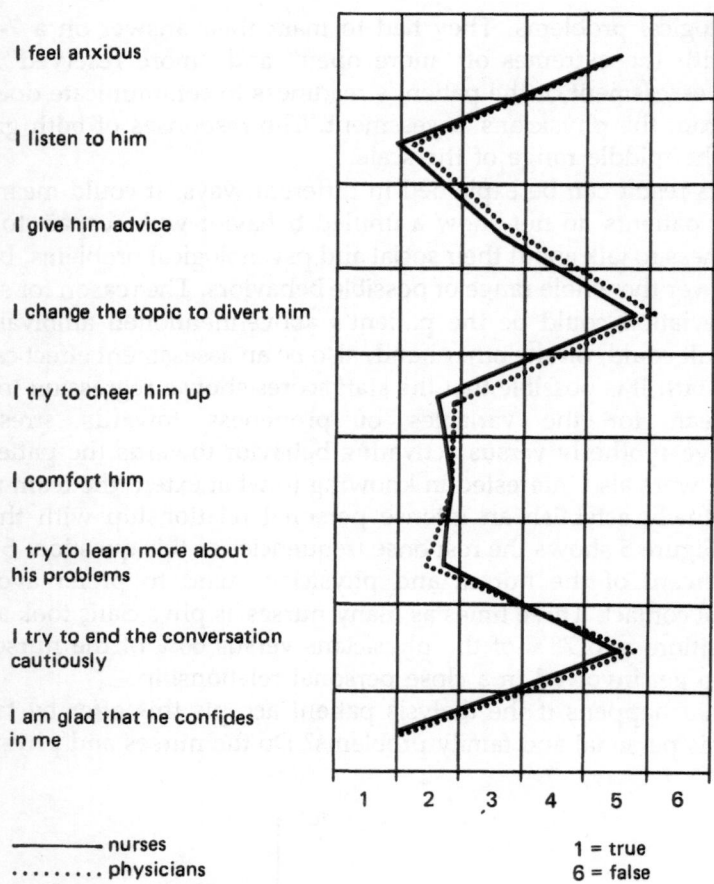

I feel anxious

I listen to him

I give him advice

I change the topic to divert him

I try to cheer him up

I comfort him

I try to learn more about
his problems

I try to end the conversation
cautiously

I am glad that he confides
in me

1   2   ,3   4   5   6

——— nurses   1 = true
········ physicians   6 = false

FIG. 6. Reactions to patients' personal problems.

react differently (Figure 6)? Our results show no significant differences between the two groups. They both start to listen to the patient, they are glad that the patient confides in them, and they try to learn more about his problems. Here we observe again the kind and accepting behavior that is also shown by the nurses in response to the patient's dependence. Also in this instance both nurses and physicians indicate a protective–motherly reaction and the patient gets comfort and encouragement. It is remarkable that in this context the physicians prove to be as protective and comforting as the nurses, whereas in response to the patient's dependence they show this behavior less frequently.

While accepting the patient by listening to him and posing questions to him could lead to a deeper relationship and could help him to find solutions to his problems, we assume that the protective–motherly behavior tends to reduce patient attempts to cope with problems in an active way.

SUMMARY

The study of stress within a team demonstrates clearly the various sources: the organization of the clinic, the ties the team members have with the team, and each team member's interdependence with the patients.

As part of these stress sources, the actual working conditions (for example, time pressure), the atmosphere and tensions within the dialysis team, the deterioration of the patient's physical condition, and finally his death are experienced as stress factors. As stress-relieving factors some members of the staff mention their positive vocational experience as well as talking to colleagues. A large part of the staff members want more opportunity to talk about events on the dialysis ward.

The response to stress on the dialysis ward is a friendly–accepting and motherly–protective behavior. We assume that this behavior is a defense against aggressive tendencies. The nurses' tendencies to promote measures which guarantee a smooth routine on the dialysis ward more than to promote measures which enhance the patient's activity point in the same direction. The ambivalence between the team members' desire to give the patients a greater amount of affection and their actual reserved behavior becomes obvious when they express their wish for more intensive personal talks with the patients on one hand, but on the other hand try to inhibit discussion about problems by their motherly–protective behavior once the patient opens up to them.

To sum up our findings it can be stated that the staff, when confronted with the stress resulting from its daily work routine in the clinic and problems within the team, seems to respond with ambivalence, alternately approaching the patient and withdrawing from him. This ambivalence appears to be intensified by the long time staff and patients work together.

The question about the generalizability of these findings to other medical units cannot be answered. We assume, however, that similar stress factors and reactions will be encountered on clinical wards and rehabilitation units where patients stay for a longer time, where the opportunity for more intensive personal contact is high, and where the patients because of their chronic illness are confronted with death.

REFERENCES

1. ABRAM, H. S. Psychiatric reflections on adaptation to repetitive dialysis. *Kidney International*, 1974, *6*, 67–72.
2. CRAMOND, W. A., KNIGHT, P. R., and LAWRENCE, J. R. The psychiatric contribution to a renal unit undertaking chronic hemodialysis and renal homotransplantation. *British Journal of Psychiatry*, 1967, *113*, 1201.

3. CZACZKES, J. W., and KAPLAN DE-NOUR, A. *Chronic hemodialysis as a way of life.* New York: Brunner/Mazel, 1978.
4. LIPOWSKI, L. J. Physical illness, the individual and the coping process. *Psychiatry in Medicine,* 1970, *1,* 91–102.
5. ABRAM, H. S. The psychology of chronic illness (Editorial). *Journal of Chronic Disease,* 1972, *25,* 659.
6. GAUS, E., and KÖHLE, K. Die Therapie der chronischen terminalen Niereninsuffizienz aus psychosomatischer Sicht: Hämodialyse und Transplantation. In T. Uexküll, *Lehrbuch der Psychosomatischen Medizin,* München, 1979, 789–807.
7. FREYBERGER, H. Psychotherapeutische Möglichkeiten und psychosoziale Rehabilitationsprozesse bei chronisch Nierenkranken im Dauerdialyse-Programm. *Fortsch Med,* 91 Jg., 1973, 3, 93–95.
8. DREES, A. Möglichkeiten und Grenzen einer Psychotherapie bei der Rehabilitation chronisch-organisch Kranker am Beispiel des Dialysepatienten. *Niedersächs Ärzteblatt,* 1976, 17, 564–570.

3

Staff–Patient Interaction

ATARA KAPLAN DE-NOUR

The interaction of the patients and staff of dialysis units is a fascinating subject and probably also an important one. Its importance stems from two sources at least. One is the often-described finding that staff–patient interaction is a main source of stress for the staff. The second reason is that staff–patient interaction can influence or modify the patient's behavior and adjustment. The present report will summarize some ideas and findings about these two aspects of staff–patient interaction.

METHODS

Over the years a number of methods and instruments were used for studies included in the present report (Table 1). Clinical observations were used, of course, both to assess staff behavior and patients' condition. In some instances, however, some aspects of patients' behavior, for example, compliance, were also rated by strict biochemical criteria. In other instances patients' reports on the Psychosocial Adjustment to Illness Scale of Derogatis[1] were used.

In a series of studies, an expectations questionnaire was used (Table 2). Each item was composed of a 5-point scale ranging from "irrelevant" to "good patient adjustment" scored as 0, to "very high" expectations scored as 4. For example, good patients gain not more than a pound in weight between dialyses, or work full time, or have no sign of psychopathology. It was repeatedly stated that the expectations from good and not ideal patients were studied.

Morgan and Cheadle's questionnaire, originally used in psychiatric units, is composed of 20 items.[2] The staff member is given an alphabetical list of the patients and has to put down the names of the most cooperative or the most interesting patients to talk to (preference items), or the most ungrateful ones (rejection items; Table 3).

The ward atmosphere was developed by R. Moos[3] and modified for dialysis units by Rhodes (Table 4). It is composed of 100 statements with

ATARA KAPLAN DE-NOUR, M.D. • Chairman and Professor, Department of Psychiatry, Hebrew University and Hadassah Medical Center, Jerusalem, Israel.

TABLE 1
Methods of Study

Clinical observations
Clinical (and biochemical) assessment of patient's condition
Derogatis PAIS (self-report)
"Expectations"—good patient
Morgan and Cheadle questionnaire
Moos–Ward Atmosphere Scale

TABLE 2
Expectations
"Good" Patient Behavior

Adjustment items:
    Fluid restriction
    K restriction
    Vocational rehabilitation
    Social rehabilitation
    Psychopathology
    Mood
    Anxiety on dialysis
    Nonexaggeration
Obedience items:
    Punctuality
    Argument about orders

TABLE 3
Morgan and Cheadle's
Questionnaire (1972)

Ten questions eliciting preference
Ten questions eliciting rejection

Scoring +1 for every patient name—preference question.
Scoring −1 for every patient name—rejection question.

TABLE 4
Ward Atmosphere Scale[a]

1. Involvement	6. Personal problems
2. Support	7. Anger/aggression
3. Spontaneity	8. Order
4. Autonomy	9. Clarity
5. Practical	10. Staff control

[a] R. Moos

false/true answers which are divided into ten subscales. It should be added that "involvement" measures patient (and not staff) involvement in the unit, but "support" measures mostly staff support. "Spontaneity" measures to what extent the environment encourages patients to express their feelings, while subscale 7 measures the same but is specific for anger and aggression. Maybe it should be added that "personal problems orientation" measures the extent to which patients are encouraged to be concerned with their feelings and to discuss them.

Staff–Patient Interaction—Stress for Staff

After working for some time in dialysis units, it did seem quite obvious that the continuous interaction with the patients is stressful for the staff.[4-6] Gradually the following theoretical outline was developed and over the years an effort was made to gather evidence about it (Figure 1). One could say that the source of all the trouble is the fact that the staff

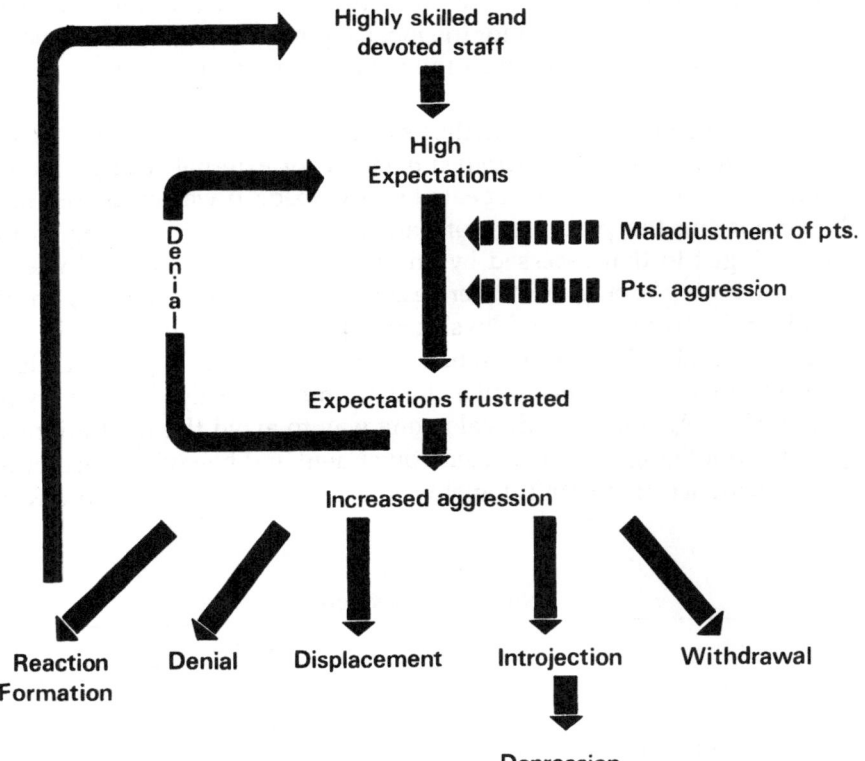

FIG. 1. Medical staff reactions.

members are highly skilled, hard working, and devoted. This, naturally, leads to high expectations that the patients will do well and at least sometimes be somewhat grateful. These expectations are very likely to be frustrated, which leads to disappointment and anger. In our culture anger towards patients is nearly a taboo. Thus the staff members now have to handle their own increased aggression and the main options tend to be as outlined above.

What proof is there, then, for the various points of this vicious circle?

There is proof that at least some staffs have extremely *high expectations* (Table 5).[7] The expectations questionnaire was administered to nurses of four dialysis units. The expectations about obedience were very high indeed in Units A, B, and D. Expectations about adjustment were very high in Unit A. Recently gathered information indicates that the medical staff indeed regard the patients as *aggressive*. The mean score of 108 physicians and nurses in seven units on the subscale of aggression on the Moos questionnaire was 6.75. There were differences between units (analysis of variance was highly significant) but all units described the patients as aggressive; the mean score for the least aggressive unit was 5.3 and for the most aggressive unit, 8.31, compared to an oncological unit in which the mean score on aggression was just under 5.

It has been possible to gather evidence about another part of the outline, that is, about *mobilization of denial* (of external reality). Denial used by the staff has been repeatedly described.[8] It was measured here by comparing the percentage of patients doing well according to the nephrologist to that assessed by an outside team of experts (Table 6). The criteria for "doing well" were exactly defined and agreed upon. By dividing the two members (Physician/Objective) an index of denial was calculated (Table 7). Thus it can be seen that the nephrologists of Units A and B used a lot of denial, while Units D and especially C used very little.[9] Such mobilization of denial is one way to avoid the frustrations of patients not living up to expected adjustment and behavior. Further indirect evidence about staff denial was recently gathered from the ward

TABLE 5
Nurses' Expectations

	Unit			
	A	B	C	D
Mean for adjustment items:	3.30	1.92	2.65	2.95
Mean for obedience items:	3.30	3.41	2.56	3.30
Theoretical range for items 0–4.0				

TABLE 6
Physician's and Objective Assessments

| | | Percentage of patients doing well in: | | | | | |
| | | Compliance | | Rehabilitation | | Psychological condition | |
Unit	No. of patients	Phys.	Object.	Phys.	Object.	Phys.	Object.
A	20	40	20	75	15	55	15
B	23	50	15	60	10	90	70
C	21	70	65	40	40	95	70
D	15	45	25	25	25	65	40

TABLE 7
Physician's Denial[a]

Unit	Compliance	Rehabilitation	Psychological condition
A	2.00	5.00	3.66
B	3.33	6.00	1.29
C	1.08	1.00	1.36
D	1.80	1.00	1.62

[a] 1.00 = no denial.

TABLE 8
Ward Atmosphere Scale: Subscale—Involvement

Unit	Staff assessment	Patients' assessment	t-test
1	6.2	3.9	Significant
2	5.1	3.8	Significant
3	7.5	5.9	Significant
4	5.6	4.9	N.S.
5	5.0	4.7	N.S.
7	5.5	4.5	Significant
8	4.4	3.1	Significant

atmosphere scale on the subscale of involvement (Table 8). This subscale measures how active and energetic patients are in the day-to-day social functioning of the ward. Patients' attitudes, such as pride in the ward, feeling of group spirit, and general enthusiasm are assessed. As can be seen, the staff rated these attitudes in the patients higher than the patients themselves in all the units, and in five of the units the difference was of statistical significance. In other words, the patients were much less involved in the unit than the staff believe them to be.

Thus we are in the position that parts of the outline (Figure 1) are supported by evidence; that is, the high expectations, patients' aggression, and denial of external reality were measured. The methods of handling the increased aggression were clinically described but not usually measured.

Staff–Patient Interaction—Influence of Patients' Adjustment

The second and maybe even more important part of the question is whether staff–patient interaction does indeed influence or modify patients' adjustment. There is indeed some available information that supports the suggestion that staff–patient interaction does influence patients' adjustment.

As to the possible influences of physician's denial, Table 9 presents some of the results from studies of medical staff expectations. On the whole, the following tendency can be found: When the physicians use denial one or two things happen to the nurses' expectations. Sometimes they develop very high and unrealistic expectations; for example, in Unit A expectation of absolute lack of psychopathology or lack of team opinion was found. In such an environment the patients are faced with double- or actually multibind communications. The next question is whether such attitudes indeed influence patients' adjustment. There does seem to be a relationship between staff expectations and patients' adjustment, though it is certainly not the only factor influencing adjustment. For example, patients' psychological condition (Table 10): The predictions were done on the basis of the patients' personality only. This table presents a calculation of to what extent the patients did or did not fulfill the prediction and, it seems that especially unrealistic expectations

TABLE 9
Physician's Denial and Nurses's Expectations

	Unit A			Unit B			Unit C			Unit D		
		Expectations			Expectations			Expectations			Expectations	
	Denial	Phy.	Nurse	Denial	Phy.	Nurse	Denial	Phy.	Nurse	Denial	Phy.	Nurse
Fluid restriction	2.00	2	D[a]	3.33	3	D[a]	1.08	2.8	2.6	1.80	3	D[a]
Vocational rehabilitation	5.00	3	D[a]	6.00	3	D[a]	1.00	3.0	2.6	1.00	4	3
Lack of psychopathology	3.66	2	4	1.29	4	D[a]	1.36	3.0	3.0	1.62	3	D[a]

[a]D = disagreement

TABLE 10
Patients' Psychological Condition

Unit	No. of patients	Team opinion	Better than predicted	As predicted	Worse than predicted
			% of patients		
A	20	Unrealistic	0	65	35
B	23	No	4	83	13
C	21	Yes	5	85	10
D	15	No	4	83	13

TABLE 11
Patients' Compliance

Unit	No. of patients	Team opinion	Better than predicted	As predicted	Worse than predicted
			Percentage of patients complying		
A	20	No	0	65	35
B	23	No	9	70	21
C	21	Yes	24	71	5
D	15	No	7	67	26

result in worse adjustment than predicted. An even more clear-cut relation was found about compliance (Table 11). It seems that when there is a clear and realistic team opinion, patients comply even better than predicted on the basis of their personality. Thus it seems that there is some evidence to support the suggestion that unrealistic expectations or lack of team opinion hamper adjustment. One has to stress, however, that the studies were carried out in small samples[10,11] and further study is highly indicated.

The next focus for investigation was the clinical observation that the emotional involvement of the staff with the patients is very high. The Morgan and Cheadle questionnaire was used and the results compared to those gathered in psychiatric units.[12] Table 12 presents the average number of preference and rejection answers. The number of answers in the dialysis unit was much higher than in the psychiatric units which indeed can be regarded as an indication of involvement. In the unit that was studied, there was a very high intrastaff agreement about which patients are accepted and which are rejected. It also provided information about what makes staff, or rather the specific staff in question, accept or reject patients (Table 13). It seems that the patient's actual behavior in the unit determine whether he was accepted or rejected; the behavior of the accepted and rejected groups showed great differences indeed.

TABLE 12
Number of Preference and
Rejection Answers[a]

	Preference answers (average)	Rejection answers (average)
Dialysis	154	82
Admission unit	70	25
Progressed unit	75	32

[a]Morgan and Cheadle.

TABLE 13
Characteristics of Accepted and
Rejected Patients

"Accepted patients"	"Rejected patients"
Well behaved	Attention-seeking
Credit to the unit	Troublesome
Cooperative	Uncooperative
Interesting to talk to	Disliked

TABLE 14
Adjustment of Accepted and Rejected Patients

	"Accepted patients"	"Rejected patients"
Physical complications	Few and light	Many and severe
Compliance with the diet	Fair	Poor
Psychological complications	Few and light	Many and severe
Vocational rehabilitation	Fair	Fair

The adjustment of the five most accepted and the five most rejected patients was assessed (Table 14). A great difference was found in the condition of the accepted patients compared to that of the rejected patients. However, it is not known what is cause and what is effect. In other words, we do not know whether being accepted led to better overall adjustment or whether being adjusted led to being accepted. We suspect that staff acceptance or rejection is the cause, but this cannot be proven from the available data.

The ward atmosphere is another highly informative method to study the staff–patient relationship. Not all the data gathered in that way can be presented, but some points should be discussed (Table 15). Here we are dealing with seven units. The number of staff members is 108 and includes nearly all the staff; the number of patients is 127 and

TABLE 15
Ward Atmosphere Scale

Subscale	Staff		Patients	
	Analysis of variance	$\bar{X}$	Analysis of variance	$\bar{X}$
Involvement	Significant	5.3	Significant	4.5
Support	Significant	7.0	Significant	6.5
Spontaneity	N.S.	6.3	Significant	6.0
Autonomy	Significant	3.9	Significant	3.1
Practical orientation	Significant	5.5	N.S.	4.4
Personal problems orientation	N.S.	5.6	Significant	4.8
Anger and aggression	Significant	6.8	Significant	3.8
Order and organization	Significant	8.1	Significant	8.0
Program clarity	Significant	8.3	Significant	7.6
Staff control	N.S.	3.8	Significant	4.2
TOTAL	Significant	60.6	Significant	55.1

does not include all patients as many were excluded because of language problems and some because of cooperation problems. Analysis of variance was significant for seven of the subscales in the staff report and nine in the patients' report, indicating that there are differences between the units as perceived by patients and by staff. The means for the total populations do not mean much, but still it is worthwhile to note that except for "staff control" the patients scored lower on all subscales and especially so on "anger and aggression."

Much more interesting, however, is the comparison of staff and patients' opinion of the same unit. As an example, some of the results from two units were compared (Table 16). The staff of Unit Y do not think that their patients are involved, they rate them as very aggressive, and feel they support them a lot. The patients, however, do not feel supported and on the total score the patients indicated a significantly lower opinion

TABLE 16
Ward Atmosphere Scale

Subscale	Unit X		Unit Y	
	Staff	Patients	Staff	Patients
Involvement	7.5	5.9[a]	5.0	4.7
Support	7.5	7.7	7.8	6.4[a]
Autonomy	5.1	5.1	4.1	5.2[a]
Anger and aggression	7.8	5.0[a]	8.3	4.4[a]
Program clarity	8.5	8.6	8.5	7.8
TOTAL	66.3	61.4	64.3	57.3[a]

[a] t-test significant.

TABLE 17
Psychological Distress

	None	Some	Quite a lot and extreme	
Worry				
Unit X	9	11	—	$x^2 = 5.04$
Unit Y	3	19	—	$h = 0.025$
Body image distortion				
Unit X	14	5	1	$x^2 = 10.77$
Unit Y	5	12	5	$h < 0.005$
Self-devaluation				
Unit X	11	6	3	$x^2 = 10.50$
Unit Y	3	15	5	$h < 0.005$

TABLE 18
Vocational Rehabilitation—% of Patients[a]

Unit	No.	Full-time work	Half-time work	None
X	21	43.0 (33)	33.0 (38)	24.0 (29)
Y	24	12.5 (0)	37.5 (33)	50.0 (67)

[a]( ) according to patients' own assessments.

of the unit. The patients in Unit X, however, do feel supported and on the total score the difference was not significant. Are these differences important? Maybe. On the Health Care Orientation section of the Derogatis scale, the patients of Unit X score significantly lower than those of Unit Y (6.82 compared to 8.95), indicating better adjustment and greater satisfaction with the treatment than the patients in Unit Y. The results of the section on psychological distress are presented in Table 17. The patients of Unit X reported significantly less psychological distress on some of the items, indicating better psychological condition. At the same time the vocational rehabilitation of the patients of Unit X (Table 18), whether assessed by the physician in charge or by the patients themselves, was significantly better.

Once more, the sample was small and the results should be regarded as only preliminary. Yet the results do seem to suggest that there is a strong relationship between staff–patient interaction, as assessed by the ward atmosphere scale and the patients' adjustment.

SUMMARY

Some evidence about staff–patient interaction was presented as well as the influence of that interaction on the emotional welfare of the staff and on patients' adjustment to chronic dialysis. All the data should be regarded as preliminary only, indicating the strong need for further study. These preliminary results strongly suggest that patients' adjustment might be improved by indirect work with the staff and by change in some staff attitudes.

REFERENCES

1. MORROW, G. R., CHIARELLO, R. J., and DEROGATIS, L. A. A new scale for assessing patients' psychosocial adjustment to medical illness. *Psychological Medicine*, 1978, *8*, 605–610.
2. MORGAN, R., and CHEADLE, A. J. Staff versus patients: The phenomenon of rejection. *British Journal of Psychiatry*, 1972, *121*, 627–634.
3. MOOS, R. H. *Evaluating treatment environment—A social ecological approach*. New York: John Wiley and Sons, 1974.
4. KAPLAN DE-NOUR, A., and CZACZKES, J. W. Emotional problems and reactions of the medical team in a chronic haemodialysis unit. *Lancet*, 1968, *2*, 987–991.
5. KAPLAN DE-NOUR, A. and CZACZKES, J. W. Professional team opinion and personal bias—A study of a chronic hemodialysis unit team. *Journal of Chronic Disease*, 1971, *24*, 533–541.
6. KAPLAN DE-NOUR, A. The hemodialysis unit. In H. Freyberger (Ed.), *Advances in psychosomatic medicine*. Vol. 10. Basel: Karger, 1980, 132–150.
7. KAPLAN DE-NOUR, A., CZACZKES, J. W., and LILOS, P. A study of chronic hemodialysis teams: Differences in opinions and expectations. *Journal of Chronic Disease*, 1972, *25*, 441–448.
8. SHORT, M. J., and WILSON, W. P. Roles of denial in chronic hemodialysis. *Archives of General Psychiatry*, 1969, *20*, 433–437.
9. KAPLAN DE-NOUR, A., and CZACZKES, J. W. Bias in assessment of patients on chronic hemodialysis. *Journal of Psychosomatic Research*, 1979, *18*, 217–221.
10. KAPLAN DE-NOUR, A., and CZACZKES, J. W. Team–patient interaction in chronic hemodialysis units. *Psychotherapy and Psychosomatics*, 1974, *24*, 132–136.
11. KAPLAN DE-NOUR, A. The influence of physicians' behavior and teams' attitudes on adjustment of chronic patients. In F. Antonelli (Ed.), *Therapy in psychosomatic medicine*, Roma: Edizione Luigi Pozzi, 1975, 120–128.
12. KAPLAN DE-NOUR, A., and CZACZKES, J. W. Nurses' rejection and acceptance of patients—A study of a chronic hemodialysis unit. *Mental Health Society*, 1977, *4*, 85–94.

4

A Patient's Perspective on Patient–Staff Interaction

JOHN NEWMANN

My first hemodialysis treatment was on September 30, 1971. I had to wait 4 months before a home training position was available, and I began dialyzing at home in mid-March 1972. I have two daughters (12 and 13 years old) who have often seated themselves on my lap while I'm dialyzing. During dialysis we would play cards or checkers, talk about their day at school, and have dinner together. They enjoy helping with the treatment and explaining it to their friends. My wife and I did dialysis together at home for 3 years until it became too much of a strain after a full day's work for each of us. I'm fortunate to have a home-aide paid by Medicare (a pilot project), which has resulted in my getting needed rest on the treatment. I was divorced in 1978; one issue among many leading to the divorce was the kidney failure and the uncertainty it brings.

Dialysis no longer limits my exercise, travel, or life style. I swim, play tennis, climb New England's mountains, go canoeing and camping, and go traveling in this country and in Asia. One adjusts to the diet over time—but it does take time. I never liked liver very much, and kidney failure gives me an excellent excuse to politely refuse when it's offered by a well-intentioned host.

There are two purposes of this presentation. First, I am delighted to share my thoughts and experience concerning patient and staff interactions. I will limit my remarks to patients of chronic uremia (I prefer to call them consumers) maintained on long-term hemodialysis. Second, and more importantly, I plan to direct the discussion toward issues I've found to be essential when pursuing complete rehabilitation while on maintenance dialysis in terms of regaining the enjoyment and involvement in predialysis life activities, and quite conceivably improving on that pre-kidney-failure life style.

JOHN NEWMANN, PH.D., M.P.H. • President, National Association of Patients on Hemodialysis and Transplantation, Brookline, Massachusetts.

In discussing patient–staff interaction, I will briefly address the importance of staff members working with each patient to be certain that adequate dialysis is being received. Given the absence of a well-defined and accepted medical definition of adequate dialysis, let me suggest it include, in addition to acceptable blood chemistries, a stable and well-functioning mind and body during and in between treatments. Cramps, headaches, chest pain, weakness, exhaustion, impotence, light-headedness, excessive thirst, and so forth should not be assumed to indicate the patient "doesn't tolerate" dialysis well. He may be dialyzed with too large or too little a surface area, too long or not long enough, with acetate or bicarbonate, untreated water, poorly preserved dialyzers, too much or too little sodium or potassium in the dialysate, and so forth (a reason to avoid central delivery systems since *all patients are not the same*). Staff should try to develop with the patient the optimal treatment conditions and specification for adequate dialysis confirmed by the way the patient feels on and off the treatment and by his blood chemistries. Kinetic modeling research currently underway may lead to effective dialysis prescriptions for each patient.

At the outset I must state clearly the critical assumption I make: Any significant rehabilitation and adjustment to chronic uremia requires a strong acceptance on the patient's part of responsibility for his physical, mental, and emotional health. This implies regaining, or in some cases, establishing for the first time substantial control and independence in living one's life, a major component of which has become the thrice-weekly dialysis treatments. As we are all painfully aware in the dialysis setting, this is no small challenge. As implied above, the patient should eventually work with his doctor and dialysis staff to establish the most beneficial dialysis routine for *his* mind, body, circulatory system, level of activity, remaining renal function, employment, and family responsibilities.

STAGE I—INITIATION OF DIALYSIS AND THE IMPORTANCE OF SELF-CARE

During the first few months of dialysis, it is often safe to assume the patient is: scared, worried, resentful, angry, tired, weak, and in a hurry to get on and off that machine which is tying him down. We are all aware of the spoken and unspoken fears of death, pain, the uncertain future, and the consequences of cheating "just a little" on the restrictive diet. These feelings and attitudes are common and normal for someone attempting to live through a major life crisis which often calls into question the viability and stability of one's entire life.

Against this charged atmosphere in which the new dialysis patient is immersed, staff begin to know the patient and have the extraordinarily complicated task of:

- Helping to keep the patient alive.
- Educating the patient and his family about what has happened and what changes must be made for him to survive.
- Encouraging the patient to recognize those areas where he can gain control to insure a quality of life which is worth the effort of compliance with the seemingly endless list of dietary restrictions and initial physical limitations.

Ten and fifteen years ago we were all justifiably impressed with medical advances which insured survival for those with renal failure. Staff and patient efforts seldom addressed the qualitative life issues other than blood chemistries, bone disease, and respiratory and cardiovascular function. Since then, increasing attention is being devoted to full rehabilitation in terms of psychological and emotional stability, stamina, endurance, mobility, mental acuity, sexual normalcy, and employability.

This initial period of introducing dialysis appears to be critical in determining the quality of life to be enjoyed or regained by the new dialysis consumer. I view the first few months with the same importance as many ascribe to the first year of marriage. New patterns are set and attitudes developed which strongly influence the future. Staff opportunity to encourage patient responsibility and control is at its height. Yet it is also a contradictory time: patients and family facing the new crisis are less likely to retain all advice and information at this time than they may later. Medical staff may be reluctant to share their responsibility with patients. Nevertheless the patterns, attitudes, and signals given by staff in the beginning have a tendency to become written in stone by the patient and his family. It is an art, not a science, to know intuitively what combination of caring, empathy, education, training, encouragement, and (sometimes) pushing are necessary as staff assist with survival and plant the seeds for patient assumption of responsibility, control, and independence. There is no question in my mind that a medical and support staff actively oriented toward self-care, whether in-center or at home, will find higher rates of rehabilitation than will the staff that simply points to options, but does not actively provide education, training, and encouragement toward the objective of self-care and the goal of full rehabilitation. Self-care *can be* for nearly everyone. Hospitals and centers with strong self-care programs include at the outset a comprehensive medical and psychological diagnostic evaluation filtering out those patients with serious medical complications and emotional conditions which would not lend themselves to effective and safe self-care.

In October 1980, the Rogosin Kidney Center at New York Hospital had 260 chronic dialysis patients: 25% of them were on home dialysis and 23% dialyzed themselve in the self-care unit of the hospital. A total of 48% were taking care of themselves—compared to the national average which was in the neighborhood of 13%. In the province of Manitoba, 79% of the 168 chronic patients assumed self-care in-center or at home (October 1980).

Suggestions for Staff in Stage I

I don't think it is possible to overemphasize the critical importance of staff encouragement of self-care with patients and family during this initial stage. Countless issues must be introduced and worked with at this time. One can only hope that the medical director takes the time to coordinate care and responsibility between doctor, nurse, technician, dietician, psychologist, and social worker. Confusion and disservice arise when patients are presented with unnecessarily conflicting views or something is left out. In addition to the necessary repetition about diet, this period is an important one to establish clearly two important realities about one's life with chronic uremia.

First, the loss is real. I often think of it as if "my kidneys failed me. I can't depend on them anymore. To survive I must not only compensate for the loss, but it's natural and healthy to grieve that loss." The grieving process never really ends. Initially much self-pity, sorrow, and jealousy of others will be experienced and should be supported. To mourn the loss of something normally taken for granted, yet essential for life, is healthy and needed. Staff, especially the doctors, ought to be able to empathize with their patients.

Second, staff should strive to remind the patient that being tired, weak, depressed, out of work, and away from sex need not be the blue print for the future. It is constructive to identify rehabilitated role models (with similar life situations to that of the patient) leading active, productive lives. Staff can and must work with the patient to identify areas in which the patient is dissatisfied and note those in which he can have some control, and those in which he does not. The type of dialysis and the setting, diet, work, energy level, and sex are all areas in which responsibility can be assumed. Through learning and sensitive experimentation one's capacity to experience them optimally can be achieved. Each patient can choose which side of the statistics he'd like to be on. The patient is naturally tempted to give up and leave his fate in the hands of busy, overworked staff, and settle for disabled status. This must be countered by a strong, positive orientation toward gaining, or regaining, control and quality in one's life.

Interdependence and inseparability of mind and body are rapidly becoming recognized and accepted in this country. For example, depressed persons don't initiate much interaction. However it is quite common for one's mental and emotional attitude to improve radically after a full body massage, a good swim or run, a tennis game or sex. Others find a good therapy session or personal talk with an understanding friend picks them up, relieving them of headaches, stomachaches, depression, or fatigue. Dialysis consumers have more reason to become aware of their bodies and emotions than others. But dialysis consumers spend so much time and effort on dialysis and being conscious of the diet, and blaming any fatigue or dysfunction on dialysis; few of them are likely to spend additional time and effort improving the quality of their lives, which in their minds have been so strongly compromised due to kidney failure. Here is where most staff have the greatest opportunity to help in the true healing process; and where many staff miss that opportunity.

There is no set formula describing which kidney disease and personality types do best under the variety of nondialysis therapies available. Just as in psychotherapy, a number of approaches must be tried until the constructive, effective combination is found for each person at his particular stage of development. The real issue is finding the unique pattern of interventions which (1) help the patient decide to "take charge of his life," and (2) bring positive results physically, mentally, and emotionally once the decision to assume responsibility has been made by the patient.

Below is a list of factors which I consider essential for rehabilitation and which should be introduced either during the initial period when dialysis commences or as soon as signs of physical adjustment to the dialysis treatment are noticed:

1. Self-care on dialysis either in-center or at home.

2. Regular availability and encouragement of psychotherapy from a *psychiatric* social worker, psychologist, or psychiatrist. This doesn't mean waiting until a psychological crisis becomes serious enough for referral. It means easy access to psychological professionals to prevent these crises by dealing with issues early. We cannot expect the unit social worker to assume this task, although some units do provide psychiatric social workers trained in this kind of work. One unit in New York City has its psychologist meet all new patients and personally inform them of his availability in the office, away from the dialysis machine. This therapy is also available to family members. Some units have

formed spouse groups that meet with psychologists to discuss common problems.

3. Availability and encouragement of a regular exercise program to increase and maintain circulation, aerobic breathing, and muscle tone. This should be preceded by a medically supervised stress test and individually tailored exercise routine. No one has studied the long-term effects on the circulatory, muscular, and respiratory systems resulting from thrice-weekly dialysis. Muscular wasting is often reported. There are studies which are looking at the benefits of exercise to these systems for persons on dialysis. I would include in this exercise program both aerobic conditioning and stretching such as yoga exercises as well as diaphragmatic (stress-reducing) breathing.

4. Balanced nutritional and dietary counseling is needed, not just pointing to the negative, that is, the restrictions. Emphasis should be placed on consuming sufficient calories and the full complement of essential amino acid proteins.

5. Counseling and guidance to assist the patient in resuming full- or part-time work and/or normal life routines are terribly important. The strengths and weaknesses of private and public sources for rehabilitation and employment should be well known by someone in the dialysis unit.

A few thoughts might be explored regarding nutritional problems associated with hemodialysis and staff attempts to deal with them. The initial and pervasive life-threatening scare of kidney failure is compounded by the threat (while maintained on dialysis) of cardiac arrest and pulmonary insufficiency caused by excessive potassium and liquid consumption. Dietary management of potassium and liquid intake, plus restriction of sodium, calcium, and phosphorus often leaves the new patient afraid of eating. Protein/calorie malnutrition and muscle wasting are commonly experienced in mild form. Staff members need to educate the new patient concerning the components of food and quantities one can safely consume. This often is interpreted by the patient as extremely negative restrictions. "Don't eat this, don't eat more than this amount of that each day." Naturally a strong psychological incentive to disobey newly imposed restrictions arises. When we are told we can't have something we're accustomed to having, we want it even more.

Therefore, staff members face two nutritional challenges. The first is to balance the negative/restrictive guidelines with a positive approach to a healthy, nutritious diet. Various dialysis units, National Kidney Foundation Affiliates, and the Mayo Clinic have published renal cook books. These should be brought to the attention of new dialysis consumers. More important is the recognition of gradual adjustment to a radical change in one's daily habits. The notion of moderation in eating must be stressed. One lesson well-learned by long-term dialysis consumers which is applicable to the entire population is: the good qualitative life is that which is lived by moderation in all activities.

Second, staff must help patients to insure adequate intake of high biologic protein along with adequate calories to prevent muscle and weight loss. Passing out protein, sodium, and potassium exchange charts for rote memorization is useful but not always effective. Meetings with long-term patients who have adjusted to the diet and can answer questions and share frustrations and experiences are often very helpful.

The five suggestions listed above as essential for rehabilitation are not new to dialysis. Effective programs including most, or all, of them are available in units in Los Angeles, Cleveland, St. Louis, and New York, to name a few. They are, however, not widely publicized and require a staff and leadership which is committed to rehabilitation of the patient through passing on considerable control and responsibility to the willing and interested patient. Medicare and/or third-party insurers will pay for self-care training and limited prescribed psychotherapy. Hospitals, dialysis centers, and consumers may have to share the costs of exercise programs.

Naturally, all of this cannot be accomplished during the first few months of dialysis. Yet it is essential to introduce this approach at that time. Staff can then follow through with those suggestions most appropriate for each patient.

STAGE II—TRANSITION TO ACCEPTANCE OF CHRONIC UREMIA

While many of the Stage I emotions, feelings, and problems may carry on to Stage II—the transition—there will be some sense of getting accustomed to the radical changes of a few months ago. The newness will be reduced, as will the fears of treatment, though diet problems, resentment, weakness, and dissatisfaction with the necessary sacrifices and restrictions may remain.

It is during this second stage that a strong push for patient control and responsibility is essential. Self-care training for home or in-center dialysis is a natural objective to emphasize. This is also a good time to introduce an exercise program. Psychotherapy, available in Stage I, may still be desired and is important to provide. As stability on dialysis is increased, return to employment, school, and/or housekeeping should be encouraged.

The transition period is one in which nurses and technicians may begin to assume the (formerly new) patient is now stable and doesn't require the personal attention and interest initially shown by staff. This is a mistake. The staff should wait for the patient to suggest or imply that he really doesn't need their ear, interest, or care. Unfortunately many free-standing dialysis units are reducing staff/patient ratios from 1 : 2 or 1 : 3 to 1 : 4 or 1 : 5 in an attempt to maintain earlier profit margins. This reduction, causing greater responsibility for staff and less time for staff–patient contact, may also be causing very high staff turnover rates. The successful self-care sections of dialysis centers I've seen have the self-care physically separated and out of sight of the full- or partial-care patients. Self-care sections seem to manage quite well with 1 : 4 or 1 : 5 staff/patient ratios. Full-care units with those ratios are findings excessive staff turnover and serious patient discontent. Staff (of full-care units) I've spoken to have not complained of salary and fringe benefits as much as they do complain of scheduling inflexibility, too much responsibility, and pressure to care for four or five patients at once. Staff have little time to spend with patients in an understanding way due to the rush to get people on and off machines, treat emergencies, and cover when other staff members take breaks.

A review of the literature of successful American business and corporate management over the past 5 years contains an important lesson for hospital and free-standing dialysis units. The IBMs and Polaroids have learned: executive management often finds quality of work maintained and profits stable or increasing over the long term when staff from the bottom up not only participate in reforms affecting their services or products, but also have a sense of their worth and top management's dependence upon them.

Suggestions for Staff in Stage II

During the transition stage, staff members would be wise to continue to assess with the patient any obstacles inhibiting the patient from enjoying an acceptable life style and pursuing goals and objectives for the future. If not accomplished previously, the identification of a role model for the patient and facilitating some interaction between the patient and role model will be very constructive. At this stage it is important to clarify the causes of patient discontent: experience on the treatment, diet problems, general fatigue, depression over changed life, and so forth. Once causes are identified, the staff and patient can set objectives for changing those areas of discontent which are amenable to change. Without full support from the attending physician, this clarification may never take place, as nonphysician staff may simply not be given the opportunity to work with the patient in this way.

The psychologist, social worker, nurse, and technician may have to discuss with the attending physician the reasons why patients are not doing well. The possible dialysis and nondialysis solutions which may lead to greater rehabilitation should be considered. There is an extraordinary opportunity for the staff to identify the large numbers of persons on dialysis who haven't yet decided to live life to its fullest. As *health care providers* it is up to the staff to introduce these patients to ways in which they can improve the quality of their lives.

STAGE III—ACCEPTANCE OF AND ADJUSTMENT TO CHRONIC UREMIA

This introduces the third stage, acceptance of kidney failure and the necessity of long-term dialysis or transplantation. No longer does the patient fight or deny what has happened or what is necessary to survive. However, he will continue to go through periods of anger, frustration, and depression—often due to recurring problems on dialysis, postdialysis fatigue, difficulty in maintaining the restrictive diet, or feeling so well and strong that dialysis becomes a very inconvenient, constant interruption in an otherwise rich and exciting life. It may be useful to divide those in the acceptance stage into three groups:

1. The well-adjusted, stable, strong-willed consumers know what they want and are working toward getting it. They still need staff encouragement to continue striving for full rehabilitation. Continued emphasis on self-care, proper nutrition, exercise, stress reduction, and getting back to work may prove beneficial to both patients and staff who can witness the results of their work. The adjusted patients can be introduced to the notion of assuming some responsibility for helping new patients when needed, just as they may have been helped by other role models.

2. Then there is the poorly adjusted, noncompliant patient, who appears to have accepted his fate and seems to thrive on complaining, being pitied, and barely surviving. If the patient has clarified his problems and those over which he can assume control, yet chooses not to, staff can make clear to the patient what he is choosing to do. That is, he is choosing deterioration, injury to his mind and body, self-destruction. If there is no interest in changing, then the staff at best has a responsibility to tolerate the noncompliant one in terms of doing their job to assist in survival, but hopefully not at the expense of other patients.

3. The most difficult are those on the borderline, in between the two, on the fence, having neither decided to make the big push to gain control, nor to give up in hopes that staff, family, and friends' pity will sustain them. There is nothing more physically and emotionally exhausting for patient and staff than a patient on the fence, and indecisive

about choosing self-responsibility or leaving his fate in the hands of others.

One serious problem in assisting this type of patient is the patient is not always aware that he is on the fence. The option of the active, full, rehabilitated life may not have been clearly shown or described. Appropriate role models may not have been identified. Steps necessary for rehabilitation may not have been effectively offered. As suggested above, these are critical responsibilities of staff, if patient–staff interaction is to go beyond patient survival.

It is not at all clear what variety of approaches works in different contexts resulting in a patient's decision to take charge of his life. The suggestions listed: active staff orientation toward self-care, psychotherapy, exercise, stress reduction, and nutritional and employment counseling are essential elements, in my view, of a comprehensive and successful rehabilitation effort. One additional avenue to encourage patient rehabilitation is to introduce him to NAPHT, the National Association of Patients on Hemodialysis and Transplantation (156 William Street, New York, NY 10038). NAPHT is the largest kidney patient organization in the United States with over 10,000 members dedicated to rehabilitation of those which chronic uremia. NAPHT publishes a quarterly magazine, sponsors various conferences, represents patients' interests in Washington, and serves patients as an excellent resource and support system.

Conclusion: What about Staff?

This discussion of patient–staff interaction and patient rehabilitation has not been very sensitive to or concerned about staff needs, attitudes, ups, and downs. The well-managed dialysis units do provide psychotherapy group sessions and other release and support mechanisms for staff members to understand better the emotional and psychological dynamics of their work and experience. Patients are seldom worried about the staff. Yet staff members have been working to keep patients alive. Those of us who have survived, and have insisted on a high quality and richness in our survival, are incapable of extending appropriate appreciation to staff who have made much of this possible. My hunch is: those staff members who have experienced the inner joy and ecstasy of seeing one of their patients really take charge of his life, know well the feeling of human accomplishment in not only saving a life, but being a part of that extra qualitative effort which makes all the difference.

5

The Impact of Renal Failure and Dialysis Treatments on Patients' Lives and on Their Compliance Behavior

ROGER J. SHERWOOD

Mr. B., a 50-year-old black male whose kidney failure was caused by glomerulonephritis, had been gainfully employed as a salesman prior to his illness. Because his job required standing most of the day, he was too physically exhausted to continue in this capacity. His wife had to begin working to meet the financial needs of the family.

Mr. B. suffered a loss of self-esteem in that he could no longer provide for his family. His marital relationship was adversely affected by his depression and sexual problems developed after he began dialysis treatments three times a week. He had great difficulty following dietary and fluid restrictions. While his wife and family attempted to help him monitor his diet, this became a "bone of contention" and created further disharmony within the family. Mr. B. reported that almost every area of his life had been greatly affected by his illness and dialysis treatments.

Which major life areas are most affected by renal failure and dialysis treatments? Are serious disruptions more frequent in males, blacks, or older patients? If the patient's life is greatly affected by the illness, will he or she be less compliant with the medical and dietary regimen? These are some of the questions we sought to elucidate in this study.

In this chapter, we first identify those areas in which patients reported being most affected by the illness and required treatments. Second, we examine how the illness and subsequent treatment impacted differentially upon various subgroups of patients. Finally, we analyze the relationship between the patients' reports of the impact of the illness and their compliance with the medical and dietary regimen. It should be noted that since we did not think that patients would be able to differentiate clearly between the impact of the illness and their response to dialysis treatments, we addressed them as a single phenomenon. Thus,

ROGER J. SHERWOOD, D.S.W., A.C.S.W. • Assistant Professor, Hunter College Graduate School of Social Work, City University of New York, New York, New York.

throughout this chapter, when discussing the impact of illness, we are also including the impact of the dialysis treatments and the medical and dietary regimen.

METHODS

This article presents one facet of a broader research project conducted between January 1979 and June 1979 at the Brooklyn Kidney Center, a free-standing satellite dialysis center. The purpose of this project was to identify variables associated with patients' compliance with their medical and dietary regimen. It was hoped that these findings would highlight areas which might be modified in order to increase compliance behavior and assist in the development of more effective interventions on the part of the staff. Understanding the impact of the illness on the patients' lives and its relationship to compliance behavior was one aspect of this larger study.

In February 1979, the population of the Brooklyn Kidney Center consisted of 131 patients. Prior to the selection of a sample for this study, 12 patients were excluded—6 because they could not understand English adequately, 2 because they were blind, 2 because they were deaf, and 2 because they had severe psychiatric problems. From the remaining population of 119 patients, a random sample of 60 was selected with equally represented patients from morning, afternoon, and evening shifts. Of the 60 patients, 55 were inteviewed for this study. The 5 patients who refused to be interviewed and the 12 excluded patients did not differ markedly on demographic characteristics or levels of compliance behavior when compared to the group of interviewed patients.

The sample interviewed ($N = 55$) was comprised of 66% males and 34% females. The mean age of the sample was 46 with a range from 22 to 72 years of age. Seventy-three percent of the sample was black, 18% white, and 9% Hispanic. The mean length of time on dialysis was 48 months, and the median time was 42 months. The patients' length of time on dialysis from 6 months to 11½ years.

We utilized a 30-page questionnaire to collect data on variables thought to be associated with patients' compliance behavior. Data was gathered through personal interviews averaging 1 hour and 40 minutes while the patient was being dialyzed. The majority of questions were constructed as a 5- or 7-point Likert-type response scale although open-ended questions were selectively utilized to elicit more in-depth information.

To provide objective measures of compliance, laboratory data from January 1979 to June 1979 were obtained for the patients with respect to serum phosphorous levels, serum potassium levels, and for between-dialysis weight gains. Phosphorous levels indicate compliance with medication and dietary instructions whereas potassium is a reliable indicator of dietary compliance. Between-dialysis weight gains reflect the patient's compliance with respect to the fluid restrictions. We constructed an overall compliance index by standardizing the scores on these three measures and then combining them into a single index. The patients' self-reports of how closely they followed instructions regarding their medications, diet, and fluid intake as well as the staff's general instructions were also utilized as another measure of compliance behavior. These five measures of phosphorous and potassium levels, between-dialysis weight gains, the overall compliance index, and patients' self-reports constituted the dependent measures used in this study.

MAJOR LIFE AREAS AFFECTED

While we knew that kidney failure and the subsequent adjustment to dialysis treatments presages pervasive change in patients' lives, we wanted to further understand the specific areas and the degree to which illness and treatment impacted on each. The domains covered were eating habits, leisure time pursuits, sexual activity, social contacts, family relationships, vacation activities, friendships, employment activities, self-esteem, sense of security, and the ability to enjoy life. Patients were

TABLE 1
Self-Described Impact of Kidney Disease on Different Areas of Patient's Life[a,b]

Different life domains	Degree of impact of the illness (percentaged across)				
	Greatly affected	Moderately affected	Mildly affected	Not affected at all	Totals
Employment activities	45.5	20.0	14.5	20.0	100.0
Vacation activities	41.9	14.5	20.0	23.6	100.0
Leisure time pursuits	32.7	23.7	30.9	12.7	100.0
Eating habits	25.5	30.9	18.1	25.5	100.0
Sexual activity	30.9	21.8	14.6	32.7	100.0
Ability to enjoy life	21.8	18.2	20.0	40.0	100.0
Self-esteem	14.5	21.8	25.5	38.2	100.0
Sense of security	9.1	27.3	29.1	34.5	100.0
Relationship with friends	20.0	10.9	23.6	45.5	100.0
Social contacts	16.4	23.6	25.5	34.5	100.0
Family relationships	14.5	14.5	18.3	52.7	100.0

[a]$N = 55$.
[b]Note: Instruction to the respondent: "Now I would like you to rate the impact of your kidney disease on these different areas of your life. For example, how has being a kidney patient affected your eating habits, self-esteem, etc.?"

asked to indicate whether each of these areas was greatly, moderately, mildly, or not at all affected.

Table 1 lists the eleven specific areas affected by the illness ordered from the most affected area (1) to the least affected area (11). As seen in Table 1, the five areas most affected by the illness and dialysis treatments were employment activities, vacation activities, leisure time pursuits, eating habits, and sexual activity. These we categorized as behavioral activities. Fifty-three percent or more of the patients in this survey reported that these five areas were greatly or moderately affected as a result of becoming a dialysis patient. The next three areas conceptualized as affective include ability to enjoy life, self-esteem, and sense of security. The last three domains categorized as relational encompass relationships with friends, social contacts, and family. In order to determine if the impact of the illness differentially affected various subgroups of patients, each of the above eleven domains was statistically analyzed with various demographic variables, such as sex, age, race, education, marital status, income, time on dialysis, socioeconomic status, place of birth, and religion.

Behavioral Activities

Let's turn first to a discussion of the impact of the illness on the five behavioral activities in an attempt to illuminate whether certain subgroups are differentially affected by the kidney disease and its treatment requirements. Some of the patients' individual comments will be in-

TABLE 2

Impact of Illness on Behavior Life Areas as Differentiated by Sex,
Marital Status, and Religion

Demographic variables	Behavioral areas (t values)				
	Employment activities	Vacation activities	Leisure time pursuits	Eating habits	Sexual activity
Sex					
Males (N=36)	1.38	⁓1.11	2.64^a	2.14	0.30
Females (N=19)					
Marital Status					
Married (N=26)	−1.46	−0.57	0.73	1.11	−2.19*
Other (N=29)					
Religion					
Protestant (N=32)	0.0	0.83	0.0	−1.76*	−0.25
Catholic (N=16)					

$^a p < 0.05$, one tail test.

TABLE 3
Correlations between the Impact of Illness on Behavioral Areas
and Selected Demographic Variables

Demographic variables	Behavioral areas				
	Employment activities	Vacation activities	Leisure time pursuits	Eating habits	Sexual activity
Income (N=47)	−0.03	−0.18	−0.04	−0.02	−0.26[a]
Education (N=55)	0.28[a]	0.16	0.26[a]	−0.01	0.29[a]
Length of time on dialysis (N=55)	0.10	−0.16	0.23[a]	0.11	0.21

[a]Sample size correlation was significant at the 0.05 level.

cluded in order to clarify how they experienced the impact of their illness on these different areas. Tables 2 and 3 display the patients' reports of the impact of the illness on behavioral activities differentiated by selected demographic variables.

Employment

Employment was the area which patients reported being most affected. Sixty-five percent of the patients said employment activities were either greatly or moderately affected by being a dialysis patient. When employment was analyzed by the demographic variables, education and socioeconomic status were significantly correlated. The higher the educational level, the less the reported impact of illness on employment activities ($r = 0.28$). One explanation for this finding relates to the type of employment opportunities available to those with higher levels of education. Many white-collar, desk-type positions require higher levels of education, while unskilled manual-type labor requires less education. These latter positions tend to be more physically demanding, and would be more adversely affected by limitations imposed by renal failure.

This explanation seems to be supported when this sample is viewed in terms of the socioeconomic status distribution. The Hollingshead[1] formula was used to calculate the socioeconomic statuses for the sample. We obtained data on both the educational level and occupation for 46 of the 55 patients. When the patients' reports of impact on employment activities was analyzed by social class, there was a significant negative trend. The lower the socioeconomic class the more the patients reported their employment activities had been affected ($r = 0.23$, $N = 55$, $p = 0.06$).

If patients reported that areas of their lives had been greatly or moderately affected by their illness, the interviewer asked in what ways. In terms of employment activities, 36 patients reponded to this question. Thirty-three of their comments could be classified as negative, for example, "I had to quit work"; "I don't have the physical strength for my job, home, or children"; "I can't walk up steps and am tired"; "My boss isn't sensitive to my feelings and my limits." Two patients had strokes prior to their kidney failure and they felt that the stroke is what affected their employment activities. One patient seemed more optimistic, stating, "My illness sets limits and guidelines, but I can manage it."

Vacation Activities

Fifty-six percent of the patients stated that vacation activities had been greatly or moderately affected by their illness. When the area of vacation activities was analyzed by various demographic variables, there were no statistically significant associations. When patients reported that their vacation activities had been greatly or moderately affected, we asked them to tell us in what ways their illness had affected them. A number of patients stated they were afraid to go to a new center at a vacation site some distance from home because they did not know the staff. Other patients identified the limited time available for travel. One patient said: "It's hard to go anywhere. I'm tied down three nights a week." Other patients noted the fact that there were no dialysis centers in other countries they wished to visit, for example, Panama, or even in some rural areas of the United States.

Leisure Time Pursuits

Fifty-six percent of the patients stated that their leisure time pursuits had been greatly or moderately affected by their illness. When the impact on these activities was analyzed by demographic variables, sex, education, and length of time on dialysis showed significant results (see Tables 2 and 3).

Males reported that their leisure time pursuits were less affected than females. One might speculate that males would experience a greater disruption in their leisure time pursuits because of a general inclination toward sports and physical activities. However, because the sample mean age is 46, physically oriented activities may not have had the significance they would have had if a younger sample of patients had been studied.

Another possible explanation for the difference between males and females relates to the amount of time and energy available for leisure time pursuits. Twenty-four males in the sample classified themselves as unemployed or retired, whereas only four females fell into these two categories. It seems plausible that retired and/or unemployed individuals would have more time and energy for leisure pursuits than those patients who are employed or are homemakers. Of 19 women, 11 listed themselves as homemakers. The role of homemaker or mother is somewhat fixed and the responsibilities may remain even after the occurrence of illness. Also the responsibilities of managing a house and/or child care may deplete the energy of these women leaving less for leisure time pursuits. This idea was partially substantiated by the comments of 29 patients. Six of the respondents, five of whom were women, used words like "tired," "weak," or "no energy." Some stated, "I'm too tired or weak to do things" and "I can't go dancing and do things because I'm tired." The majority of the other 23 respondents noted a general decrease in activities.

The impact of renal failure and dialysis treatments on leisure time pursuits was also significantly associated with educational level. The higher the levels of schooling, the less the impact of the illness ($r = 0.26$). One explanation for this finding is that people with more education may select activities which are more intellectual or cultural. When confronted with an illness that limits physical energy, the illness would not conflict as radically with their normal leisure time activities.

Length of time on dialysis was also significantly associated with the patients' reports of the degree of impact on their leisure time pursuits. The longer a patient had been on dialysis, the less the leisure time activities were reported affected ($r = 0.23$). This finding probably reflects adjustment to the limitations of the illness. Patients who have been on dialysis longer may have been able to develop activities that are within the limitations imposed by their illness and consequently feel that their leisure time pursuits have been less affected.

Eating Habits

The impact of kidney failure and dialysis treatments on the patients' eating habits was another area explored in the interview. Fifty-six percent of the patients reported their eating habits were greatly or moderately affected by their illness. When the area of eating habits was analyzed by different demographic variables, sex and religion showed a significant associations (see Table 2).

Males reported their eating habits were less affected than those of females. One possible explanation for this finding is that the males in the study do not adhere to their dietary regimen as rigorously as females, and therefore feel less of an impact. This explanation was not supported by the concrete dietary measures of potassium and phosphorous compliance, as males and females did not significantly differ on these two measures. However, males and females may differ on eating habits in other ways. For example, males may use more salt or eat food with higher levels of sodium than women. This would result in increased fluid intake and retention. This premise was somewhat substantiated by the finding that males were significantly less compliant with respect to between-dialysis weight gains ($t = 4.81$, $df = 53$, $p = 0.000$).

The other significant finding differentiated subgroups by religion. Catholics reported less of an impact on their eating habits than Protestants. We have no ready explanation for this finding.

We asked the patients to comment about the ways in which their eating habits had been affected. Many patients noted a loss of appetite, while others reported that they ate less and could not eat their favorite foods. One patient commented: "I had to give up a lot of foods and give up my usual restaurants." Another patient stated: "I've had a good appetite all my life and now it's really hard to stick with a diet." In general, patients identified the marked changes and difficulties encountered in making a healthy adjustment to the prescribed renal dietary regimen.

Sexual Activity

The last of the behavioral variables to be discussed here is the patients' reports of the impact of illness on their sexual activity. Fifty-three percent of the patients said their sexual activity had been greatly or moderately affected by their kidney disease and dialysis treatments. The three demographic variables of education, marital status, and income were significantly related to the extent of the impact of illness on sexual activity (see Tables 2 and 3).

Patients with higher levels of education reported less of an impact on their sexual activity than those with lower levels of education ($r = 0.29$). One possible explanation for this finding is that patients with higher levels of education may have been exposed to alternative ideas for dealing with sexual problems and a broader spectrum of values with reference to sexual behaviors. When confronted with the limitations imposed by renal failure, that is, a decrease in physical energy and less sexual drive, they may be able to modify previous sexual behavior patterns as a means of coping with the new situation.

Married patients reported their sexual activity was more affected than those not married. This may in part be explained by the dissonance created by the disruption of stable, ongoing sexual activity patterns. Patients' normal sexual activity would be markedly affected particularly during the acute stages of the illness. Patients with a consistent pattern of sexual activity may have more difficulty denying the changes which are concomitant with decreased physical energy and desire for sexual activity. Awareness of changes in sexual activity might be less and the tendency to deny easier among those patients without regular sexual partners or with those for whom opportunity for contact was less frequent than in ongoing, living-together arrangements such as marriage.

Patients with higher incomes reported their sexual activity was more affected than those with lower incomes ($r = -0.26$). We have no ready explanation for this finding.

Thirty patients who stated that their sexual activity had been greatly or moderately affected responded to further inquiry with only negative comments. Thirty percent of the patients stated that they had no desire for sex. Twenty-seven percent of the patients mentioned decrease in stamina and lack of energy.

Affective Areas

The next three areas, ability to enjoy life, self-esteem, and sense of security relate to the patients' sense of well-being and are conceptualized as affective areas. Table 4 displays the patients' report of the impact of the illness on these areas as differentiated by selected demographic variables.

Ability to Enjoy Life

Forty percent of the patients stated that their ability to enjoy life had been greatly or moderately affected by their renal disease. Generally, the patients stated that they were unable to engage in many previous activities because of physical limitations. One patient stated: "I can't do the things I want like take vacations and go to restaurants." Another patient

TABLE 4
Correlations between the Impact of Illness
on Affective Areas and Selected
Demographic Variables

| | Affective areas | |
Demographic variables	Ability to enjoy life	Self-esteem
Education (N=55)	0.20	0.26[a]
Income (N=47)	-0.26[a]	-0.11

[a]Sample size correlation was significant at the 0.05 level.

summarized many of the difficulties encountered by dialysis patients, saying: "I get tired a lot, and don't enjoy things with other people. The buses, subways, and shopping are all hassles now, and I can't afford to take a taxi. I also need someone with me because I can't carry the packages."

When the ability to enjoy life was analyzed by various demographic variables, income was the only one that showed a significant association (see Table 4). Patients reporting less income stated that their ability to enjoy life had been less affected by their illness than those reporting higher incomes ($r = -0.26$). One explanation for this finding is that patients with lower incomes may not have experienced as severe a change in their financial resources as those in the higher income group. Patients living on marginal incomes prior to their kidney failure would have about equivalent incomes when becoming eligible for Social Security Disability or Supplemental Security Income. Patients who had been earning better incomes may experience greater relative changes in their financial standings, which would probably affect their life styles to a greater extent. For example, if one has had the available income to take long vacations to other countries, and so forth, this activity may be considerably decreased with subsequent loss of income. Another change has to do with eating habits. Often individuals with higher incomes can afford to, and do, go out to eat at restaurants more often. Patients usually decrease the frequency of eating out, because of the difficulty of eating foods which are compatible with their renal diet.

Self-Esteem

We also inquired about the impact of the patients' illness on their feelings of self-esteem. Thirty-six percent of the patients indicated that their self-esteem had been greatly or moderately affected by their illness. When the patients' report of the impact of their illness on their self-esteem was analyzed by demographic variables, education was the only statistically significant association (see Table 4).

Patients with higher levels of education reported that their self-esteem was not as greatly affected as those with lower educational levels ($r = 0.26$). One possible explanation for the correlation between education and self-esteem has to do with the person's sense of self-esteem prior to experiencing kidney failure. Patients with higher educational levels may have had greater self-esteem prior to illness because of their educational accomplishments and concomitantly more prestigious employment and higher incomes. Even when faced with drastic life changes due to their illness, they may still have greater reserves of positive feelings to draw upon. While we did not have data on the patients' levels of self-esteem prior to illness, we did find a significant correlation between educational levels and levels of self-esteem as measured by Rosenberg's Self-Esteem Scale[2] at the time of the interview. Patients with higher levels of education had higher levels of self-esteem ($r = -0.38$, $N = 55$; $p = 0.00$).

Another explanation for this finding is that patients with higher educational levels may be more readily able to continue their life styles including employment and intellectual and cultural interests. The idea of self-esteem being related to continuing a certain life style is given credence by the findings that patients with higher education levels reported their employment activities were less affected ($r = 0.28$), and their ability to enjoy life was less affected ($r = 0.20$, $p = 0.07$).

When patients who reported that their self-esteem had been greatly or moderately affected were asked to elaborate, they related that they felt less capable, independent, and productive than before their kidney failure. Some patients felt they could no longer take care of their family and meet the expectations of various roles, for example, husband, employee, mother, and so forth. One patient's comment reflected the potential impact of this illness on one's self-perception and self-esteem. He said: "I don't feel like a normal human being anymore."

Sense of Security

We thought that a life-threatening illness, such as kidney failure, would have considerable impact on a patient's sense of security. When patients were asked to rate the impact of their illness on this variable, surprisingly, only 36% of the patients indicated that their sense of security had been greatly or moderately affected as a result of their kidney failure. When the impact of the illness on the patients' sense of security was analyzed by the demographic variables, there were no statistically significant associations.

When we asked the patients who had reported being greatly or moderately affected how their sense of security had been affected, 31% said they felt more vulnerable financially. Other comments related to the unpredictability of the illness and feelings of emotional insecurity.

Relational Areas

The last three areas to be discussed, relationship with friends, social contacts, and family relationships are conceptualized as relational areas. Tables 5 and 6 show the patients' reports of the impact of the illness on these areas as differentiated by selected demographic variables.

TABLE 5
Correlations between the Impact of Illness on Relational Areas
and Selected Demographic Variables

Demographic variables	Relational Areas		
	Relationship with friends	Social contacts	Family relationships
Education (N=55)	0.38[a]	0.07	0.15
Income (N=47)	0.24[a]	−0.05	−0.02
Time on dialysis (N=55)	−0.04	0.09	0.26[a]

TABLE 6
Impact of Illness on Relational Life Areas

Relational areas	Demographic variables
	New York City born (N = 19) vs. born outside New York City area (N = 36)
Relationship with friends	−2.24[a]
Social contacts	−1.11
Family relationships	−2.08[a]

[a]$p < 0.05$, one tail test.

Relationship with Friends

Thirty-one percent of the patients reported that their relationships with friends had been greatly or moderately affected by their illness. When the impact of the illness on relationships with friends was analyzed by the demographic variables, education, income, and place of birth showed statistically significant associations (see Tables 5 and 6).

The higher the patients' education, the less they reported that their relationships with friends had been affected ($r = 0.38$). This again may reflect friendships developed around more intellectual or cultural interests which are more readily maintained in the face of illness and treatment requirements. Another possibility is that persons with higher levels of education may have broader interests and more alternatives around which they can develop and sustain friendships.

Patients with higher incomes reported that their relationships with friends were less affected than those patients with lower income levels ($r = 0.24$). This may reflect greater financial resources and a certain life style which may be less disrupted by dialysis treatments. Individuals with higher incomes can afford various types of transportation which would allow them to visit friends outside their specific locale. People with limited incomes may have to forego visiting if it means the rigorous task of negotiating public transportation.

Patients who were born outside the New York City area reported that their relationships with friends were less affected than those patients born in the New York City area. One possible explanation is that people who migrate develop a larger network of friends as part of coping with the relocation, and that these bonds are less disrupted by the impact of their illness. This explanation is somewhat substantiated by the finding that patients born in places other than New York City reported having more friends ($t = 1.41$, $df = 53$, $p = 0.09$). These two groups of patients did not differ on the amount of time they spent with their friends or on the patients' reports about how well their friends understood their kidney disease and treatment requirements.

Patients who stated that their relationships with their friends had been greatly or moderately affected were asked to elaborate. They reported that they see their friends less, and cannot participate in many of their previous activities, such as drinking, partying, engaging in physical activities, and so forth. Nearly a third of the patients who responded to our in-depth inquiry indicated that they had stopped seeing friends, and not vice versa.

Social Contacts

We also inquired about the impact of the patients' kidney disease on social contacts. Forty percent of the patients stated that their social contacts had been greatly or moderately affected by their illness. When this area was analyzed by the different demographic variables, no significant associations were found. Of those patients who said their social contacts had been greatly or moderately affected, 75% said they do not go out at all or go out less. Many of the patients' comments suggested a movement toward isolation and indicated experiencing a general sense of loss. However, one patient seemed to have a somewhat philosophical view of his situation, stating: "Life has stopped somewhat. This illness slows your life down. You learn that a lot of different things become important. It makes you feel sorry for people who take things for granted."

Relationship with Family

The last relational area investigated was the impact of the illness on the patient's relationships with her/his family. Twenty-nine percent of the patients stated their relationships with their families had been

greatly or moderately affected by their illness. When this area was analyzed by different demographic variables, the variables of length of time
on dialysis and place of birth showed significant associations. Patients
who had been on dialysis longer reported their relationships with their
families had been less affected by their illness than those patients on dialysis for a shorter period of time $(r = 0.26)$. This finding probably reflects an adjustment to dialysis by both the patient and the family. After
the initial crisis of the illness, patient and family would likely reestablish
a certain level of equilibrium.

Patients born outside the New York City area reported that their relationships with their families were less affected than those patients
born in the area. One possible explanation for this finding is that individuals or families that migrated to this area tended to have a greater
reliance on the family. Those patients who migrated to this area were
black patients from the Caribbean islands or the southern parts of the
United States. The sense of family may have been stronger for this
group of patients, thus the impact of the illness on family relationships
was felt less.

We asked those patients who stated that their relationship with
their families had been greatly or moderately affected to elaborate. Of
the 15 patients who responded to this inquiry, 80% felt that the impact
on the family had been negative. Problems included difficulties with
children, divorce, sexual problems, and less contact with the family. For
the three patients who felt that their relationships with the family improved, one felt the family was closer, another said they treat him nicer,
and the third patient just said it was better.

IMPACT OF ILLNESS AND COMPLIANCE BEHAVIOR

One may speculate on the association between impact of illness and
compliance behavior in several ways. For example, one might argue that
the more negative the impact of the illness, the more the person would
comply in order to attempt to reestablish an equilibrium closest to the
pre-kidney failure level of functioning. On the other hand, one could argue to the contrary that the greater the impact of the illness, the more
discouraged a patient would become leading to increased apathy and
lack of caring as to whether or not the medical and dietary regimen were
followed. For those patients who felt that the illness had not greatly affected their lives, one might expect to see a trend toward continued
noncompliant behavior prompted by the feeling that there was no need
to modify their behavior. On the other hand, one could also argue that
these very patients might worry about the potential hazards of

noncompliant behavior and therefore try to be more compliant to avoid having their lives greatly affected.

We did an inter-item correlational analysis in order to ascertain the degree of relatedness of the eleven areas previously discussed. The alpha level of internal reliability for these eleven areas was 0.82. We then summed each patient's scores on the eleven items in order to construct the overall impact scale. We correlated this overall impact scale with the dependent measures of phosphorous and potassium levels, between-dialysis weight gains, an overall compliance index, and patients' self-reports of compliance. Surprisingly, there were no statistically significant associations ($p = 0.05$). One possible explanation for the absence of significant findings is that the extent of the impact of illness may differentially affect patients. As we speculated earlier, the extent of the impact of the illness may act as a motivator or inhibitor of compliance behavior.

Our next step was to look at each of the eleven areas and the measures of compliance behavior. Correlational analysis of each of the areas with the five dependent measures showed a total of only six statistically significant associations (see Table 7). We must add a cautionary note that given the small number of significant correlations, it is possible that some of these findings are a result of probability.

There were significant negative correlations between the impact of the illness on family relationships and three of the dependent measures of compliance behavior. In other words, the greater the negative impact on family relationships, the less the compliance with respect to phosphorus ($r = -0.23$), between-dialysis weight gains ($r = -0.23$), and the overall compliance index ($r = -0.25$). As family relationships become disrupted by role reversals, increased financial pressure, and the

TABLE 7
Correlational Analysis of Selected Life Areas and Five Measures of Compliance

Life areas	Measures of compliance				
	Phosphorous levels	Potassium levels	Between-dialysis weight gain	Overall compliance index	Self-report of compliance
Family relationships	−0.23[a]	−0.10	−0.23[a]	−0.25[a]	0.14
Relationships with friends	−0.03	−0.01	−0.26[a]	−0.13	0.08
Social contacts	−0.10	0.19	−0.09	−0.00	−0.25[a]
Sense of security	−0.06	0.26[a]	0.06	0.17	−0.09

[a]Sample size correlation significant at the 0.05 level.

stresses of the treatment requirements, the family may have greater difficulty in supporting the patient's adaptation to the medical and dietary regimen. Compliance may also become a control issue over which the family expresses its dysfunctional adaptation to the illness. For example, families may become overly zealous in wanting the patient to rigidly follow the medical and dietary regimen with the patient subsequently rebelling by being noncompliant.

Another significant finding was the relationship between the impact of the illness on friendships and compliance behavior. The greater the negative impact on friendships, the less the patient's compliance with respect to between-dialysis weight gain ($r = -0.26$). While we have no ready explanation for this finding, this area warrants further attention by the health care team, as this appears to be one which could be influenced by professional interventions.

The other significant finding was that patients who identified themselves as compliant experienced a greater disruption in terms of social contacts ($r = -0.25$). Patients have identified and/or may anticipate social events as difficult because other people often do not realize their need to restrict their sodium intake, amount of fluids, certain foods, and so forth. Hosts may either not provide the proper food substitutes or may enourage the patient to be noncompliant in terms of saying "have another drink," and so forth. Because of these stresses, the patient who wants to be compliant may avoid these social events. While this behavior may assist them in being more compliant with their medical and dietary regimen, the results may be deleterious to their social life.

We also found that patients who reported less of an impact on their sense of security were less compliant with respect to potassium levels ($r = 0.26$). This finding may be viewed from the perspective of the dysfunctional utilization of the defense mechanism of denial. Realistically, renal failure poses many potential problems and assaults to one's sense of security. If a patient denies the limitations and potential problems of the illness, then one could also deny the need to follow the diet, which could result in noncompliant behavior.

SUMMARY

Renal failure has a pervasive impact on patients' lives. In this study we found that the behavioral areas, employment activities, sexual activities, eating habits, vacation activities, and leisure time pursuits were the aspects most affected by renal failure and the subsequent adaptation to a dialysis regimen.

Less educated, married, female patients, new to dialysis, seem to be hit the hardest by the impact of renal failure and dialysis treatments. Pa-

tients with less education reported more of an impact regarding employment activities, leisure time pursuits, sexual activity, self-esteem and relationships with friends. Patients with lower socioeconomic status felt a
greater impact on their employment activities. Higher educational levels
seem to mediate the impact of the illness on the patient. Perhaps patients in these categories have greater internal and external resources to
draw upon while making changes necessitated by the illness and treatment regimen.

Female patients reported a greater disruption with respect to leisure
time pursuits and eating habits than male patients. Being a relatively
new patient to dialysis seems to impact greatest on the areas of leisure
time pursuits and family relationships. Married patients experienced a
greater upheaval in terms of their sexual activity than those patients not
married.

The lack of an abundance of associations between the impact of the
illness and the compliance behavior lends some credence to the idea of
differential reactions to illness. As discussed previously, we feel that the
degree of impact of the illness may act as a motivator or inhibitor with
respect to adjusting and complying with the medical and dietary regimen; however, this warrants further research. Understanding which
groups of patients are most affected by the impact of renal failure will
assist the health care team in providing the maximum support.

ACKNOWLEDGMENTS. The author expresses his appreciation to M. M.
Avram, M.D., F.A.C.P., Chief, Division of Nephrology, and the staff at
the Brooklyn Kidney Center for their support and assistance in conducting this research project.

REFERENCES

1. HOLLINGSHEAD, A. B. *Social class and mental illness; a community study.* New York:
   Wiley Press, 1958.
2. ROSENBERG, M. *Society and the adolescent self image.* Princeton, New Jersey: Princeton
   University Press, 1965.

6

Liaison Psychiatry Considerations in Renal Hemodialysis Patients with Acute Organic Cerebral Disorders

RICHARD A. FAMULARO AND CHASE P. KIMBALL

Renal personnel are trained and equipped to deal with medical emergencies but have little training in the management of acute behavioral, cognitive, and emotional changes. The disoriented, combative, noncompliant, or paranoid patient presents a host of problems. The main focus of this discussion is the recognition that acute alterations of personality and mentation often herald an organic cerebral disturbance. Patients with chronic renal disorders are particularly susceptible to a variety of severe physiological disturbances and subsequent cerebral disorders (Table 1). Typically, emergency psychiatric consultation is requested following an abrupt change in the patient's behavior. At the University of Chicago hospitals, as high as 50% of all emergency psychiatric consults were ultimately found to be related to patients with organic cerebral disorders. This indicates that there is both a difficulty in recognizing organic causes of confusion and delirium and an inexperience in managing such disturbances. This combination of factors places the renal liaison psychiatrist in an important role due to his training in evaluating mental status, his ability to understand the interpersonal concerns between staff and patient, and his understanding of abnormal behavior.

An extended mental status exam is indicated for all patients with suspected organicity. It is the purpose of this discussion to present various bedside techniques requiring only simple questions, paper and pencil, and neurological physical exam when indicated. These evalua-

RICHARD A. FAMULARO, M.D. • Clinical Instructor of Child Psychiatry, Harvard Medical School, Boston, Massachusetts.   CHASE P. KIMBALL, M.D. • Professor of Psychiatry and Medicine, Division of Biological Sciences and Professor in the College, University of Chicago, Chicago, Illinois.

TABLE 1
Renal Disorders and Complications
Which May Contribute to or Cause
an Organic Cerebral Disorder

Renal Failure:
Uremia
Hyperkalemia
Hyponatremia
Hyperphosphatemia
Hypocalcemia, hypercalcemia
Metabolic acidosis
Complications of Renal Failure:
Anemia
Arrhythmias
Congestive heart failure
Stroke
Hypertensive encephalopathy
Sepsis
Seizures
Endocrine disorders
Other CNS abnormalities
Complications of Treatment:
Dialysis dysequilibrium syndrome
Dialysis dementia
Medication
Infection
Bleeding disorders

tions are helpful in identifying organic cerebral disorder (Table 2). However, the absence of positive signs does not, by definition, rule out organicity.

Organic cerebral disorders are always complicated by the patient's personality and emotional reaction to the disease. Rarely does one find an organic deficit without concomitant psychological changes. In certain respects, a distinction between "organic" and "functional" is artificial. The expressed behavior, affect, and cognition is determined by common final neuropsychological pathways. Identification of etiology assumes significance because organic factors are potentially amenable to medical intervention.

LEVELS OF CONSCIOUSNESS

The first and perhaps the most important evaluation of the mental status is a determination of the patient's level of consciousness. The term consciousness is difficult to define precisely and is frequently am-

TABLE 2
Indicated Evaluations in an Extended Mental Status Exam When
Cerebral Disorders Are Suspected

Evaluation of/for	Signs and symptoms
Level of consciousness (see section on levels of consciousness)	A true decrease in arousal is indicative of a brain stem lesion or diffuse brain function depression. Minor impairment of consciousness has no pathognomic signs and detection is based on clinical judgment.
Onset of illness (by presentation and history)	A rapid onset of behavioral, emotional, and cognitive changes may suggest an organic cerebral disorder.
Lability of mood (excessive emotional responses)	Rapid changes of mood are seen frequently in cerebral disorders as well as acute manic delirium.
Orientation (to person, place, and time)	The inability to recognize person, place, and time is consistent with cerebral disease.
Aphasia (dysphasia) (the inability of the patient to understand or express words, even though the mechanisms of articulation, sensory systems, and sensorium are intact) Disorders are classified as expressive (speaking and writing) and receptive (reading and listening). Expressive aphasia is tested by having the patient write something spontaneously. Receptive aphasia is tested by giving a simple command to follow or having the patient read silently and then explain the passage.	Generally, these disorders implicate a lesion in the left parasylvian region with the expressive disorder more anterior and the receptive more posterior.
Language dysfunctions (other than aphasia) Common disorders are: articulation (dysarthria), word omissions, inaccuracies of grammar (paragrammartisms), echolalia, and neologisms.	The presence of these language dysfunctions is correlated with cerebral disease to a greater degree than to a schizophrenic thought process.
Apraxia (dyspraxia) (the inability to perform a volitional act even though the motor tracts and sensorium are intact) Some of the more useful and practical tests include: copying figures (circle, square, cross, triangle, diamond, or cube) and the construction of objects (clock, bicycle, or house).	In a person with normal cerebral integration (providing there has been no previous lesion or retardation, and the person has at least a fourth-grade education), no errors are expected on tasks of copying geometric figures. The overall integration of the constructed objects may give valuable information regarding the lesion site.

(continued)

TABLE 2 (*continued*)

Evaluation of/for	Signs and symptoms
Agnosia (the inability to understand the significance of sensory stimuli even though the sensory pathways are intact) Testing includes the naming of common objects placed in the hand (astereognasia) and naming a number written in the palm (agraphognosia).	Providing sufficient premorbid skills were present, no errors are expected in persons with normal cerebral integration.
Topographical sense and R–L orientation (the performing of simultaneous tasks, such as placing the left hand on the right ear and placing the right hand on the left elbow)	Patients with an intact brain are expected to perform without error.
Disturbance of body image Face–Hand Test: Patient with hands on knees and eyes closed sits facing examiner who simultaneously touches the cheek and dorsum of the subject's hand. The procedure by Bender, Fink, and Green as modified by Kahn and Pollach includes the following order of stimulation: 1. R ch & L h 6. R h & L h 2. L ch & R h 7. R ch & L h 3. R ch & L h 8. L ch & R h 4. L ch & L h 9. R ch & R h 5. R ch & L ch 10. L ch & L h	Providing the sensory pathways are intact, no errors are expected. Errors may include: displacement (touch reported on untouched body parts); extinction (patient does not report touch); and exosomethesia (reports touch outside himself).
Test for finger agnosia: Touching two of the patient's fingers and asking him to state how many fingers lie between them.	This is a sensitive test for dominant parietal lobe lesion.
Memory and recall Common methods for testing include digit span and historical information.	The loss of recent memory is greater than the loss of past memory in organically impaired patients.
Arithmetical operations Testing includes the performance of simple addition, subtraction, multiplication, and division.	Taking into account the patient's school history and achievements, no errors are expected.
Alternating sequences Tests include: alternately drawing circles and crosses; or having the patient predict which of the clinician's hands is hiding a coin.	This tends to be a sensitive test of frontal lobe dysfunction.
Human figure-drawing (for children) The diagnostician asks the child to draw a person.	Figures with stick arms, stick legs, incorrect number of fingers, no pupils, no neck, poor integration of parts, and a figure angled more than 15%, are statistically significant indicators of organic cerebral disorder.

(*continued*)

Table 2 (continued)

Evaluation of/for	Signs and symptoms
Physical exam	The presence of a Rhomberg sign, wide base gait, lack of manual precision, sucking reflex, palmomental reflex, glabella reflex, babinski, and others indicate significant neurological disease but usually are not as fine a measure nor as early an indicator as some of the previously mentioned tests.

biguous. It often tends to be more of a literary or philosophical term than a medical term. In its narrowest form, consciousness may be defined as a normal reaction of the self to the environment. A more global explanation would include the perception of one's entire mental, cognitive, and emotional self, as well as his perception of his surroundings. Neurophysiologically, normal waking consciousness is expressed by the electrical potential of the brain through regular waves of alpha rhythm (8–15/sec) and beta rhythm (16–25/sec). With the exception of mild clouding and confusion, all disturbances of consciousness are reflected by some variation in brain wave activity. An evaluation of consciousness must include a definition of the patient's "content" of consciousness (sum of mental functions) and "arousal" of consciousness (associated with wakefulness). The content component is structurally related to the cerebral hemisphere whereas the arousal element is a function of the brainstem (diencephalon, midbrain, pons). Impairment of arousal or content may present separately (as found in a localized aphasia without changes in arousal level) or together (such as an acute metabolic delirium). The various levels of consciousness include:

1. Normal consciousness: This is the state of awareness of self and environment in the normal waking adult.

2. Clouding of consciousness: A patient in this state presents with irritability and excitability, alternating with drowziness. Reaction time increases, clarity of thinking decreases, and the patient appears easily distracted, startled, and hypervigilant.

3. Confusional state of consciousness: Within this state there is a more intensive and progressive clouding. Mild disorientation and memory impairment, especially recent memory, is observed. The patient appears confused, and has difficulty following commands and performing simple tasks (such as figure drawing, writing, reading, and recall). One's attention span is short, stimuli are less clearly understood, and the significance of previously understood concepts may be lost. Drowziness and agitation may both be prominent and alternating. Emo-

tional lability, anger, sadness, suspiciousness, fearfulness, and uncooperativeness are evident. The ability to express oneself either verbally or in written form, and the ability to receive and process words may be diminished.

4. Delirium: Delirium represents a much more intensive and volatile state. The patient may be loquacious, loud, and verbally assaultive. Fear, agitation, disorientation, and significant confusion may alternate with lucid periods (which demands the liaison psychiatrist to perform sequential evaluations). Hallucinations, delusions, illusions, loose associations, derailment, flight of ideas, paranoia, thought control, thought broadcasting, and ideas of reference can occur. Affective disturbances, rapid mood changes, poor impulse control, lability, depression, and a sense of euphoria may appear. Variations in level of arousal may be prevalent and electroencephalogram changes are noted. The inability to perform various tasks, as mentioned in the confusional state, persists.

5. Stupor: In this state of consciousness the individual can only be aroused by intense, repeated stimulation.

6. Coma: Coma is the state of complete unresponsiveness to stimuli, during which time the patient cannot be aroused.

The presentation of stupor or coma is the necessary result of an injury or insult to the brainstem activating structures (directly or by compression), or a diffuse, global depression of the brain. Numerous neurophysiological states may produce stupor and coma, and only rarely do psychiatric disorders present in a coma-like state (psychogenic unresponsiveness). Psychogenic unresponsiveness lasting more than 5 minutes is uncommon. Pupilary reflexes, dolls-eyes, caloric testing, resistance to passive movement, plantar reflexes, and most reliably, the EEG, aid the physician in a determination of the presence of psychogenic unresponsiveness. Stupor and coma obviously are in the realm of the neurologist and neurosurgeon, however the liaison psychiatrist is often called upon by the renal service to evaluate the hypervigilant, clouded, confused, or delirious patient. It is within this context that the psychiatrist can offer the most assistance because of his expertise in evaluating mental status and suggesting the appropriate treatment.

REPORT OF A CASE

The patient, a 65-year-old female was admitted to the university hospital with a provisional diagnosis of FUO. For many years she had been maintained on three/week chronic hemodialysis secondary to polycystic kidneys. Admitting physical exam was positive for mild CHF, fever, and anemia. There were no focal neurological findings, and chemistries revealed no significant changes from her normal baseline. In addition, the admitting notes stated that she seemed depressed, uninterested, fatigued, and uncharacteristically noncompliant with the medical regime. The day following admission, the liaison psychiatrist was consulted on an emergency basis "to comment on the patient's confusion, agitation, and possible depression." The initial psychiatric mental status revealed: drowziness; minimal spontaneous speech; fluctuating periods of agitation; and sadness without despair, hopelessness, or futility. Though interaction with the interviewer was generally appropriate, she had difficulty fully appreciating the nature of her situation. Thought process and content revealed none of the following: hallucinations, delusions, illusions, ideas of reference, paranoia, loose associations, derailment, flight of ideas, thought control, thought broadcasting, nor self-destructive ideation. The sensorium was judged to be mildly clouded with decreased attention span, disorientation to data, and poor 1-minute recall. Extinction and displacement were noted in face–hand test, although performance was normal on two simultaneous tasks. Retesting in 6 hours revealed constructional apraxia (unable to draw a triangle), astereognosia (misnamed a quarter), and expressive dysphasia (dysgraphia). In addition, the patient mislabeled the hours of the clock and drew a very distorted representation of a bicycle. During these 6 hours there had been no change in wakefulness, but increasing lability was appreciated. Approximately 1 hour later, significant peripheral perfusion changes were noted and ABG revealed hypoxia. The patient was begun on oxygen (and increasing doses of digoxin) with subsequent physical and neuropsychological improvement. This was witnessed by a normalization of face–hand, constructional, and language tasks; a decrease in agitation; and an increase in compliance. This case illustrates some of the alterations of mentation early in the course of a cerebral insult (in this patient, a diffuse metabolic process).

MANAGEMENT AND TREATMENT

Optimal treatment implies knowledge of the etiology. As previously mentioned, the presence of clouded consciousness, confusion, and delirium may be related to different disease processes. Repeated observation and testing over time may prove to be the only course to follow when the etiology is unclear. The liaison psychiatrist is a valuable consultant and teacher to the medical personnel, especially when the patient is delirious. The patient may be hostile, noncompliant, and generally disruptive to the smooth flow of management desired by the staff. The renal staff may become frightened, concerned, and angered at the confused and delirious patient. Concern for the individual's welfare and anger at the patient's behavior are reactions that may coexist within the staff. It is possible that a staff member may unconsciously act out his anger at the patient (dispensing medication off-schedule, trying to transfer the patient to another unit, less intensive observations, and so forth), resulting in less than optimal care. During this time, a psychiatrist's role may become that of a mediator, teacher, consultant, and group leader. The goal is to aid the staff in developing a true sense of empathy for the patient and his disease process. Medical personnel need to understand the natural behavioral and emotional consequences of the organically impaired patient.

Acute changes in personality and cognition constitute a psychiatric emergency (and perhaps a medical emergency). Consistency, ready availability, and a working knowledge of the unit's ongoing activities are vital qualities the liaison psychiatrist must possess. Weekly seminars with the staff serve the function of lessening staff anxiety and increasing empathy towards the patient.

Immediate management of the delirious patient should include: (1) never leaving the patient alone; (2) speaking to the patient in simple, orienting, and repeated statements; (3) keeping change and unusual stimuli to a minimum; (4) repeated sequential mental status evaluations; (5) indicated diagnostic procedures (serum chemistries, CAT scan, EEG, and so forth); and (6) psychopharmacological treatment. (The level of arousal must be clearly assessed since certain psychotropics can be CNS depressants. Minor tranquilizers should be avoided in the delirious patient.)

SELECTED BIBLIOGRAPHY

1. BENJAMIN, S., and SHERWIN, I. Organic brain syndromes: An empirical study and critical review. *American Journal of Psychiatry*, 1978, 135(1), 13–21.
2. BENSON, D. F., and BLUMER, D. (Eds.), Psychiatric aspects of neurological disease. New York: Grune and Stratton, 1975.
3. BOND, T. Recognition of acute manic delirium. *Archives of General Psychiatry*, 1980, 37, 553–554.
4. CHARATAN, F. B. Acute confusion and the elderly. *Hospital Physician*, 1975, 12, 8–10.
5. FAUMAN, M. A. Treatment of the agitated patient with an organic brain disorder. *Journal of the American Medical Association*, 1978, 240, 380–382.
6. HALL, R. C., Physical illness manifesting as psychiatric disease. *Archives of General Psychiatry*, 1980, 37, 989–995.
7. KIMBALL, C. P. Liaison psychiatry. *Psychiatric Clinics of North America*, 1979, 2(2), 201–210.
8. KOPPITZ, E. M. *Psychological evaluation of children's figure drawing*. New York: Grune and Stratton, 1968.
9. KRAKOWSKI, A. J. Liaison psychiatry in North America. Bibliotheca Psychiatrica, 1979, 159, 4–14.
10. LEZAK, M. A. *Neuropsychological assessment*. New York: Oxford University Press, 1976.
11. LISHMAN, W. A. Organic psychiatry. In *The psychological consequences of cerebral disorder*. Oxford: Blackwell Scientific Publications, 1978.
12. MCFIE, J. *Assessment of organic intellectual impairment*. New York: Academic Press, 1975.
13. PETERSON, H. W. and MARTIN, M. J. Organic disease presenting as a psychiatric syndrome. *Postgraduate Medicine*, 1973, 54, 78–82.
14. PLUM, F., and POSNER, J. B. *The diagnosis of stupor and coma*. 3rd Ed. Philadelphia: F. A. Davis Company, 1980.
15. SCHRIER, R. W. (Ed.), *Renal and electrolyte disorders*. Boston: Little, Brown and Company, 1976.

7

Patient Self-Reported Adjustment and Health Beliefs in Compliant versus Noncompliant Hemodialysis Patients

STEPHEN ARMSTRONG AND ANNE WOODS

INTRODUCTION

It is universally assumed among health care professionals in nephrology that compliance to diet and fluid restrictions predicts survival on chronic dialysis. The consequences of noncompliance are more immediate and potentially lethal than in every other chronic disease syndrome. In one of the first clinical studies in this area, eight of the ten fatalities were patients who abused the fluid and dietary regimens.[1] Inasmuch as the suicide rate is noted to be far higher than that of the healthy adult population and that nearly all patients abuse their restrictions, noncompliance is tacitly or explicitly linked to patient suicide.[2]

To assay a patient's compliance to restrictions or to therapy is no mean feat.[3] We could arbitrarily define patients as "compliant" who meet certain criteria, but we may not be able to generalize such definitions (for example, "all patients who gain less than 1.5 kg between dialysis treatments" does little for the 115-kg man versus the 45-kg petite woman at the clinic). We could "index" compliance, for instance with metabolites, specific substances in the blood, or markers, but individuals differ in absorption and metabolism, and such markers or metabolites can give only ranks-within-a-group of compliance, not degrees of it. We could also use expert clinicians' ratings of compliance, but these are not especially valid, mainly because experts (physicians) systematically tend to overestimate compliance, no matter how much (or little) contact they have with patients.[4,5] Finally, we could depend

STEPHEN ARMSTRONG, PH.D. • Associate Clinical Professor, Tufts University School of Medicine; Pediatric Psychology, Baystate Medical Center, Springfield, Massachusetts. ANNE WOODS, M.S.W. • Nephrology Social Worker, Baystate Medical Center, Springfield, Massachusetts.

on patients' self-report, but patients' statements do not correspond well with other measures of compliance,[6,7] and one gets widely different results depending on how one asks a patient.[3] As one can see, there is no single best way (operationally) to define compliance. The previous attempts in the hemodialysis literature reflect these alternative, disparate, and not entirely effective methods: expert statement,[2,8] absolute levels of biochemical markers,[1,7,8] or patient report.[2,10]

In an attempt to shed some light on what is said to be an important problem when we knew methods of forming "compliance groups" would be looked at carefully, we did the following study.

METHODS

Enumerating a Sample

For all 127 Springfield, Massachusetts, medically stable patients, we collected six consecutive readings on three biochemical markers which usually are taken as important measures of the patients' condition: weight, phosphorous, and potassium. We then calculated five interdialysis slopes for each measure and calculated the mean slope value for each marker. We deleted from the sample all patients who had experienced a major medical crisis or hospitalization during the enumeration period. Then we ranked all remaining patients on the mean slopes for each marker. We assume in this study that small slopes reflect better adherence to the treatment and restrictions than large slopes, which indicate rapid shifts (that is, large relative gains) in important markers unrelated to intercurrent medical distress. We also assume that slopes are satisfactory proxies for absolute values, which could reflect girth or sex rather than adherence.

We then selected 20 patients for each group who had the lowest mean slopes ("compliant" group) or highest mean slopes ("noncompliant" group). Since a person hypothetically could be "good" on one marker and "terrible" on another, we also identified 10 patients with widely discrepant ranks ("crazy-quilt" compliance group), that is, rank differences of more than 80 places on the 127-patient list for any two markers.

We also asked six health care professionals to rate all 127 patients on 5-point Likert scales of compliance, thereby having a set of "subjective" ratings.

With informed consent and without inducements, we asked these 50 people selected on "objective" criteria compliance to be interviewed. Interviewers were blind as to which group the person belonged, and the interview order was randomized.

Interviews

There are three models of compliance currently extant in the nephrology literature. The first is psychodynamic and uses constructs, loosely operationalized, from personality theory.[1,2] Since the operationalization of these constructs is so difficult, especially in short, non-therapeutic interviews, we dismissed the model as regrettably untestable.

The second model is called the "ecological adjustment" model; it is essentially a stress–diathesis conceptualization currently in vogue in social work. Briefly stated, the patient is seen as a complex biopsychosocial person in a complex medical system in which component parts can fail by virtue of poor feedback or stress. For our purposes, we chose five areas of a patient's life we wished to know more about: (1) his/her interpersonal adjustment, (2) his/her control of health and restrictions, (3) his/her beliefs about one's place in the "life cycle," (4) his/her relations among the medical staff, and (5) his/her adjustment within the family, which is a topic especially strongly linked to compliance in a recent study.[12]

The third model is called the "health beliefs" model. It is an empirically "strong" social and psychological model of attitude formation and activation, most cogently articulated by Becker in a number of studies.[13,14] The core propositions are that patients are motivated to comply with treatment when there is a proper mix of (1) health attitudes about personal vulnerability to an illness, (2) awareness of severity of consequences of noncompliance, (3) belief in the benefits of compliance and capability to absorb costs, (4) expectation of personal control over the health care, and (5) an absence of barriers to health care. Parts of the model have been tested in a wide range of illnesses and compliance behaviors,[14] including chronic hemodialysis.[8]

Both the ecological adjustment and the health beliefs models are expressed in terms of patients' perceptions, so we constructed a 30-item questionnaire to measure five ecological adjustment scales and four health beliefs scales. We also asked patients to respond to a 53-item psychiatric symptom inventory, as a control measure for psychopathology (the Brief Symptom Inventory, a derivative instrument from the Hopkins Symptom Check List and Symptom Check List—90).[15,16] The interviews took approximately 45 minutes and were done while patients were receiving hemodialysis treatments.

FINDINGS

Since the compliance literature is so frought with results dependent on sample selection and reliability, we present the results of objective and subjective compliance measures first; then, reliability of the nine scales, second; then, the scales which "predict" membership in the three compliance groups.

Objective Measures of Compliance

At an intuitive "eyeball" level we noticed that patients could have widely discrepant rankings on mean slope values for weight, potassium, and phosphorous levels, but statistically the rankings are concordant, suggesting that we can trust that our three patient groups are "pure spectrum" compliers, noncompliers, or crazy-quilters. (Kendalls' Concordance [W] = .37, χ^2 = 142.6, df = 126, p > .14.)

Subjective Measures of Compliance

Basically, there are three ways to evaluate the six experts' ratings, and we are including all three as an illustration of the "trickiness" of compliance research methodology. First, the subjective ratings look "copacetic" because the Pearson correlations are all positive and range from .22 to .75 (Table 1). Yet the statistically inclined among us will appreciate that Pearson correlations conceal significant differences between rater pairs,[17] and for illustration we have shown that the two physicians differ from the four nonphysicians, and each other, on six out of nine rater-pair combinations (Table 2). The direction and magnitude of the differences are not readily predictable, but they are (usually) within one point of a five-point scale (Lawlis and Lu's χ^2 values) and average about 50% better than the ratings that chance alone would pro-

TABLE 1
Pearson Correlations between Clinicians' Ratings of Compliance

Rater	1	2	3	4	5	6	All non-MDs	MDs
1	1.00	0.62	0.73	0.38	0.70	0.46	0.82	0.59
2		1.00	0.60	0.22	0.60	0.42	0.66	0.49
3			1.00	0.37	0.74	0.45	0.85	0.64
4				1.00	0.42	0.34	0.57	0.39
5					1.00	0.75	0.52	0.93
6						1.00	0.74	0.87
All non-MDs							1.00	0.69
MDs								1.00

TABLE 2

Comparison of Compliance Ratings of Specified Rater-Pairs: 1 Point or Less Disagreement

Rater pair	Number of joint ratings of patients			Lawlis and Lu χ^2		Tinsley and Weiss t	Paired t-test				
	Patients	Agree	Disagree	Value	p	Value	t-value	p(2-tail)	Correlation	Mean difference	Std error
Dr. A—Rater 1	43	33	10	10.53	0.01	0.52	−1.95	0.06	0.71	−0.35	0.18
Dr. A—Rater 2	42	32	10	9.83	0.01	0.52	−5.55	0.00	0.60	−1.00	0.18
Dr. A—Rater 3	41	36	5	21.02	0.01	0.75	−1.91	0.06	0.73	−0.29	0.15
Dr. A—Rater 4	36	23	13	2.05	ns	0.25	−2.96	0.01	0.42	−0.67	0.22
Dr. B—Rater 1	36	23	13	2.05	ns	0.25	0.56	ns	0.46	0.14	0.24
Dr. B—Rater 2	35	24	11	3.85	0.05	0.34	−2.98	0.01	0.42	−0.60	0.20
Dr. B—Rater 3	35	27	8	8.85	0.01	0.52	0.96	ns	0.46	0.20	0.21
Dr. B—Rater 4	32	26	6	10.95	0.01	0.61	−0.98	ns	0.35	−0.22	0.22
Dr. A.—Dr. B.	36	32	4	19.50	0.01	0.77	3.61	0.00	0.75	0.53	0.14

TABLE 3
Intraclass Correlation of Expert Raters of Patient Noncompliance
under Varying Assumptions

Rating group	If raters are adjusted (e.g., by using Z- scores) or if a set of observations is used to classify patients	If individual raters' ratings only are used to classify patients	If composite ratings from a set of raters are used to classify patients
All Springfield dialysis patients			
All six experts	0.32	−0.15	0.74
Physician raters only	0.39	−0.93	0.56
Nonphysician raters only	0.30	−0.27	0.63
Only interviewed patients			
All six experts	0.58	−0.28	0.77
Physician raters only	0.56	−0.70	0.72
Nonphysician raters only	0.27	−0.49	0.60

vide us (Tinsley and Weiss's T values). Our third evaluation of the reliability of the subjective ratings is the Intraclass Correlation, which clearly shows that we can depend on subjective ratings only if we use more than one rater (in fact, in this study, all six subjective raters) (Table 3). The implication is obvious: subjective compliance ratings should be made only by teams of raters, not by single observers. Of the 46 patients we selected on objective measures, there would have been an 80% overlap and had we used composite ratings from all six raters, but the sample would have been very different had we used single raters' subjective judgments.

Scale Reliability

As part of our study we wanted to look at how reliable and homogeneous our nine scales are. We adopted this rather labored stance because we found no previous evidence that the constructs are metrically reliable. Basically, we found positive but widely varying item-scale correlations for all nine scales (Table 4), indicating some "lumpiness" in the patients' responses to individual items that we tried to put together into smooth measures; the "lumpiest" scales are the Control of Health and Susceptibility to Consequences scales, which are measures of a patient's perception of internal control over diet, fluids, health, and side effects (Table 5). Despite these comments about the internal inconsist-

TABLE 4
Scale Composition and Item–Scale Correlations for Five "Ecological
Adjustment" and Four "Health Beliefs" Scales

Scale name	Item	Item–scale correlation	Squared multiple correlation
"Ecological Adjustment" scales			
Interpersonal Adjustment	Husband–wife–parents make it a lot easier.	0.15	0.14
	Many family problems.	0.61	0.37
	Kidney disease makes it a lot harder.	0.49	0.31
	Kidney disease really changed family relationships	0.37	0.24
	I worry family may fall apart, because of my kidney disease.	0.56	0.32
Control of health	To feel OK, I have to watch diet closely.	−0.11	0.05
	I can control what happens to my health.	0.18	0.04
	To feel OK, I have to watch my fluids closely.	−0.01	0.08
Life cycle	Kidney disease makes these "big jobs" more difficult.	0.77	0.59
	I have changed my expectations about these "big jobs."	0.77	0.59
Medical Staff relations	Doctors here deserve some criticism.	0.29	0.08
	Even so, doctors and nurses here work well as part of total team.	0.29	0.08
Family adjustment	I have a lot of family problems.	0.52	0.28
	(If disagree) Even so, kidney disease makes it a lot harder.	0.50	0.28
	Kidney disease has really changed family relationships.	0.42	0.18
"Health Beliefs" scales			
Severity of consequences	I worry a lot about my kidney disease.	0.55	0.30
	Family–friends react to fistula's looks.	0.55	0.30
Benefits of compliance	To feel OK, I have to watch my fluids closely.	0.40	0.16
	I actually do follow fluid limits closely.	0.50	0.27
	I actually do follow my dietary limits closely.	0.53	0.29
Barriers to compliance	I worry a lot about my kidney disease.	0.36	0.13
	I sometimes don't buy a prescription or drug or go to the doctor because of cost.	0.36	0.13
Consequences	I am a lot healthier than other people with kidney disease.	−0.04	0.01
	To feel OK, I have to watch my diet closely.	0.14	0.05
	The odds of having these side effects are low.	0.02	0.07
	My health will be worse in the future.	−0.09	0.05

Table 5
Scale Reliability and Homogeneity of Variance

Scale name	Number of items	Mean	SD	Standardized alpha	Homogeneity of variance[a]	
					Cochran C	Bartlett-Box
"Ecological Adjustment" scales						
Interpersonal adjustment	5	21.11	5.90	0.68	ns	ns
Control of health	3	11.58	2.90	0.03	ns	ns
Life cycle	2	8.41	3.60	0.87	ns	ns
Medical staff relations	2	9.16	2.14	0.45	0.03	0.06
Family adjustment	3	11.23	4.31	0.67	ns	ns
"Health Beliefs" scales						
Benefits of compliance	3	13.28	4.00	0.66	ns	ns
Barriers to compliance	2	7.23	3.21	0.52	ns	ns
Severity of consequences	2	7.76	3.56	0.71	ns	ns
Susceptibility to consequences	4	14.81	3.64	0.01	ns	ns

[a]Degrees of freedom for tests of homogeneity of variance: Cochran's C = 16, 2; Bartlett-Box = 1, 3040.

Table 6
Analysis of Variance of Scale Composition

	Source of variation between measures		Nonadditivity	
	F	p	F	p
"Ecological Adjustment" scales				
Interpersonal adjustment	21.46	0.00	2.25	0.13
Control of health	20.67	0.00	0.39	ns
Life cycle	7.34	0.01	4.49	0.04
Medical staff relations	59.46	0.00	15.05	0.00
Family adjustment	28.92	0.00	2.28	ns
"Health Beliefs" scales				
Benefits of compliance	1.11	ns	0.14	ns
Barriers to compliance	39.18	0.01	0.39	ns
Severity of consequences	1.23	ns	0.18	ns
Susceptibility to consequences	7.98	0.00	0.08	ns

our nine scales, the items do generally form linear additions to each other (Table 6) and contribute to the overall (psychometric) stability of our findings about compliance.

Can We "Predict" Compliance from a Patient's Self-Reported Adjustment?

Here, we cannot let the statistics speak for themselves. Basically, no single scale, ecological or health belief model, isolates our three groups (Table 7). This is a uniform and invariably disappointing null result and should not be readily dismissed (or argued against, as null results inevitably are). Yet, when we modify the analysis to include combinations of scales, we can better predict group membership, at least on a statistical basis. When combined into a "multivariate predictor," three of the ecological scales and three of the health beliefs scales are "more or less" significant. These multivariate predictors of scales are not exceedingly potent (Wilks' Lambda = .73 for the ecological adjustment scales; Lambda = .80 for the health belief scales), but they do border on significantly discriminating "objective" compliance group membership (Table 8). We take heart in the fact that these scales do better on the "objective" criteria of compliance than they do on the physician-defined "subjective" compliance groups, that is, that patient attitudes are reflected more closely in biochemical markers than in physician ratings, a finding that conforms to both the ecological and health belief predictions and our own sense that patient attitudes are slightly more reliable indices of objective compliance than are physicians' statements.

In all forthrightness, however, we can demonstrate easily the confusing nature of the positive relationship between patients' self-reported adjustment and compliance. Consider, first, the ecological ad-

TABLE 7
Post Hoc Univariate Analysis of Variance of Specific Scales

Scale name	SS hyp	SS error	MS hyp	MS error	F	D
Ecological adjustment scales						
Interpersonal adjustment	2.68	52.71	2.68	1.64	1.63	ns
Control of health	1.59	24.86	1.59	0.78	2.04	ns
Life cycle adjustment	9.88	125.73	4.94	3.14	1.57	ns
Medical staff relationships	1.10	47.36	0.55	1.18	0.47	ns
Family adustment	3.31	83.31	1.66	2.08	0.80	ns
Health beliefs scales						
Severity of consequences	2.46	130.95	1.23	3.28	0.38	ns
Susceptibility to consequences	2.34	32.44	1.17	0.81	1.44	ns
Benefits of compliance	2.73	71.99	1.36	1.79	0.76	ns
Barriers to compliance	9.51	98.90	4.76	2.47	1.92	ns

TABLE 8
Stepwise Discriminant Analyses of "Objective" Group Membership for
Ecological Adjustment and Health Belief Scales[a]

Scale name	Step entered into analysis	Wilks' Lambda	Significance
Ecological adjustment scales			
Life cycle	1	0.88	0.08
Medical staff relations	2	0.81	0.09
Control of health	3	0.73	0.06
Health beliefs scales			
Barriers to compliance	1	0.91	0.16
Severity of consequences	2	0.85	0.18
Benefits of compliance	3	0.80	0.19

[a]Scales not included because of stepwise minimum tolerances: Family Adjustment, Length of Time on Dialysis, and Susceptibility to Consequences.

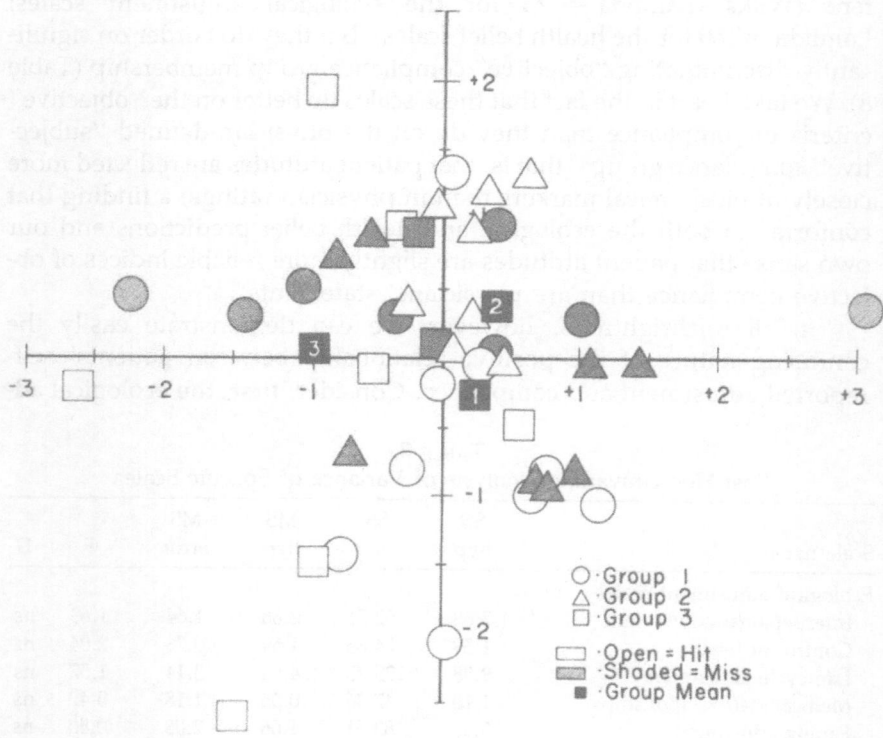

FIG. 1.   Three compliance groups (1 = high, 2 = low, and 3 = "crazy-quilt") discriminated in a two-dimensional "ecological adjustment" multivariate space composed of life cycle adjustment, medical staff relations, and control of one's health.

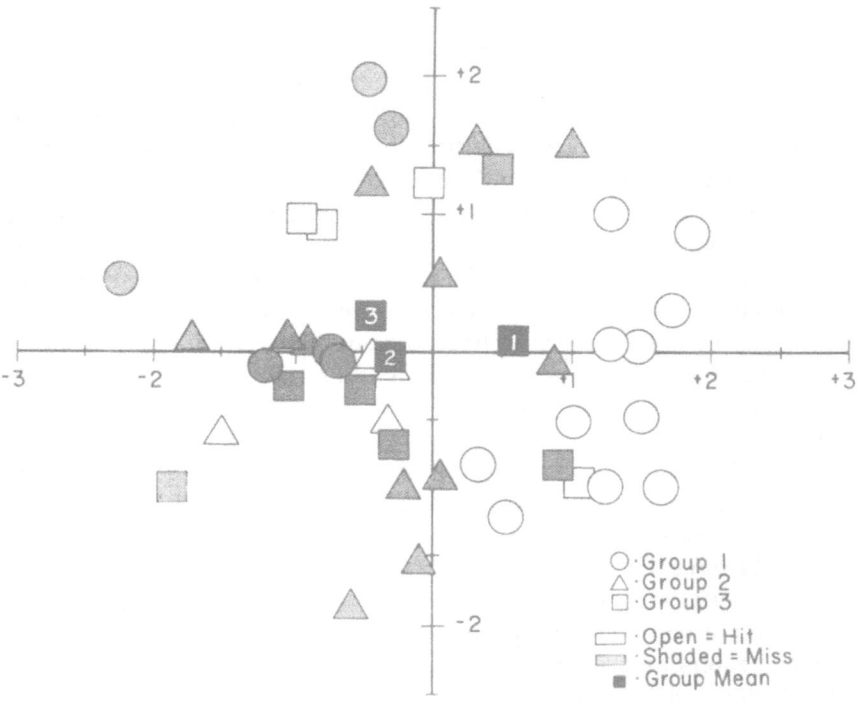

FIG. 2. Three compliance groups (1 = high, 2 = low, and 3 = "crazy-quilt") discriminated in a two-dimensional "health beliefs" multivariate space composed of barriers to compliance, benefits of compliance, and severity of consequences of noncompliance.

justment scales, which correctly predict group membership for 60% of our sample, which is a prediction 44% better than random predictions (Cohen's Kappa = .44). These predictions are better than those from the health beliefs scales, which allow for a similar proportion correctly classified (60%) but in which the groups are "closer together" in the "multivariate space" (cf. Figure 2) and there are, therefore, more "misclassifications" into the "crazy-quilt" group: the health beliefs measures do only 30% better than chance (Cohen's Kappa = .30). On a statistical basis, then, the ecological model is stronger, until we look at the group means in the ecological adjustment "multivariate space" (Figure 1): the scales fail to separate high from low compliance groups; they separate only the highs-and-lows from the "crazy-quilt" compliance groups (F test, $p < .05$)! Thus, in moments of (statistical) analytic candor, we see one model (ecological) does not segregate the two groups we are most interested in, while the other model (health beliefs) does only 30% better than chance. All of this is on pure spectrum groups with psychometrically valid instruments.

DISCUSSION

We have tried to incorporate a number of methodological refinements into our quest for some explanation for hemodialysis patient noncompliance. In modesty we cite first the limitations of this study. First,
while we used "pure spectrum" compliance groups based on biochemical markers, we had no behavioral indices of compliance as, for example, one would have through pill counts or more controlled assays of
fluid or diet intake. Second, we had no *in vivo* measures of interpersonal
adjustment, medical staff interaction, family adjustment, and so forth,
so our report is limited entirely to patients' perceptions, no more.

Nevertheless, we added a number of refinements to the study
which had not occurred before. First, we selected our compliance
groups on the simultaneous basis of three, not one, biochemical markers
of medical distress, independently of any health professional's subjective assessment. Second, we controlled for psychopathology, and no
group, not even the noncompliant group, was found to be significantly
different from each other or from national norms for medical patients on
measures of psychiatric distress. Third, we showed that subjective assessments of compliance typically obscure significant mean differences
between raters and are not well-related to objective measures. Fourth,
we selected "pure spectrum" groups, thereby achieving better assessment of the "crazy-quilt" compliance patient, who resembles more the
"low-compliance" patient on a number of ecological adjustment and
health belief attitudes than he/she does a "high-compliance" patient.

Our study compares favorably to the three other extant
hemodialysis survey studies[8,9,18] in the following ways. First, we similarly found difficulty defining *compliance* empirically, even though we
finally settled on a reasonably robust procedure. Second, we found
somewhat less agreement with the two models than we had hoped to,
but we did find roughly consistent results, in that compliant patients say
they have better adjustment than noncompliant and crazy-quilt patients
in the areas of control of their health; relations with medical staff, satisfaction with life stage adjustment; and better adjustment in terms of seeing fewer barriers to compliance, more severity of consequence of noncompliance, and more benefits in compliance.

Selecting an appropriate psychosocial treatment strategy for the
noncompliant patients is our next task. We are encouraged that patients'
statements of adjustment seem to predict compliance (somewhat), and
that the best subjective classification method must involve consensus
from several clinicians. An "ecological" intervention strategy presumably would focus on the patient's change or stress in terms of life cycle
adjustment and how much a part of the treatment team they see themselves being. Within this context we think it reasonable for the patient to

be instructed in the benefits of compliance and the severity of the consequences of noncompliance.

We offer a final comment here: We note that all of the noncompliance-in-hemodialysis literature is predicated on the notion that noncompliance decreases one's chances of medical survivorship. We know of no study that documents this presumption based on a survivorship analysis.

SUMMARY

From the entire sample of Springfield, Massachusetts, dialysis patients, we selected three groups of patients on "objective" criteria of compliance, and compared these 43 patients on their self-reported adjustment and health beliefs. We also assessed "subjective" ratings of compliance made by the treatment staff. The "objective" measures had higher reliability than the subjective assessments, even though the objective measures were far from statistically laudable. The subjective measures were one notch less satisfactory and failed to separate "low-compliance" from "crazy-quilt compliance" patients who were "good" on one or more objective measures but not so good on others.

Using a multivariate discriminant analysis, we could statistically isolate our three compliance groups on two sets of patient attitudes: The first analysis, from the "ecological adjustment" literature, correctly classified 60% of our patients by their attitudes about medical staff relations, family adjustment, and life cycle adjustment. We used a second set of attitudes, from the "health beliefs" literature, to correctly classify a similar percentage of our patients by reference to their beliefs about the benefits of compliance, barriers to compliance, and severity of the consequences of not complying to dietary and fluid restrictions. We conclude that, while both the health beliefs and ecological adjustment models help us understand something about patient compliance, what the patients say is not necessarily reflected in objective measures of compliance; the patients say one thing about their attitudes and this is only one turn in the road to compliance. Nevertheless, we also point out that the patients' attitudes are stronger predictors of their objective compliance measures than are physicians' own ratings of compliance; so, by implication, any treatment program should include patients' attitudes as much as physicians' dicta.

ACKNOWLEDGMENTS. We wish to acknowledge Roger Sherwood's encouragement in this research, the professional staff at Baystate Medical Center (John Fitzgibbons, M.D.; Judy Mains, R.D.), and the 43 interviewed patients.

REFERENCES

1. KAPLAN DE-NOUR, A., and CZACZKES, J. W. Personality factors in chronic hemodialysis patients causing noncompliance with medical regimen. *Psychosomatic Medicine*, 1972, 34, 333–344.
2. ABRAM, H. S., MOORE, G. I., and WESTERVELT, F. B., Jr. Suicidal behavior in chronic dialysis patients. *American Journal of Psychiatry*, 1972, 127, 1199–1204.
3. DUNBAR, J. Issues in assessment. In S. J. Cohen (Ed.), *New directions in patient compliance*. Lexington, Massachusetts: D. C. Heath and Company, 1979.
4. CARON, H. S., and ROTH, H. P. Patients' cooperation with a medical regimen. *Journal of the American Medical Association*, 1968, 203, 120–124.
5. ROTH, H. P., and CARON, H. S. Accuracy of doctors' estimates and patients' statements of adherence to a drug regimen. *Clinical Pharmacology and Therapeutics*, 1978, 23, 361–370.
6. PARK, L. C., and LIPMAN, R. S. A comparison of patient dosage deviation reports with pill counts. *Psychopharmacologia*, 1964, 6, 299–302.
7. ROTH, H. P. Problems in conducting a study of the effects on patient compliance of teaching the rationale for antacid therapy. In S. J. Cohen (Ed.), *New directions in patient compliance*. Lexington, Massachusetts: D. C. Heath and Company, 1979.
8. HARTMAN, P. E., and BECKER, M. H. Non-compliance with prescribed regimen among chronic hemodialysis patients: a method of prediction and educational diagnosis. *Dialysis and Transplantation*, 1978, 7, 978–981; 984; 986; 988–989.
9. BLACKBURN, S. L. Dietary compliance of chronic hemodialysis patients. *Journal of the American Dietetic Association*, 1977, 70, 31–37.
10. LEVY, N. B. The psychology and care of the maintenance hemodialysis patient. *Heart and Lung*, 1973, 2, 400–405.
11. GERMAIN, C. B., and GITTERMAN, A. *The life of social work practice*. New York: Columbia University Press, 1980.
12. STEIDL, J. H., FINKELSTEIN, F. WEXLER, J. FEIGNENBAUM, H., KITSEN, J., KLIGER, A. S., and QUINLAN, D. M. Medical condition, adherence to treatment regimen, and family functioning. *Archives of General Psychiatry*, 1980, 37, 1025–1027.
13. BECKER, M. H. The role of the patient: social and psychological factors in noncompliance. In L. Lasagna (Ed.), *Patient compliance*. Mount Kisco, New York: Futura Publishing, 1976.
14. BECKER, M. H. Understanding patient compliance: the contributions of attitudes and other psychosocial factors. In S. J. Cohen (Ed.), *New directions in patient compliance*. Lexington, Massachusetts: D. C. Heath and Company, 1979.
15. DEROGATIS, L. R., LIPMAN, R. S., RICKELS, K., UHLENHUTH, E. H., and COVI, L. The Hopkins Symptom Checklist (HSCL). In P. Pichot (Ed.), *Psychological measurements in psychopharmacology*. S. Karger, Basel, 1974.
16. DEROGATIS, L. R., and CLEARY, P. A. Factorial invariance across gender for the primary symptom dimensions of the SCL-90. *British Journal of Social and Clinical Pathology*, 1977, 16, 347–356.
17. TINSLEY, H. E. A., and WEISS, D. J. Interrater reliability and agreement of subjective judgments. *Journal of Counseling Psychology*, 1975, 22, 358–376.
18. SHERWOOD, R. J., and AVRAM, M. M. The ecological approach to compliance behavior: A realistic model for assessment and intervention. Unpublished manuscript, Long Island College Hospital, 1980.

8

Children of Dialysis Patients

ROBERT JOEL FRIEDLANDER, JR., AND MILTON VIEDERMAN

INTRODUCTION

The poignancy of a child's confrontation with stressful life experiences has engaged the interest and concern of many people. With respect to physical illness, previous study was focused almost exclusively on the sick child and his family, while little attention has been given to the well child of a physically ill parent. Our pilot study was motivated by an interest in the impact of chronic hemodialysis of a parent on the children living at home and on their relationship with the sick parent. We were interested in understanding how children perceived their parent's illness and treatment by obtaining some knowledge of their fantasy life. We studied both center and home dialysis patients and their families in order to assess the impact of home therapy on the child.

Rutter[1] has described an association between chronic physical illness of a parent and psychiatric disorder in the children. His study of children with a psychiatric disorder attending the Maudsley Hospital revealed a significantly increased incidence of chronic parental physical illness in that population as compared to matched groups of controls. Arnaud[2] used the Rorschach to compare children of parents with multiple sclerosis with children whose parents were not ill. In her study the children of MS parents showed higher levels of body concern, dysphoric feelings, hostility, dependency longings, constraint in interpersonal relations and a pattern of false maturity. Pynoos, in a study of the early responses of children to parental suicidal behavior, noted that some of

ROBERT JOEL FRIEDLANDER, JR., M.D. • Former Fourth-Year Medical Student, Cornell University Medical College, New York, New York. Present affiliation: Resident Physician in Medicine, New York Hospital, Cornell Medical Center, New York, New York. MILTON VIEDERMAN, M.D. • Professor of Clinical Psychiatry, Cornell University Medical College; Director, Consultation–Liaison Division, Department of Psychiatry, New York Hospital, New York, New York. This work was supported in part by NIMH Grant #5 TO1 MH14747 04. A shorter version of this paper has been published in *The American Journal of Psychiatry*.

these children reveal "the use of denial, defensive and pathological identification, rage, reversal of roles and pseudomaturity."

There is little information about the psychological impact of chronic hemodialysis of a parent on the children. Friedman et al.[3] found that the majority of parents assessed their childrens' reactions toward dialysis as positive. Mass and Kaplan De-Nour[4] reported that children of center dialysis patients were restricted in bringing home friends because "father had to rest," and that some children were ashamed to tell their friends about their father's illness.

In a study of 15 children of six families in which one parent was on home dialysis, Tsaltas[5] found that all the children showed depressive and hypochondriacal MMPI patterns. Figure drawing revealed emotional constriction, anxiety, depression, and bodily concern. Two-thirds of the children had been referred for counseling or psychiatric evaluation because of behavioral problems in school. These children also showed disorders of psychomotor activity and reduced academic achievement.

SUBJECTS AND METHODS

To select families for this study, the charts of all center and home dialysis patients affiliated with the Rogosin Kidney Center of the New York Hospital were reviewed. Patients on dialysis for more than 6 months, with at least one child between the ages of 7 and 14 living in an intact family were considered as potential subjects. Thirteen of 70 home dialysis patients met these criteria, but 6 of these patients were unable to participate since their children were unavailable when the study was being done. The remaining 7 patients readily agreed to participate. Of 150 center dialysis patients, 11 qualified for the study; 5 of these patients refused to participate, 5 agreed, and 1 was unable to since his child was away.

Five of seven home dialysis families and two of five center dialysis families were seen at home. The remaining families were interviewed in out-patient facilities of the New York Hospital. Each family session began with a loosely structured interview with the sick parent and spouse when possible, conducted by the senior author meeting the family for the first time. These interviews focused on how parents presented the illness and treatment to their children and on their views of how their children had been affected by chronic illness in the home.

When possible all children in the dialysis families between the ages of 7 and 14 were interviewed. The children were seen individually, in the absence of other family members, and the same format was followed with all the children. Each child was asked to draw a picture and then to tell a story about the picture. The child was encouraged to elaborate on the style and content of the drawing and narrative through free associations. All children were then asked a standard set of questions designed to explore in an explicit manner the child's understanding of the parent's illness and treatment; the way in which information about the illness and treatment was presented; the extent to which such information is discussed with friends; the child's reaction to the treatment, including feelings about participation in the case of home dialysis; the child's dreams; and the child's aspirations for the future. A roughly matched control group of six children was selected in order to provide us with a sense of how children without ill parents would express themselves when confronted with the same unstructured task of drawing a picture and then telling a story about it.

It would appear that nonparticipation in the center dialysis group was correlated with parental anxiety that information about the illness and exploration of feelings in the child would be damaging. It is likely that the amount of communication about the illness was less in these families than in the study group. Paranoid character traits in a few families contributed to the refusal. The husband of one center dialysis patient would allow his family to participate only if he was presented in advance with a list of all questions to be asked of his children, and if he or his wife were permitted to be with the children throughout the interview. His wife, anxious to participate and embarrassed by her husband's demands, expressed concern about the effects of her illness on her young son; at school he had drawn a mural of the New York City skyline in which a hospital towered over the other buildings.

RESULTS

The Sick Parent's Perspective

All center and home dialysis patients expressed guilt over becoming sick. Restricted employment and educational opportunities, dependence on a time-consuming treatment, decreased energy, mood swings, and the necessity of involving other family members in their care all contributed to a feeling of uneasiness and concern about their ability to parent.

One-half of the sick parents had at times been afraid that their children might develop renal disease, another potential source of guilt. This manifest anxiety was not limited to parents with inherited disease; those with glomerulonephritis and pyelonephritis rapidly sought medical attention when their children developed symptoms suggestive of a strep throat or a urinary tract infection. Latent anxiety was evident in the diabetic father who persistently became upset at the sight of a scar near his son's wrist from a minor injury. He may have associated the scar with his own fistula scar, with subsequent guilt over the fantasy of his son as a dialysis patient. Moreover, his concern that "people will think [his] son tried to slit his wrist" would appear to be a projection of latent suicidal ideation.

Most sick parents stressed that it was the spouse who had explained the treatment and prognosis of renal disease to the children; of the few who had discussed these issues only one, a 32-year-old woman on center dialysis, was able to recollect her explanation. She had told her two sons that her arm would be "bionic" by virtue of the fistula, reflecting her attempt at mitigating the impact of her illness on her children.

The sick parents almost all reported a lack of awareness of their children's thoughts and feelings about chronic illness in the home. Several parents asked the interviewer to share his findings with them and make recommendations for psychological counseling if deemed necessary. Despite this apparent lack of communication, the majority of the sick parents were very involved with their children. They described with a sense of pride how well their children were able to assume additional responsibilities in the home as a result of their own limitations. It became clear that they found their children's compassion and efforts at parenting very gratifying, and above all encouraged and rewarded precocious behavior. Some parents tended to overindulge their children in an attempt to perpetuate these special relationships. The sick parent often selected one child to be his principal caretaker as well as the recipient of an inappropriate amount of his attention, occasionally incurring the resentment of the siblings.

Sick parents who had greater difficulty accepting their illness and treatment generally invested more energy in such intimate relationships with their children, suggesting the importance of these relationships as a potential source of strength to the parent. Two mothers on dialysis who experienced frequent depression emphasized that their daughters "really keep them going."

Only one parent on dialysis, a man with polycystic disease enraged over his genetic illness and fate, derived satisfaction from the aggressive behavior of his children. He spoke with pride about his 10-year-old son's violent outbursts at home and in school.

Children's Drawings and Behavioral Correlates

Children from all three groups were equally receptive to the task of drawing a picture. Support and encouragement relieved any initial concern about the unstructured nature of the request. In general this projective technique proved much more effective in promoting a dialogue with the child than the set of explicit questions. Since no significant differences were found between children of center and home dialysis patients with respect to the five categories detailed below, these results will be combined and described together.

Dialysis and "Connection" Imagery

Of the 14 drawings from children of dialysis patients, 1 contained a manifest representation of a fistula while another depicted, by virtue of a clear association on the part of the child, a skyscraper as a symbol of the dialysis machine. It was possible to infer the presence of dialysis imagery in 8 of the remaining 12 drawings; 5 of these drawings contained examples of "connection" imagery in which a figure associated with the sick parent is literally connected to a protective machine such as a plane or ship (see Figure 1).

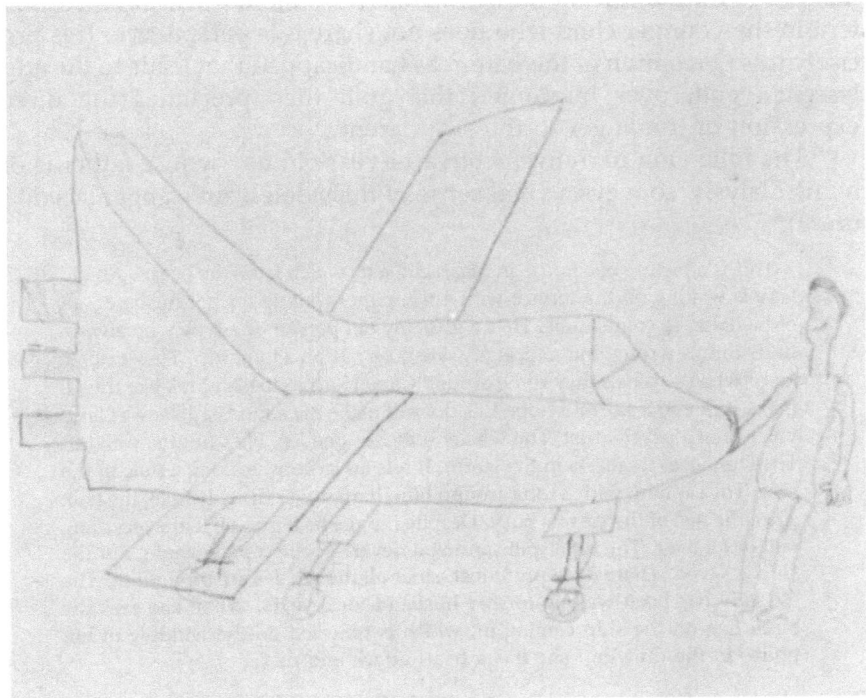

FIG. 1.

Aggression

While only the 13- and 14-year-old children in the study verbalized aggressive feelings toward the sick parent, evidence for such feelings was found in the drawings and narratives of children from ages 8 to 14. Eleven of 14 drawings suggested latent aggressive impulses toward the sick parent or a figure associated with the sick parent; 8 of these 11 drawings depicted the sick parent or a sick parent surrogate on a potentially dangerous voyage.

Children between the ages of eight and ten appeared well adjusted to their parent's illness and treatment on the surface; they were content if not enthusiastic to make sacrifices for the sick parent. Eleven- and 12-year-old children, in contrast to the younger children, expressed a growing awareness of how different their sick parent was from other healthy parents. Their most common complaint related to restricted family travel, yet they accepted all sacrifices as being in the best interest of the sick parent. The 13- and 14-year-old children began to question sacrifices they made for the sick parent and expressed varying degrees of anger about the effects of chronic illness in the home. It appears that the recognition of the sick parent as being different from other parents justifies to the adolescent his overt anger, an emotion which remains latent in the younger child who does not share this perspective. It is precisely this perception of the parent as handicapped that leads to the adolescent's guilt over his anger; this guilt then precludes the direct expression of the anger to the sick parent.

The following narrative, from a 14-year-old boy whose father is on home dialysis, conveys a vivid sense of this adolescent's anger (see Figure 2):

> This is a picture of a house in Massachusetts which faces the ocean. An old lady is waiting on the terrace with a telescope, waiting for her husband, an old whaler, to come home. He's a grumbly old person, the type who always finds things wrong, but a nice guy. He goes out on a long trip. They catch a lot of whales. When they come around Cape Horn it doesn't look like they'll make it due to a storm. I hope this doesn't make me sound sadistic—at least you're not a psychiatrist. The whaler only has one leg. He's not too well off. The ship loses its masts in the storm. It hits an iceberg, making a hole in the side. The captain, with a rope around him, hangs over the side to fix the boat since the rest of the crew is busy. Despite his age he has to do it or everything will be all over. The rope splits and you never see the captain again, but the ship is saved. There is no profit lost, since all the whales are brought in. The old lady has been waiting for her husband for 3 years. When she sees the black flag on the ship coming in, which is reflected on the window of her house in the drawing, she has a heart attack and dies.

The whaler is a clear reference to the father who had been on dialysis for 3 years and was described by his son as being demanding, critical, and

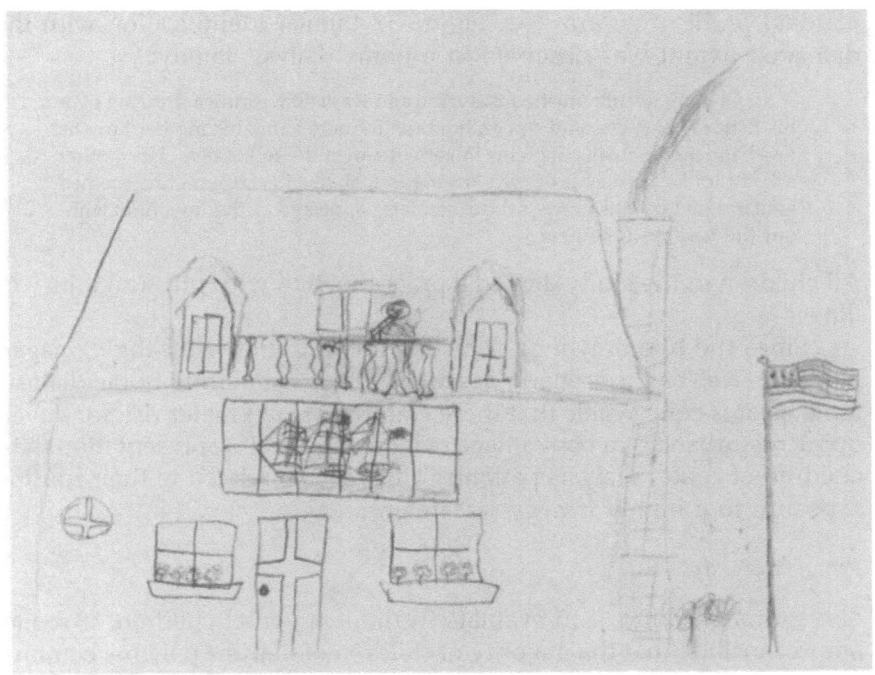

FIG. 2.

overly active despite his illness. The whaler as an amputee reflects the son's view of his father as being physically damaged. This adolescent begrudgingly initiates his father's dialysis 3 days a week. He feels "tense, serious and less mischievous" as a result of this obligation, yet has never expressed his anger to his father for fear of appearing disloyal.

While 2 of 14 children of dialysis patients had behavioral disturbances marked by poor impulse control requiring professional intervention, causality is difficult to determine, although in one case the temporal continuity between onset of home dialysis and the onset of delinquency is intriguing. Both cases involved latency age sons of fathers on dialysis; whether this relationship predisposes to the development of delinquent behavior in early adolescence needs further investigation.

The Child's Identification with the Sick Parent

One example of identification with the sick parent was observed in the behavior of the children, while 5 of 14 drawings contained evidence for this. The 12-year-old son of a diabetic on home dialysis drew a picture of his family including the needle holes on his father's arm and a

bandaid on his own arm (see Figure 3). Similar identification with the
damaged parent was observed in a home dialysis family:

> Mr. X had recently finished dialyzing and was still wearing a dressing over
> his fistula. His 9-year-old son entered the room to show his mother how he
> had bandaged a small cut on his finger with an entire roll of tape. His mother
> asked him facetiously if he was "trying to look like his father." She seemed
> embarrassed by this behavior; the son later appeared at the interview with-
> out the tape on his finger.

All children in the study denied a preoccupation with physical injury or
illness.

Since the two drawings depicting identification with the damaged
parent as well as the scenario described above come from home dialysis
families, it is conceivable that these children are at greater risk for developing disturbances in body image or a damaged self-representation than
children of center dialysis patients. This may be related to their routine
exposure to a highly invasive treatment.

Pseudomaturity

Although difficult to evaluate in the less verbal children, it seems
fair to conclude that the majority of children of dialysis patients communicate a sense of maturity, wisdom, and experience inappropriate to
their years. This finding was particularly striking in two families. The
drawing of the 11-year-old son of a man on center dialysis depicted a
meeting with his father upon his return from the hospital (see Figure 4).
The son, carrying his father's bag, bears a stronger resemblance to the
father or to a doctor than to a child. This child is in fact called on to assume a great deal of responsibility in life. He must return home from

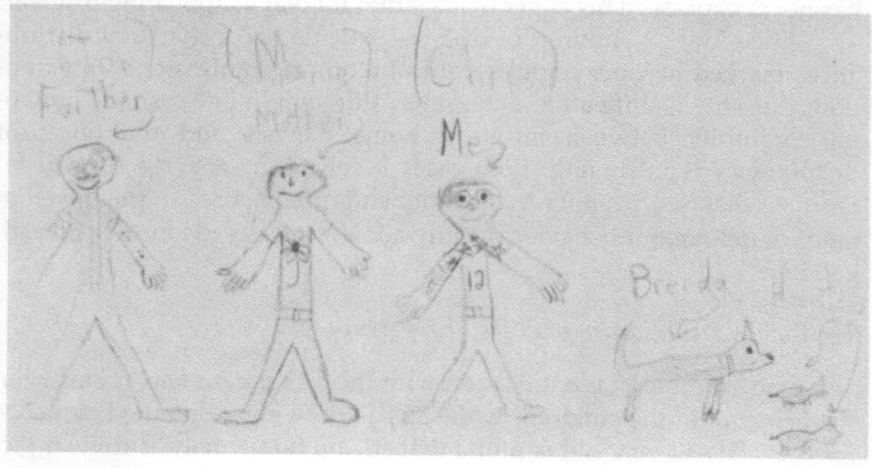

FIG. 3.

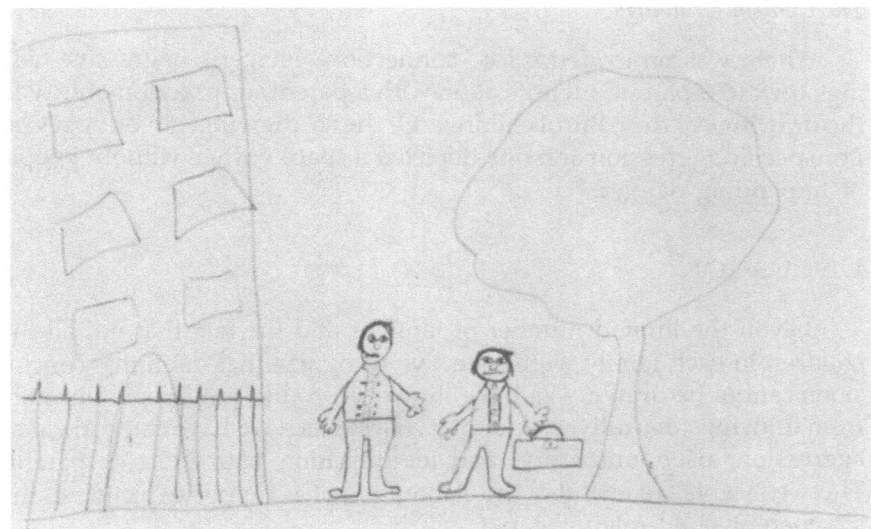

FIG. 4.

school at noon 3 days each week to care for his younger siblings while his father is at the hospital and his mother is at work.

The 8-year-old daughter of a woman on home dialysis also displayed a striking degree of pseudomaturity. She has assisted her mother with the dialysis treatment from the age of five. A home visit during the mother's dialysis revealed a poised, slightly reserved but articulate girl constantly fussing over her mother.

Many children of dialysis patients expressed a desire to become a doctor or nurse. The 8-year-old girl wants to become a nurse so she can dialyze her mother when her father is too old to do so. The 11-year-old boy discussed at the beginning of this section wants to be a doctor because he is afraid of becoming sick and having no one to take care of him. This may be related to the actual or perceived absence of a protective parental figure in his life.

Formal Aspects of the Drawings

Formal equivalents of both aggression and pseudomaturity are present in the drawings of children of dialysis patients. Six of 14 drawings contain prominent jagged lines similar to the teeth of a saw; this representation of aggression does not appear in the control drawings. The greater complexity of the drawings of children of dialysis patients, in terms of the number of figures, the interaction between the figures, the background elements, and the attention to detail is consistent with the prevalence of pseudomaturity in this group.

The Control Drawings

There was no evidence for "connection" imagery, aggressive feelings toward a parent, identification with a parent, or pseudomaturity in the drawings of the control children. Of the six drawings, two suggested nonspecific aggression and one depicted a space voyage without people or impending danger.

DISCUSSION

Given the limited number of families and the fact that not all the children in each family were seen, we recognize that definitive conclusions cannot be drawn. We have, however, found patterns in our data from drawings, narratives, and interviews which we have categorized as aggression, pseudomaturity, and identification with the sick parent. These concepts are useful in the elaboration of a composite picture of the sick parent–child relationship.

It is interesting that so many of the drawings of children of dialysis patients were related, either by manifest content or by associative connections, to the dialysis of the parent. We understand this to be a reflection of the children's awareness of the goals of the study. The children seem to have directed their fantasy production as if they wished on some level to help us understand the experience of having a chronically ill parent.

The repeated theme of the sick parent on a potentially dangerous voyage may be understood on several different levels. It may literally represent the child's desire for the sick parent to take a trip as other parents do. In fact the children's most common complaint about chronic illness in the home was the restricted family travel. It is easy to infer that the child wishes the parent to be independent, thus freeing him from the emotional burden and added responsibilities imposed by the parent's illness. The metaphor may also represent the child's wish that the parent be away, and on the most primitive and aggressive level, that the parent be dead. "Departing on a journey is one of the commonest and best authenticated symbols of death," according to Freud.[6]

The pseudomature behavior assumed by these children serves two purposes.

First, it acts as a defense against aggressive impulses, and second, it permits the child to deal with the feared loss of the parent by establishing protective control. Pseudomaturity in the extreme is represented by the child's fantasy of being the doctor or the nurse. This is a common fantasy in normal children which reflects an attempt at mastery and an identification with the aggressor.

The model child who never strays from his role as caretaker of the sick parent compromises the gratification of many dependency needs. This raises the general question of whether children who grow up with added responsibilities from either illness or poverty in the family will be prepared to face crisis situations later in life such as their own illness or the illness of a family member. Retrospective and prospective studies are needed to follow the fate of children who live under these circumstances. The impact of these demands on the adolescent who is attempting to establish his own separate identity requires further study.

Sick parents who experience guilt over their ability to parent become threatened by their children's dependency needs and by the possibility that their children may have been adversely affected by chronic illness in the home. They positively reinforce the natural inclinations of their children, that is, pseudomaturity, in order to assuage this guilt and vicariously experience a renewed sense of independence. The tendency of the less well-adapted parent to give meaning to his own life by fulfilling the needs of a child may reflect his vicarious identification with the child who represents an idealized image of himself prior to his illness.

Children may also defend themselves against aggressive feelings by displacement, resulting in delinquent behavior which, like precocious behavior, is not without encouragement from the sick parent. Johnson[7] first described the concept of superego lacunae, by which parents find vicarious gratification of their own poorly integrated forbidden impulses in the acting out of the child, most often through an unconscious permissiveness of certain behaviors by the child.

Although we found less evidence for identification with the sick parent than for both aggression and pseudomaturity, we feel that this issue may have a particularly profound impact on the development of many of these children. Follow-up studies of these children are necessary to determine whether they retain unconscious self-representation of damage.

Parsons and Fox[8] have presented an interesting perspective on the resources the American urban family has for undertaking major responsibility for care of the sick. They write that:

> The optimal balance between supportive–permissive and disciplinary facets of treating illness is peculiarly difficult to maintain in the kind of situation presented by the American family. Medico-technical advances notwithstanding, therefore, therapy is more easily effected in a professional milieu, where there is not the same order of intensive emotional involvement characteristic of family relationships.

Our study does not reveal significant differences in adaptation between children of center dialysis and children of home dialysis patients, an unexpected finding in light of the uniqueness of the home dialysis situation, in which children are routinely exposed to and often participate in a highly invasive life-sustaining treatment for their parents. This suggests that at least from the child's perspective the sick parent himself is the source of major concern, not the circumstances of the treatment. In this regard it would be interesting to compare the adaptation of children of dialysis patients with children of parents suffering from other chronic illnesses.

The conclusions from this pilot study require further testing. With large numbers of subjects our findings can be verified and the following issues can be addressed—whether the sex of the sick parent and the sex of the child affects the child's adaptation, and whether the child's age at the time the parent begins dialysis is of importance. The process by which one child is selected by the parent to be the principal caretaker needs further investigation. On the single occasion the children were seen there was little evidence of manifest depression or hypochondriasis as reported by Tsaltas,[5] though formal testing was not done. These issues also should be studied.

Although few differences were found between children of center and home dialysis patients, the significantly increased nonparticipation in this study among center dialysis families may reflect their greater anxiety over the effects of chronic illness on the family. If there is an actual increase in psychological morbidity in the center dialysis population, psychological research and support should be directed to this group. Finally, we hope that the concerns we have raised in this pilot study will stimulate further research involving children of sick parents.

ACKNOWLEDGMENTS. The authors would like to thank Drs. Richard Breslow, Theodore Shapiro, and Robert Pynoos for their assistance. Dr. Pynoos was particularly helpful in suggesting the use of the projective drawing technique as a method for obtaining data.

REFERENCES

1. RUTTER, M. *Children of sick parents*. London: Oxford University Press, 1966.
2. ARNAUD, S. H. Some psychological characteristics of children of multiple sclerotics, *Psychosomatic Medicine*, 1959, 21, 8.
3. FRIEDMAN, E. A., GOODWIN, N. J., and CHAUDHRY, L. Psychosocial adjustment of family to maintenance hemodialysis: II, *New York State Journal of Medicine*, 1970, 70, 767.
4. MASS, M., and DE-NOUR, A. Reactions of families to chronic hemodialysis. *Psychotherapy and Psychosomatics*, 1975, 26, 20.
5. TSALTAS, M. O. Children of home dialysis patients. *Journal of the American Medical Association*, 1976, 236, 2764.

6. FREUD, S. *Interpretation of dreams, the complete psychological works of Sigmund Freud*. Vol. 5. London: Hogarth Press, 1953, 385.
7. JOHNSON, A. Sanctions for superego lacunae of adolescents. In K. R. Eissler (Ed.), *Searchlights on delinquency*. New York: International Universities Press, 1949, 225–245.
8. PARSONS, T., and FOX, R. C. Illness, therapy and the modern urban American family, *Journal of Social Issues*, 1952, *13*(4), 31.

9

The Patient on Renal Dialysis
Strategies for Sexual Counseling

ROSALYN JONES WATTS

A discussion of the sexual concerns of patients with end-stage renal disease must be viewed as a "quality of life" issue. Unlike other basic physiological drives such as the need for food, water, and sleep, fulfillment of sexual needs is not a necessary condition for survival. More specifically, sexual appetite and behavior differs among individuals. At polarized opposite ends of the spectrum are those with a lifetime intense interest in sex and others with low sex interest. Many persons are aware of fluctuations of sex needs which may vary with one's state of health, quality of relationship, life style and current life events. For many individuals the total love-making experience enhances the quality of life, resulting in a resurgence of energy, tranquillity, and ultimate pleasure.

In coping with a chronic illness such as renal failure (RF), sex becomes an issue for those who want it . . . value it . . . need it. Is it a self-fulfilling prophecy that this population on lifelong dialysis will exist as "sexual cripples" for the rest of their lives? A survey of the literature on sex and RF suggests that patients complain of diminished libido, erectile failure, and orgastic dysfunction. Some of the psychophysiological factors which contribute to sexual inadequacy with this population include:

1. Pathophysiologic Factors[1]

   - Anemia
   - Postdialysis "washout" or lethargy
   - Uremic neuropathy
   - Drug-induced side effects from antihypertensive medication
   - Hormonal imbalances disrupting sexual and reproductive capacity
   - aging process

ROSALYN JONES WATTS, Ed.D., R.N., • Associate Professor, University of Pennsylvania School of Nursing, Philadelphia, Pennsylvania.

2. Psychosocial Factors[1,2,3,4]

- Changes in self-esteem, self-concept, and body image
- Depression due to innumerable losses—physical functioning, body integrity, independence, economic security, and family stability
- Role reversal in the marital relationship

COMPREHENSIVE NATURE OF SEXUALITY

I would like to suggest that sexual assessment and counseling of patients on hemodialysis must extend beyond constricted physiological parameters of genital sex. Let me propose the following assumptions about the nature of sex and sexuality.

1. Sexual activity fulfills a biological need for procreation and erotic pleasure. Animal studies have shown that electrode stimulation of subcortical structures in the brain, that is, the limbic system and areas in the brain stem, result in penile erection and ejaculation.[5] Sexual activity may be generated or suppressed depending on individual needs. The pioneering research of Masters and Johnson[6] classified the physiologic components of sexual responsivity into four stages—excitement/arousal, plateau, orgasm, and resolution. This vasocongestive and myotonic response also involves a generalized extragenital response of increased respiration, pulse, and blood pressure.

2. Interpersonal sexual behavior is learned. The roots of love, trust and intimacy are learned at an early age. Sex roles are also learned. It is unfortunate in our society that adult men and women have become imprisoned and locked into stereotypic sex roles. One well-known Philadelphia marriage counselor stated that the socialized male suffers from tactile deprivation and tends to become overgenitalized whereas the erotic experience of the female is more diffuse. We must also realize that sexual value systems are also learned. A sexual value system refers to the erotic fantasies, attitudes, feelings, beliefs, and sexual behaviors which are unique to the individual. Thus, conflicting sexual value systems such as unequal sex drives or variation in expression of sexual behavior may disrupt the quality of the relationship.

3. Sexual attitudes and beliefs are shaped by cultural and religious influences. In the western world our attitudes about sexual behavior are still greatly influenced by Judeo–Christian doctrines. It's not enough to record on a chart that the individual is Catholic, Protestant, or Jewish. When discussing sexual attitudes, beliefs, and behavior it's important to determine how the individual interprets her religious teachings. This information may be important when discussing with clients the extracoital options of love-making. One person may be grief stricken about his

mastubatory behavior whereas another, without guilt, freely incorporates this activity into sexual play.

The total sexual experience is influenced by an interplay of biological, psychosocial, and cultural factors. In sex therapy clinics, for example, the clinician determines if sexual problems are caused by organic or psychogenic factors. At most reputable clinics it is estimated that 90% of sexual disorders are triggered by psychosocial causes. These include: misinformation about sex, maladaptive social behavior and erotic skills, intrapsychic conflicts, and interpersonal conflicts. For the purposes of this discussion, I would like to define sexuality as the perception of a desire for sex along with the ability to become aroused, attain orgasm, and achieve sexual satisfaction.

SCREENING FOR SEXUAL FUNCTIONING

Screening for sexual functioning should begin with the initial health history during admission. Specific questions about sexual functioning will logically flow from inquiry into reproductive status. If health care providers from all disciplines participate in the activity, that is, physicians, nurses, social workers, and counselors, patients will begin to accept questions as a normal and appropriate area of inquiry. Additionally, permission to discuss sexual issues at a future time has been extended to the client.

Since fertility may be an issue for male patients with RF, questions about number of children may be followed by inquiry into genital infection, morning erection, difficulty in achieving erection, desire for sex, and change in ejaculatory volume. I have noticed that the term "impotence" is nonspecific and conveys different meanings.

Likewise for females, inquiry about reproductive status may be followed by specific sex questions. These include: date of last period, duration of flow, intermenstrual bleeding, methods of contraception, vaginal lubrication during intercourse, coital pain, desire for sex, and ability to achieve climax.

In summary, during the initial history, a transition from reproductive status to sexual questions is appropriate, rational, and helps to identify specific problems in the desire, arousal, and orgastic stages of sexual responsivity.

GUIDELINES FOR SEXUAL INTERVIEW AND COUNSELING

If patients on hemodialysis are concerned about sexual functioning, opportunity should be given to communicate sexual concerns. The major purposes of the sexual interview are to:

1. Determine the quality of sexual functioning prior to the onset of RF.
2. Assess the current level of sexual functioning while on dialysis.
3. Ascertain both patient and partner expectations regarding ongoing sexual interaction.
4. Educate both persons about sex and sexual potential.
5. Evaluate if referral to other health professional is necessary.

The goals of sexual counseling are to:

1. Facilitate communication for disclosing sexual concerns.
2. Dispel myths and misconceptions about sex.
3. Resume sexual intimacy in the relationship.

Several approaches are helpful in learning the patient's sexual history. Asking facilitating questions tends not to increase the patient's shame or embarrassment. Conducting the interview in private and informing the patient about confidentiality of the session is essential. Direct questions should be used which focus on sexual learning, attitudes, and behavior. The sexual language used by the interviewer should be simplistic, avoiding the use of medical jargon and profanity/slang which may be offensive to the client. The interviewer should not impose his/her sexual value system on the client and should attempt to create a therapeutic climate in which the patient may express his sexual concerns in his own language.

COMPONENTS OF THE SEXUAL HISTORY

Baseline Data

The following information should be obtained during the course of the interview.
Areas of inquiry:

- Age, sex, occupation, ethnic group, religion, socioeconomic status, marital status, number of children and their ages
- Other medical/surgical or mental health complications
- Drug profile—prescription and nonprescription drugs (always include alcohol)

Rationale: Such information provides data about those factors which may positively or negatively influence sexual functioning.
Intervention: Review patient's understanding of his illness, physical limitations, and drug therapy.

Attitude about Sex and Sexuality

I usually proceed from less threatening interpersonal aspects of sexuality to more sensitive areas of autosexuality when inquiring into the pre-illness level of sexual interaction. Many patients expect you to begin with questions about intercourse.

Area of Inquiry:

• Determine if sexual interaction is an important aspect of life.

Some persons will describe sex as a soothing, tension-relieving natural experience which is fully integrated into his/her life. Others, however, convey the notion that intercourse is an anxiety-provoking or performance-oriented task which will be more stressful when the individual is sick. Such anticipatory anxiety may be reduced through effective education and counseling.

Intervention: Reinforce the potential (if desired) for incorporating previous patterns of sexual activity into the activities of daily living.

Interest and Frequency of Sex

Areas of Inquiry:

• Degree of interest in sex prior to the onset of RF
• Frequency of intercourse prior to the onset of RF
• Current interest in sex and frequency of intercourse while on hemodialysis
• Date of last sexual experience
• Duration of that activity
• Time during the day when love-making most enjoyable

Rationale: Some patients complain of excessive fatigue and a lack of interest in sex with the onset of RF and hemodialysis. Others report interest in sexual interaction but are unable to have intercourse due to lack of partner cooperation. The frequency of sexual intercourse may range from abstinence to one time per month to several times per week. Patients frequently offer explanations about diminished libido.

Intervention: Allow patient to express anxieties and fears about previous, current, and potential levels of sexual functioning; dispel myths and misconceptions about sex and renal disease.

Sexual Intercourse

Areas of Inquiry:

• Most enjoyable/comfortable coital position

- Variation in coital positions
- Ability to attain and maintain erection for vaginal entry; ejaculatory problem (males)
- Degree of vaginal lubrication; pain with intercourse; ability to reach orgasm (females)
- Satisfaction with sexual performance

Rationale: Such inquiry provides more data about pre-illness sexual capacities and/or sexual dysfunction, for example, premature ejaculation, erectile dysfunction, inadequate vaginal lubrication, or orgasmic difficulties. Such cases could be referred to appropriate professionals. It also illuminates the degree of sexual experimentation on the part of the couple.

Intervention: Continue to allow patient to express feelings; educate when appropriate.

Extracoital Options of Love-making

Areas of Inquiry:

- What sexually arouses or "turns on" client
- Initiator of sexual interaction
- Most enjoyable aspect of foreplay
- Ability of client to show affection
- Ability of client to communicate sex desire to partner
- Variations in sexual expression which are enjoyable, for example, oral–genital, mutual genital stimulation
- Use of self-stimulation/masturbation as a source of pleasure

Rationale: Many of the above questions provide a better understanding of the sexual value system of the patient/couple. Inquiry about the affective aspects of the relationship, that is, touching, holding, caressing, and pleasuring may reveal the extent to which the patient is comfortable with sexual intimacy. I will frequently notice at this point maladaptive patterns of communication and conflicting sexual value systems. I feel that such questions are essential since the extragenital options of love-making could be suggested for those persons who are comfortable with the intimate interaction. In addition, those who find coitus as a stress-provoking event may begin with the nondemanding sensual aspects of lovemaking. Masturbation may be considered as an acceptable sexual option.

Intervention: Emphasis on enhancing previous style of extragenital love-making; discuss attitudes/feelings about masturbation, oral–genital sex, and pleasuring if accepted as a sexual norm.

Quality of the Relationship

Areas of Inquiry:

- Description of other aspects of the relationship
- Changes in relationship since onset of ESRD and hemodialysis

Rationale: The quality of the sexual relationship may reflect patterns of communication in other aspects of the relationship. Previously destructive patterns of communication may continue.

Intervention: Emphasis on the need for communication of sexual feelings between partners. Extracoital options of love-making may be less fatiguing, for example, touching, holding, caressing, and non-demand pleasuring. Emphasis should be placed on resuming intimacy in the relationship, for example, extended foreplay and postcoital touching.

Upon completion of the interview several observations may be evident. For example, some persons may just need an opportunity to discuss sexual concerns/fears with an informed, nonjudgmental, and sensitive health care provider. Additionally, they may need information about impact of ESRD on sexual functioning. Finally if outstanding sexual problems are identified during the course of the interview, for example, erectile failure, orgastic dysfunction, and diminished libido, referral to the appropriate health care professional may be necessary for more extensive medical work-up, psychiatric evaluation, and relationship counseling.

CASE STUDY

Mary O'Brien is a 48-year-old married female with chronic renal failure requiring hemodialysis three times a week. Additional diagnoses were hypertension, anemia, and angina. Her medications included catapres, folic acid, and nitroglycerin prn. Mrs. O'Brien was referred to the nurse counselor after questions were raised about sexuality during the initial admission history at the dialysis center.

This individual may be described as an extremely neat, moderately obese, and articulate person who had previously worked as a legal secretary. She stated that her major loss since starting hemodialysis was the inability to work. Married a second time for 10 years to an older man, she described the relationship as one of loving companionship. These findings were confirmed by nurses and the social worker, who stated that the husband was attentive and supportive. She also stated that her network of friends and children helped her to adjust to the limitations imposed by illness.

Sexual activity (that is, arousal and orgastic capacity) did not change when comparing pre-illness and current levels of functioning. She never had a intense desire for sex and could "take it or leave it." Sex was important because it pleased her husband who enjoyed sexual interaction about once a week. She had no difficulty with vaginal lubrication and could achieve a climax if she wanted to. She particularly enjoyed touching and cuddling aspects of the love-making experience and would occasionally engage in oral–genital sex. Her major sex-related problem was coping with the lethargy and "washed out" feeling associated with hemodialysis.

Intervention

Emphasis was placed on conservation of energy.

1. Determining optimal time for sexual interaction; for example, Sunday prior to dialysis; avoiding extreme temperatures and heavy meals
2. Using previous coital position and discussing advantages and disadvantages of alternative modes
3. Easing into sexual activity, making provisions for extending the preliminaries of love-making and relaxing during the postcoital period of afterplay
4. Increasing communication with partner about level of sexual desire and feelings
5. Educating about sexual myths and potential for sexual activity when afflicted with ESRD

Discussion

Although it has been reported that females on dialysis tend to report deterioration in the frequency of sexual interaction,[4] specifically orgastic dysfunction, it appears that this patient did not experience or was not concerned about these problems. Sexual activity helped to maintain the quality of the relationship. Her role as a passive, dependent female in an emotionally and financially secure marriage changed very little. The attitude of the woman about sex and marital relationships also reflects the views of subjects in the Redbook Study.[7] For example, many of these women achieved sexual satisfaction even though they were not orgasmic with each erotic encounter. In a study with chronically ill cancer patients, Lieber et al.[8] reported that female patients expressed a greater desire for physical closeness and less desire for sexual intercourse.

In summary, this presentation focused on the holistic nature of the sexual experience, reviewed the essential components of a sex history, and described strategies for appropriate intervention. A case study was also presented.

REFERENCES

1. ABRAM, H. S., HESTER, L., SHERIDAN, W. F., and EPSTEIN, G. Sexual functioning in patients with chronic renal failure. *The Journal of Nervous and Mental Disease*, 1975, *160*(3), 220–26.
2. BROWN, T., FEINS, A., PARK, R., and PAULUS, D. Living with long term home dialysis. *Annals of Internal Medicine*, 1974, *81*, 165–170.
3. LEVY, N. B. The psychology and care of the maintenance hemodialysis patient. *Heart and Lung*, 1973, *2*(3), 400–405.
4. LEVY, N. B. Psychological studies at the Downstate Medical Center of patients on hemodialysis. *Medical Clinics of North America*, 1977, *61*(4), 759–69.
5. MACLEAN, P. Brain mechanisms of elemental sexual functions. In D. J. Kaplan and A. M. Freedman (Eds.), *The sexual experience*. Baltimore: Williams and Wilkins, 1978.
6. MASTERS, W. and JOHNSON, V. *Human sexual response*. Boston: Little, Brown and Co., 1966.
7. Redbook report on sexual relationships. *Redbook Magazine*, October 1980, 73–80.
8. LEIBER, L., PLUMB, M., GERSTENZANG, M., and HOLLAND, J. The communication of affection between cancer patients and their spouses. *Psychosomatic Medicine*, 1976, *28*, 379–389.
9. THURM, J. Effect of chronic renal disease in sexual function. *Medical Aspects of Human Sexuality*, 1976, *10*(8), 81–82.

10

Termination of Hemodialysis Treatment—Staff Reactions

SUE E. SLEVIN

The progress of hemodialysis from an experimental phase to a therapeutic stage has brought new and difficult psychological problems. Stages of patient adjustment to dialysis from honeymoon, to middle let-down phase, to acceptance, have been identified. This helps staff to understand the psychological effects of the treatment upon the patient. The availability of hemodialysis to greater numbers of people was made possible by legislation in 1972 which saved the lives of end-stage renal disease patients on a nonselective basis. This availability of dialysis has created additional problems for patients, family, and staff about the efficacy of treatment. It is not uncommon for patients with no hope of functioning or rehabilitation, who are completely dependent on society for their existence, to be dialyzed. Professionals are more actively looking at what science and the government have accomplished and many are troubled by what they see. The dialysis honeymoon is over 17 years after it was instituted as the treatment of choice for ESRD. The treatment, patients, and care-givers are in the middle let-down stage regarding the quality of life for the patient on hemodialysis. We are becoming increasingly aware that in many cases it does not improve the prospect of a normal life for the patient. We as professionals are being forced to look at our feelings and the feelings of patients as well as those of their families before we determine what our part is to be in working with patients who have not adjusted to dialysis and who wish to terminate treatment. Ways of handling this problem are few and are often unsatisfactory or of questionable legality. The patient may be considered suicidal and institutionalized in order to continue dialysis.The patient may be denied return to the hospital unless willing to comply with treatment. In other instances the patient dies alone or, if more fortunate, with family who are willing to stay with him in the absence of medical support. Patients

SUE E. SLEVIN, R.N., M.S. • Psychiatry Nurse–Clinician, Maimonides Medical Center, Brooklyn, New York.

are dialyzed after they become incoherent and can't refuse treatment. In a few instances patients are given the option to discontinue treatment and are hospitalized to receive medical support in dying. The latter occurs only with patients who happen to be treated in a hospital whose physicians have the philosophy of allowing the patient to discontinue treatment when living is untenable for them.

Much has been written on how the nurse, social worker, and doctor are supposed to treat patients, but little thought has been devoted to the psychological experience of the people treating the patient, the effects of these personal reactions upon the patients who wish to terminate treatment, or the other patients who view the staff–patient interaction regarding this issue. The purpose of this paper is to explore the clinical problem of the reactions of the staff and the subsequent effect on the patient and staff when faced with a request to terminate treatment. Data for this paper was obtained by interviews and observation of staff–patient interaction over a period of 7 months when a patient verbalized the wish to terminate treatment. Interviews were also conducted with the staff of various other units with similar problems when there was no clear-cut policy about dealing with the patient who verbalized the desire to stop treatment.

Up to now, the psychological focus has been primarily on the patient's adjustment and the neurotic problems which prevail in his decision to terminate treatment. The patient's positive or negative use of denial in his adjustment has been widely discussed . The most frequently observed staff reaction is also denial.[1] Abram[2] notes that denial may prevent discouragement among staff which can interfere with effective patient treatment. Kaplan De-Nour and Czaczkes[3] found that denial of staff interferes with patient care and that compliance with diet and vocational rehabilitation were found to be better in units with nondenying physicians. It has also been postulated by Eisendrath[4] that staff denial aids the patient in his identification with the staff and the patient is able to utilize the staff's attitude in continuing to accept his life on hemodialysis. Kaplan De-Nour and Czaczkes[5] studied emotional problems and reactions of the medical team in a chronic dialysis unit and found the main reactions of the team were feelings of guilt, possessiveness, overprotectiveness, and withdrawal from patients. They suggest that withdrawal is also evidenced by the high drop-out rate of nurses, physicians, and even psychiatrists from the field. They postulated that demands on patients to do extremely well on the treatment as well as the tendency to deny that the patients are ill, are believed to result from these emotional reactions. Foster and McKegney[6] studied group dynamics and survival on chronic hemodialysis with findings that suggest that intergroup relations between patients and staff are a critical determinant of patient survival on dialysis. Alexander[7] showed how the staff–patient relationship in dialysis fulfills the criteria of a double-bind system. She describes independent behavior as being demanded and denied and that greater patient dependency resulted in less gratitude, and more anger and frustration being experienced by the staff. Gratitude from the patient is both needed and rejected by the staff. Much evidence points to the fact that the physician-in-charge is the barometer of the unit. When the physician used denial, either the staff developed an unrealistic opinion of patients expecting them to be always relaxed and happy on dialysis, or the communication gap between the denying physician and the staff led to a lack of team opinion. In the second instance, the patient is always faced with double-bind communications emanating from the different staff members. If the physician did not use denial, the patients tended to do better and the staff developed realistic expectations about their patients.[8]

As professionals we have tried to alleviate some of the tension for ourselves by developing more medical, psychological, social, and legal criteria to ensure as far as possible a scientific reaction to and treatment plan for the patient who wishes to terminate dialysis treatments. This approach arises from a desire to reduce the emotional view, for fear of experiencing unwanted and unpleasant emotional reactions such as guilt, anger, hopelessness, helplessness, and loss of self-esteem from interfering with the patient's decision. We are acutely aware of the difficulties in approaching this issue. We have developed our medical technology to such an extent that we can maintain even the comatose patient in a state of quasi-survival to prevent death. We have developed elaborate rituals to preserve life. The scientific data leaves out the patient as an emotional being reacting to the slow deterioration of his body, unable to participate in the active process of life. Decisions to maintain life are still value-laden and made from the depths of the souls of doctors and nurses who have never been in the same arena as the patient. We have no firsthand experience with the existence of the patient unless perchance it happens to one of us or to someone with whom we are close. It threatens the very core of our existence when someone states that life is not worth living no matter what we have to offer.

The law has become involved because of the conflict of attitudes and personal values. However, there is no explicit legislation regarding the issue of discontinuing treatment. There are no clear guidelines to the patient's rights in accepting or refusing medical care. A hodgepodge of legal facts entwined with highly charged emotional reactions have done little to make the complexities of this issue clear.

Laws have transpired out of a societal need. The first laws on human death were related to body-snatching, a phenomenon originating in the nineteenth century as a result of medical schools needing human cadavers for training medical students. This law was updated with the advent of organ transplantation in the 1960s due to political pressure exerted for the advancement of medical science. The Uniform Anatomical Gift Act was instituted in July 1968. This need for organs precipitated the problem of the definition of death. Common-law definition of death has given way to many recent court decisions which accepted the neurologic definition of death. Many states have adopted this definition. The most explosive development of the law regarding death concerns termination of treatment. In response to the problems created by technology's artificial prolongation of life beyond natural limits, California became the first state to enact the Natural Death Act in 1976. Only one person was able to take advantage of the law by 1978 due to the complexity of restrictions on the ill person. Other states have passed similar laws but have equal difficulty using them. For many, termination of treatment still falls within the definition of suicide or homicide. This increases the medical profession's fear that serious legal repercussions will flow from discontinuing extraordinary care being rendered to a terminally ill patient. It is confusing when legislation such as Idaho's Natural Death Act states that adult persons have a fundamental right to control decisions relating to the rendering of their medical care, including the right to have life sustaining procedures withheld or withdrawn in instances of a terminal condition. Thus far, New York and other states wait for court cases to occur. In this day and age, doctors and nurses are forced to practice malpractice medicine.

More attention is being given to the question, "Is it a pathological depression or a rational decision when a patient verbalizes the wish to terminate treatment?" Patients are still perceived as suicidal if they decide to terminate life-supporting treatments. A patient who consents or demands that a doctor discontinue treatment may be guilty of the crime of attempting to commit suicide. The physician may be considered as aiding and abetting a suicide and thus to have committed a crime. It seems that if death has been redefined for our needs, a redefining of suicide and homicide may be necessary also.

In spite of the threat of being involved in a crime, treatment decisions are being more widely discussed in the literature. Beauchamp[8] writes that dialysis treatment is not obligatory when it offers no prospect of benefit to the patient or when its burdens outweigh its benefits for the patient. He states, "in the case of irresponsible or intentional refusals, the physician has at most a weak obligation to dialyze the patient."

Supposedly religious and moral precedents relieve a doctor from the obligation to continue the use of extraordinary means to care for the hopelessly ill patient. In 1957 Pope Pius XII declared that the prolongation of the dying process by extraordinary medical intervention is not required. The problem now occurs with the definition of extraordinary means. The American Medical Association holds that some treatments are optional and may be discontinued when death is imminent. There is confusion in the statement when it is applied to dialysis. The World Medical Association describes the condition of health as being sound in body, mind, and spirit. This is certainly questionable in the cases of many dialysis patients.

A few articles have been written indicating how different units have handled this problem. Schriener and Maher (1965)[11] described a policy of "allowing" patients to voluntarily withdraw from dialysis but considered this outcome to be a therapeutic failure at the time. McKegney and Lange[9] suggest that the possibility of death, discussed with the patient as an option would create less acting-out behavior and covert suicide attempts in patients. They postulated that talking openly about dying with a patient allows the patient to evaluate their quality of life with more objectivity. Even so, they did indicate that it was difficult to bridge the communication gap between the staff and the patients based on a different set of values regarding life and death. Patients were noted to be unable to express their feelings to staff when they did not value their present state enough to continue to live. Staff anger, withdrawal, and rejection caused the patients to have feelings of abandonment and isolation which gave them more reason to stop treatment. Discussing this option was impaired by staff reaction. In more recent years doctors have actively favored the patient withdrawing from treatment when the problems for the patient outweigh the benefits, but they do so quietly. Many units still choose to dialyze a patient despite the difficulties. The effect upon staff and patients cannot be underestimated.

Part of the difficulty for the nurse in remaining in the field lies in the immense amount of emotional involvement felt due to close contact with the patient. Working with the dialysis patient has a large social dimension. It arises out of the fact that the relationship is expected to be a long-term one. More information about our patients tend to be acquired than in the usual hospital work and more of our personal lives shared in seeing the patients an average of three times a week for years. A large part of the mystique of doctors and nursing staff is removed through this association. This prolonged and intensive contact with patients has been described as one of the major stresses of chronic hemodialysis, especially for nurses.[2]

The degree of emotional involvement with the patient varies with the doctor, nurse, dialysis technician, social worker, and other staff members. The greatest contact with the patient is experienced by the nursing personnel and the least by the physician. Yet it is the physician who holds the ultimate decision-power regarding treatment of the patient. Because of this, many dialysis units still operate without team input and joint decision-making, sticking to the traditional medical model. Along with this concept, it is not unusual to see the greatest conflicts first occurring between the nurses and the patients and then being discharged onto the rest of the dialysis staff. Intrateam tensions producing critical attitudes, especially about the physicians, have been described as displacement of aggression from the patients to the doctor and other team members.[3] In a working team of medical professionals, difficulties and conflicts between different disciplines as well as conflicts in staff–patient interaction can be dealt with directly and openly leaving the staff and patients with a feeling of personal integrity and competence within their respective roles and allowing each to maintain a sense of humanness. Without this concept, stress increases, conflicts remain unresolved, and mutual respect can be withheld or entirely missing within the unit. Patients feel threatened as does the entire team.

The patient is the person who ultimately suffers in unit conflicts. Many patients are frightened of potential ridicule at the hands of a staff for whom illness and suffering and the apparatus of treatment appear routine. Although as staff, we are employed for the sake of the patients, it is not by mistake that Kaplan De-Nour depicts the former as the center of the staff–patient interaction in her studies, and their high expectations as the primary cause of many difficulties with ensuing aggression on the part of the staff to the patient, the patient to the staff, and the staff members to each other in their mutual disappointments.[10]

In dealing with the patient who wishes to discontinue treatment, the ultimate example of noncompliance, a number of emotional reactions can be seen occurring between all members of the unit. The patient and the nursing staff experience most of the difficulty; the physician and even the social worker are better able to use denial of the problem as they are usually not directly involved with the actual treatment. Many units have not developed a mutual philosophy regarding the question of discontinuing treatment because of the confusion that exists, as shown previously in a review of the literature, and because the question is still of a very personal nature with no uniform societal values as yet determined.

The following sequence of events illustrates staff denial and the breakdown of that denial with its subsequent behavioral and emotional implications for patient and staff when the former openly verbalizes the wish to terminate treatment with the prospect of dying.

Initially, the patient's verbalizations may be perceived as a suicide wish and the patient would be instructed to discuss the wish with a psychiatrist. Nursing staff frequently experience anxiety, but just as frequently respond with compassion for the patient, admitting they themselves question the merits of dialysis. Social workers respond similarly to nursing staff. Attending physicians generally feel that the patient is seriously depressed and suicidal, using strong denial regarding the efficacy of treatment for the patient. Residents are more likely to find themselves somewhere in between the attitudes and feelings of the attending physicians and the nursing staff.

When the patient becomes more verbal in demands to discontinue treatment but continues to come to dialysis, the nurses and technicians are usually the first to experience guilt and have increasing anxiety cannulating the patient. The nurses are usually the first, often followed by the social worker, to report dreams about the patient who wishes to discontinue treatment, especially as the patient becomes more verbally aggressive. Avoidance of the patient is often observed when the staff denial of the difficulties of hemodialysis for the patient is challenged by the patient's pleas.

As a result, the patient is subject to the experience of isolation from the staff. The patient may respond with increased somatic complaints as an expression of anger and as a demand for attention. The nursing staff, more comfortable with the realm of physical complaints, inform the doctor who examines the patient willingly for a physical problem to deal with feelings of guilt and hostility about the patient's wish to discontinue treatment. The patient is generally admitted for a work-up even when a new diagnosis is doubtful. This represents an effort on the part of the physician to continue denial and overcompensate for feelings of anger towards the patient, who in turn expresses no gratitude for the medical care. Unable to find the etiology for the complaints, the resident frequently becomes the first of the doctors to openly experience frustration with the patient. In one situation the resident expressed not wanting to go see the patient, because he was angry that he couldn't make the patient feel better, and would never get any thanks or acknowledgement from the patient about the care he was giving him. He openly admitted disliking the patient and questioned for the first time his choice of a career in medicine.

Patients frequently criticize physicians, saying that they don't know what they are doing, and patients have been known to tell other patients who are new to the treatment that dialysis is terrible. Physicians, not having found the cause of physical complaints, reaffirm in their minds that the patient's problems are "all in the head" and consider the patient crazy for requesting them to discontinue treatment. However, the patient is frequently allowed to remain in the hospital, and the physicians allay their guilt by ordering more tests. It is not uncommon for the doctor to forget these patients on rounds or to do rounds without asking the patient how he feels. It is not unusual for these patients to finally refuse more tests and subsequently be asked to sign out against medical advice as the doctor can no longer justify keeping the patient in the hospital.

As the patient becomes more verbal and demanding in the unit, the other patients cannot help but become involved. Other patients have been known to criticize the patient openly to the staff or to tell the patient directly to shut up. Patients may request not to be placed next to the disruptive patient, reinforcing for the third time the sense of isolation the patient has experienced from the nursing staff and the physicians.

Frustration of the nursing staff often leads to complaints about the patient in front of the other patients when the patient is expected in the unit. This occurs as a result of dialysis units rarely having a separate nurses' station where the staff may carry out conversation about patients. Also, given the nature of the work, comments are usually done across the room and within hearing range of other patients. This is not unconscious or deliberate on the part of the staff. It can be estimated that 95% of staff communication takes place within the hearing range of other patients.

Eventually, the hostility of staff members toward the physicians for not dealing with the patient who is requesting termination is no longer hidden from each other nor from the other patients and is frequently known to the patient requesting termination. In one instance, the patient expressed a certain satisfaction that everybody was fighting because of her request. The nursing staff's anger at the physicians may be acted out in other treatment decisions such as not making room for an acute patient until after-hours, forcing the physician to stay late, or by not being available to help the physician with a treatment. Physicians' anger can equally affect the nursing staff; for example, the physician may call in a nurse in the middle of the night to do an acute patient who could have waited until morning to be dialyzed.

Hostility towards the physicians who will not discuss the issue in a team meeting and who avoid the patient may be projected back upon the patient for being difficult. Staff begin to avoid each other as well as the patient. The staff may be divided into two different camps, those who begin to agree with the patient for reasons of their own and those who adamantly believe in life at any cost.

In order to deal with their anxiety, splitting of the bad versus the good patient may occur. A patient who was having multiple problems yet was grateful to the staff was seen as an angel while the patient who was desiring to quit was seen as ungrateful and the worst patient in the unit. Patients were glad they were not like the "bad" patient. In one case, hostility of the staff was acted out when the primary nursing approach was instituted, making the one nurse in the unit whom the patient didn't like responsible for her care.

In most units, the staff members in general become angry with the psychiatric nurse or psychiatrist who cannot cure the patient. In several units, the nursing staff frequently paged the psychiatric nurse or social worker to "sit with the difficult patient during dialysis."

Factors such as the staff being close to the patient's age seemed to influence whether they thought the patient wanted to die or wanted attention. If the staff was about the same age as the patient, they felt he wanted attention. If the patient was older and senile, they felt it was more of a wish to die and get it over with. If the situation becomes an impasse between the patient and the staff, eventually the patient refuses to come for treatment. This may result from the patient getting the message from either the staff or other patients, "why come to dialysis if you wish to terminate?"

In one instance, the patient was considered suicidal by the psychiatrist and also a danger to the people in her building because she smoked in bed while by herself. Concern was for the patient and also for the apartment dwellers for fear she would set the building on fire if she became severely confused secondary to uremia. The patient was brought to the hospital by the police. The patient became angry with the psychiatric nurse, stating that she could no longer trust her. When a psychiatrist was asked to evaluate her competence to refuse treatment, she verbalized that people must think she was crazy. She stated that she felt no better than a criminal in prison and in fact requested she be taken to prison for her crime to be dialyzed there. She felt she had no rights left in the world. In this instance, the psychiatrist determined her to be able to make the decision to terminate treatment and suggested that she be told the exact consequences of her actions, including what to expect. The physicians avoided talking to the patient about termination, saying that she didn't ask them and that besides they were there to save lives. This particular patient was kept in the hospital in a private room, became psychotic, and died from unknown causes 1 month after she was admitted to the hospital.

In summary, denial was seen as the first reaction of the staff to hearing the request of a patient to terminate treatment. Denial is a defense mechanism, which operates unconsciously to resolve emotional conflict and allay anxiety by disavowing thoughts, feelings, wishes, needs, or external reality factors that are consciously intolerable. In this case, denial can be considered to be threatened by the middle phase let-down stage of treatment. Denial gives way to suppression and eventually guilt. In suppression, the staff makes a conscious effort to control and conceal unacceptable impulses, thoughts, feelings, or aggressive acts against patients or other staff.

Guilt was experienced when the staff became aware of their anger and felt that they had somehow violated their committment to curing the sick in having a patient who rejected their ministrations. The ungrateful patient should have faded into the woodwork, disappeared, or died so that they wouldn't have to be faced with their failure. Guilt may also be associated with identification with the patient and agreement with the request when they as caregivers should endorse life. Guilt is an individual feeling and cannot be so easily shared unless it is verbalized. It is very heavy when carried alone.

Withdrawal from and subsequent isolation of the patient became a way of dealing with guilt and anger. Avoidance of the patient reduced the experience of guilt felt by the staff, but only temporarily. As the unit is an intense social experience, the patient who is avoided becomes hostile, which generates more hostility from and between the staff and then is projected back onto the patient. Projection in this instance worked as a defense mechanism which operated unconsciously. The experience of anger and frustration in the staff needing an outlet was transferred back upon the most vulnerable member of the unit, the patient.

Splitting occurred within the staff and towards the patients. Splitting in psychoanalytical terms relates to an unconsciously employed reaction separating the good and bad, in this case patients, into parts with the intent of separating feelings of love and aggression. The staff has a firm faith in and love of their work. These feelings are threatened when a patient wishes to terminate treatment. Splitting occurs when primitive aggression prevents development in which "all good" and "all bad" self and object images are integrated into a concept of self and objects. Aggressiveness split from the idealized staff and others prevents integration, triggering unbearable anxiety and guilt. In other words, strong identification of staff with patients and wanting them to do well causes unbearable guilt secondary to the aggression experienced against them when they refuse to do well. Thus splitting patients into groups of bad or good arises as a defense against the aggression and guilt experienced in relating to the patients and also helps to protect their image of themselves.

This splitting leads to further isolation of the patient and his lowered self-esteem for not being able to take the treatment. Minimizing the patient's request to that of wanting attention is often a weak defense against the stronger reactions invoked, causing the process of splitting.

In any event, increased hostility and anger resulting from anxiety due to crumbling defenses, lead to different solutions. In the one instance cited, the patient who refused to come was considered to be suicidal and a danger to the other tenants in her apartment building. In other instances, the patient is forgotten or considered to be in the care of the unfortunate family. The patient is doomed to an irrevocable failure at life in these circumstances. The staff are forever guilty and the families will be forever condemned by this experience.

A post-mortem examination of units which have to deal with the patient who wishes to terminate treatment has elicited the following reactions. Usually, there is little acknowledgment in the unit that a patient has died. In one instance a nurse resigned shortly after the experience. Attempts to interview staff regarding these problems were thwarted by people forgetting appointments or by difficulty in setting a mutual time for discussion. Staff admitted becoming less interested in the emotional lives of their patients. In one hospital, a patient stated one year later that he had the same wish to discontinue treatment but was afraid to bring it up with the staff as he didn't know what would happen. Some staff have expressed relief that the patient died and expressed grief that they could not help the patient die gracefully. They felt an opportunity was lost, so to speak. In one hospital, psychiatric consultations reduced in number. Some nurses commented that they look at their work more as a job, not really sure how much they are helping people. Most of the nursing staff felt that the doctors have the problem with the issue of termination of treatment. However, no one on the nursing staff could answer directly regarding the question, "Would you be willing to tend the patient who was dying from refusal of treatment?" Most nursing staff are afraid that it will happen again and worry about what will occur.

Social workers and psychiatric nurses reported experiencing hostility, rejection, and feelings of being scapegoated by staff for not making the patients better and reestablishing their will to live. Medical staff tend to say it is the patient's depression and not his illness that make them worse, even after their condition has deteriorated as far as a stroke with the patient being unable to communicate.

Patients have reported that they felt like they were going crazy after experiencing the various reactions of staff toward them when they verbalized their wish to terminate treatment. Other patients reported relief that a patient died and was relieved of misery.

In many units, the demand from the nursing staff was for team meetings to discuss the issue of the patient who wants to terminate treatment. Usually these were not actualized. It could be postulated that these meetings threatened the medical staff's denial of death and posed to them the reality that their treatment could be seen as persecuting and undesirable. It is of interest to note that this reaction is similar to that of patients who have refused to attend group meetings with other hemodialysis patients. The realities of hemodialysis could not be endured if the denial in the service of survival is challenged. In this sense, staff denial, in the service of continuing to treat patients, allows minimal emotional involvement and becomes a source of strength to staff when it becomes necessary to repeatedly treat a patient who moans and groans, a patient screaming that doctors are barbarians and pleading with them to stop the treatment.

In conclusion, the problem of discontinuing dialysis is a difficult one, complicated by the medical, psychological, social, and legal criteria under which we all operate. We can alleviate some of this tension by developing more clear-cut criteria regarding this decision. However, as we review the experience of staff members faced with this problem, we must recognize it is not that simple. This issue provokes much stress for staff members because it is also a very personal issue. Staff reactions themselves are part of the complexities that must be sifted out in order to look at the issue more clearly.

One could also say that the psychological reactions of staff members are the same in any unit when there are conflicts about the treatment. However, it can also be said that the explosive issue of stopping treatment develops these problems in greater depth and intensity because of the ultimate issue, death. It is clear that the staff is not a closed system within the hemodialysis unit, but, as we have seen, it is a dynamic one in which each part affects the other and in which countertransferences are detrimental to effective functioning of staff and to patient care.

Research still needs to be done to determine how the staff attitudes influence or modify patients' choice concerning continuing or discontinuing treatment. Research is also needed to evaluate the effect of the team approach upon the experience of the patient and the staff. Staff conferences and group meeting were the most recommended solution for staff difficulties. Staff meetings have been noted in the literature for years as a way for reducing unit stress, yet many dialysis units still tend to minimize their importance. We not only need to further our understanding of patient experience on dialysis but also must develop a better understanding of ourselves in relation to patients and other staff members in order to achieve better satisfaction in our work. Not understanding our frustrations and other emotional reactions is an added stress leading to our sense of helplessness and impotence in the already stressful environment of hemodialysis.

REFERENCES

1. SHORT, M. J., and WILSON W. P. Roles of denial in chronic hemodialysis. *Archives of General Psychiatry*, 1969, *20*, 433–437.
2. ABRAM, H. S. Psychiatric reflections on adaptation to repetitive dialysis. *Kidney International*, 1974, *6*, 67–72.

3. KAPLAN DE-NOUR, A., and CZACZKES, J. W. Team–patient interaction in chronic hemodialysis units. *Psychotherapy and Psychosomatics*, 1974, 24, 132–136.
4. EISENDRATH, R. M. Adaptation to renal transplantation. In J. G. Howells (Ed.), *Modern perspectives in the psychiatric aspects of surgery*. New York: Brunner/Mazel, 1976, 380–389.
5. KAPLAN DE-NOUR, A., and CZACZKES, J. W. Emotional problems and reactions of the medical team in a chronic hemodialysis unit. *Lancet*, 1968, 2, 987–991.
6. FOSTER, G. F., and MCKEGNEY, P. F. Small group dynamics and survival on chronic hemodialysis. *International Journal of Psychiatry in Medicine*, 1977/78, 8, 105–116.
7. ALEXANDER, L. The double-bind theory and hemodialysis. *Archives of General Psychiatry*, 1976, 33, 1353.
8. BEAUCHAMP, T. L. Can we stop or withhold dialysis? In G. E. Schreiner (Ed.), *Controversies in nephrology*. Washington, D.C.: Georgetown University Nephrology Division, 1979, 163–170.
9. MCKEGNEY, P. F., and LANGE, P. The decision to no longer live on chronic hemodialysis. *American Journal of Psychiatry*, 1971, 128, 267–274.
10. KAPLAN DE-NOUR, A. Staff–patient interaction. This volume.
11. SCHREINER, G. E., and MAHER, J. F. Hemodialysis for chronic renal failure. Medical, moral and ethical, and socio-economic problems. *Annals of Internal Medicine*, 1965, 62, 551–563

11

Problems in Discontinuation of Hemodialysis

WILLIAM A. GREENE

Fifteen years ago we were faced with problems of whom to take on hemodialysis and whom to exclude. Federal support and available services make this selection less of a quandary today. Now, however, with patients living longer on dialysis and starting dialysis at more and more advanced ages and with more complex illnesses (diabetes, hypertension, lupus erythematosus, coronary heart disease, and so on), another quandary arises: the dilemma of when and how to take patients off dialysis, allowing them to die.

The option of discontinuing dialysis may be initiated by the patient, relatives, or staff. Such an eventuality can create problems for everyone, particularly nurses, technicians, and social workers who usually know the patients and their family members best. Who should or can take the responsibility for such a decision?

Consideration of all aspects of the problems of patients on hemodialysis can seem very complicated. The complexity of the variables involved in successful or unsuccessful dialysis often seems to be quite nebulous and difficult to appreciate in precise terms. At times it appears that there can be no scientific approach to the understanding of the multiple problems involved. Actually, one can think of the situation quite simply and presumably scientifically by talking in dimensions of MASS, SPACE, and TIME, variables dealt with by the physicist and therefore presumably the quintessence of scientific gymnastics. This perspective can be depicted in Figure 1.

This complexity may be abstracted quite simply. MASS, between the two parallel lines, shows the patient with his clinical and demographic characteristics. This MASS progresses over TIME, depicted as proceeding left to right with the point of first dialysis at 0, on through the first 12

WILLIAM A. GREENE, M.D. • Professor of Medicine and Psychiatry, University of Rochester Medical Center, Rochester, New York.

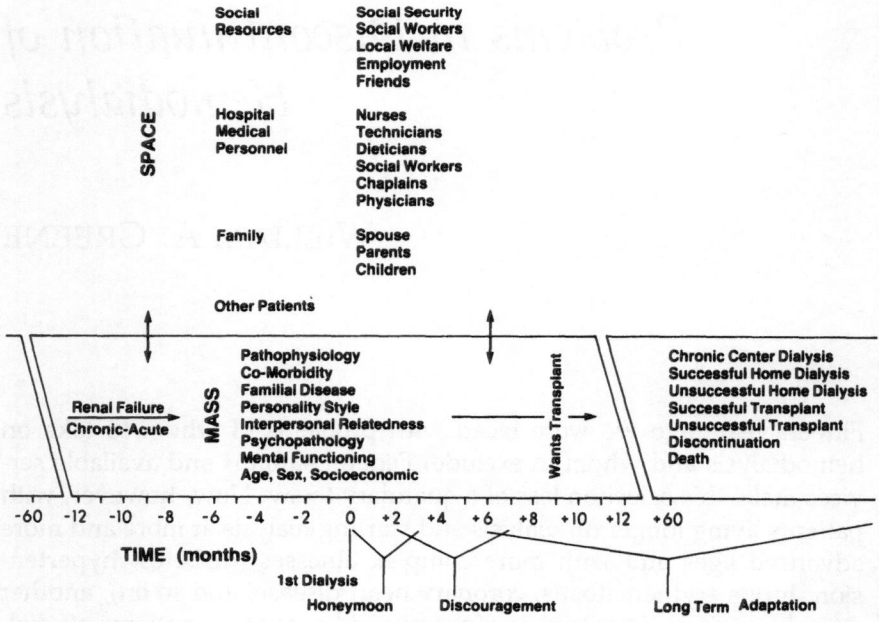

FIG. 1.   Factors in psychosocial adaptation to hemodialysis.

months of dialysis and then on to an eventual course of 5 years or more. Above is represented the dimension of SPACE, meaning the interrelationships of the patient with the many persons or agencies with whom he interacts. These constitute the variable of SPACE. The patient is MASS. This MASS in SPACE depicted over TIME is shown before and after the first dialysis. The first 3 months of dialysis are referred to as the "honeymoon" period.[1] Usually after 2 or 3 months the patient goes into a period of disenchantment or discouragement. He then settles down to a long-term adaptation phase. Within the first year, the patient generally wants to have a transplant if this has not occurred earlier in his treatment.

This dialysis processing can be depicted more simply in Figures 2, 3, and 4.

Figure 2 shows the MASS dimension; the internal components which the patient brings to his predicament and which operate for and/or against him. These include psychophysiological components, renal pathophysiology, comorbidity such as diabetes or hypertension, possible familial disease of the kidney, as well as his particular personality style. In spite of the fact that dialysis patients are said to be generally depressed, they have differing means of coping with their general life

PSYCHOPHYSIOLOGIC CHARACTERISTICS

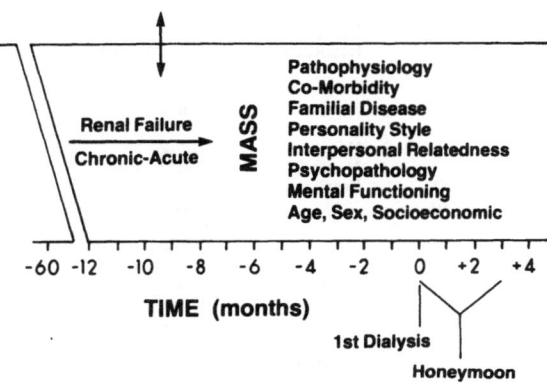

FIG. 2.   Mass or psychophysiologic characteristics.

situation once on dialysis. They also have different abilities for relating interpersonally. Occasionally, there will be gross psychopathology. Mental functioning is frequently disrupted in patients with uremia who may be acutely delirious or chronically demented. As time goes on and we see older and older patients started and perpetuated on dialysis there are more who become grossly demented. Also, patients vary according to their age, sex, and socioeconomic status. It has seemed that the patients who come to dialysis are not a random sample of the population but are generally those of lower socioeconomic status. In addition, it appears that persons coming to dialysis are those who have had more than the usual share of social disruptions in their lives, particularly, in the year or so before going on dialysis.

Figure 3 shows the SPACE dimension, the *social resources* of the patient, those persons who are often intimately concerned with how the patient does on dialysis and also are involved in major decisions which have to be made about the specific treatment to be undertaken. These persons affect the patient's course on dialysis and are in turn affected by that course—especially family members. There is evidence that patients on home dialysis do better than patients on center dialysis. This is probably mainly a function of patient selection. Those who have a home suitable for home dialysis and have a family member for back-up are generally more effective in any type of endeavor. We have to keep in mind not only what we are doing *for* the patient who goes on dialysis, but also what we are doing *to* his children, his parents, and particularly to his spouse. Whether, for how long, and how the patient continues on dialy-

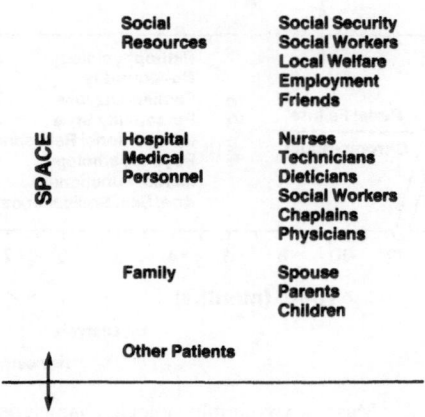

FIG. 3. Space or social resources.

sis is crucial to the spouse, who is the most common support for a patient on home or center dialysis.

Figure 4 shows the conclusions of the TIME dimension; what are called *eventualities*. The patient can continue successfully with varying degrees of rehabilitation on chronic center dialysis. He may go on to successful and effective home dialysis. In some cases it turns out that home dialysis is not feasible for the patient or the back-up or the home situation in general. He may have to go back to chronic center dialysis. Some patients, many less than the number predicted 15 years ago, go on to a successful renal transplant with a live-related donor or a cadaver kidney. Too many have an unsuccessful transplant with complications or rejec-

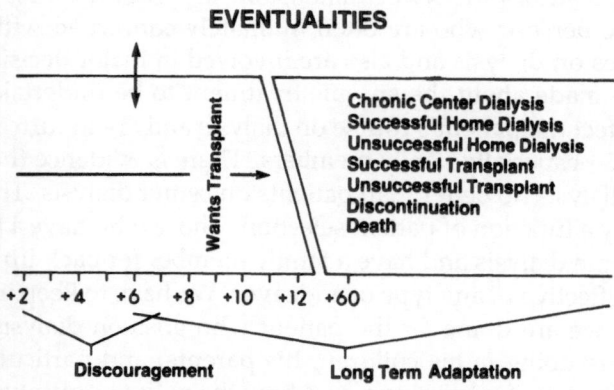

FIG. 4. Eventualities over time.

tion and have to go back on dialysis. Many patients who start on dialysis die of one of the many complications. A mortality rate of at least 10% per year is a reasonable working assumption. A few are considered for discontinuation.

We are now dealing, and have been for a number of years, with a new type of problem in eventuality: the discontinuation of dialysis. This is a difficult problem in terms of ethics, medical custom, and compassion for those undergoing hemodialysis. This is so not only in reference to the patient, but also for his family members. This can be a problem among individuals in the dialysis treatment team. It has not been publicly touched on enough. It is going to be a problem of increasing frequency and concern in the months and years to come. Who can make these decisions, presume to take such responsibility (see Figure 5)?

In the mid-sixties the Dialysis and Transplant Committee of the Medical Center at Rochester was formed to evaluate the most suitable treatment for patients with end-stage renal disease. The University Hospital, Strong Memorial, is the center for dialysis and transplantation. This Committee, 30–50 in number, meets weekly. In 1974, a subcommittee of this Medical Center Dialysis and Transplant Committee was established to appraise the question of possible criteria for *not* taking patients on dialysis, but mainly to consider the question of what might be criteria for discontinuing dialysis once it had started. This committee was chaired by Dr. Nathaniel Whitcomb, an Episcopal Canon who is the Chaplain of Strong Memorial Hospital. Also on this subcommittee was a priest, a dialysis nurse, a social worker, a nephrologist, a transplant surgeon, and myself. We met two or three times a month over 2 years to agonize about some of the problems with which we and the dialysis and transplant caretakers were wrestling.

WHOSE RESPONSIBILITY?

PATIENT

FAMILY
    Parent
    Spouse
    Child

PHYSICIAN(S)

NURSE(S)

CLERGY

SOCIAL WORKER(S)

SOCIETY (Government)

FIG. 5.   Treatment choice is whose responsibility?

While the questions of establishment of criteria for patient selection occupied much of the initial year of the deliberations, during the second year we rapidly got into the questions of criteria for discontinuing or terminating dialysis. It was evident that the consideration of termination of treatment arises from two main circumstances: first, the physiological status of the patient, and second, the psychological and social situation. The patient may request that dialysis be terminated. At times the patient's physical deterioration indicates that termination of treatment should be considered. The patient may accept the recommendation and give written consent for cessation of treatment. He may wish to continue. If the patient is psychologically incompetent to arrive at a decision by himself, a three-person committee, including two physicians, can attest to the patient's incompetence and accept the responsibility for deciding to terminate dialysis. If the patient elects to terminate treatment the medical staff must be confident that they offer all other available help, both physical and psychological, to the patient. It is also relevant to consider the degree of family morbidity incurred through excessive physical and emotional strain on family members of the chronic hemodialysis patient and to consider their degree of discomfort or comfort by the patient's continuation as compared to discontinuation of long-term hemodialysis therapy. Lawyers informed us that there is little existing legal guidance with reference to terminating a chronic treatment such as hemodialysis. The prevalent trend is to judge such actions of the physician in the hospital according to the standard of medical care in the community. This implies that once a physician begins to treat a patient, the physician is not legally permitted to abandon him and that the patient can expect to continue to receive care of a quality comparable to that which might be provided by any other qualified physician or institution in the community.

It should be emphasized that the consideration and implementation of dialysis discontinuation is not a brief consolidated maneuver by any one individual. It involves an interacting process over time by several persons: the patient, his family, and the care-taking staff. The outcome is determined by the individual patients and their characteristics (MASS) and social resources (SPACE over TIME).

From our experience and deliberation it appears that there are five main categories of dialysis discontinuation as shown in Table 1.

Other categories could be added or some of these could be collapsed. So far this has seemed a useful classification. Actually over the course of 2 years in the early 1970s, in an average population of 65 patients at any one time and 40 new patients each year, 12 patients were discontinued on dialysis. This does not count the patients who had

TABLE 1
Categories of Dialysis Discontinuation

Acute dialysis not going on to chronic dialysis
Chronic dialysis with severe pathopysiologic complications
Chronic dialysis with severe psychosocial problems
Chronic dialysis with patient and/or family request to stop
Chronic dialysis and successful renal transplant with seeming paradoxical depression in
   the patient

acute complications while on or between dialysis which led to their death.

Details of the course of these patients and the circumstances leading to discontinuation are shown in the following case vignettes. These are arranged according to the five categories of discontinuation.

ACUTE DIALYSIS NOT GOING ON TO CHRONIC DIALYSIS

Case 057

This 70-year-old man was put on acute dialysis when he developed cardiac failure with renal failure. The patient was a bachelor who had lived alone in a nearby town. He had one living relative, a sister, who was also over 70. She lived nearby and had helped him to shop and did some of his cooking. After being dialyzed acutely for 3 weeks and feeling, to be sure, appreciably better, it was felt necessary to continue him on chronic dialysis if he would survive. He himself indicated that he did not wish to continue on the machine. At a meeting of three physicians, the sister, and the patient, it was decided to let him go home to a local hospital for supportive care. This was warmly endorsed and agreed to by his local physician who had known him for many decades.

This is an example of a patient's decision not to go on to chronic dialysis after acute dialysis.

Case 030

This 81-year-old man was acutely dialyzed for 3 weeks. It was impossible to adequately interview him because of severe dementia and apathy. He had always been a very active, outgoing, independent farmer. The staff felt that it was too traumatic to try to inflict chronic dialysis on him. We met with his very devoted and understanding wife and their two daughters and sons-in-law, without the demented patient. It was decided among the group that we would not continue the procedure. This was again very definitely done with the understanding that we were making the decision rather than the members of the family.

This is a patient who was not continued from acute to chronic dialysis.

CHRONIC DIALYSIS WITH SEVERE PATHOPHYSIOLOGIC COMPLICATIONS

Case 003

A 49-year-old former laundry worker had a 30-year history of diabetes requiring insulin. He had been blind because of retinopathy for 1 year and could only see shapes vaguely. He had also had a gastrectomy many years before for a peptic ulcer. He had been adopted and knew nothing about his parents and had no known siblings. He had been married for 14 years. His 43-year-old wife was extremely anxious. They had no children. They lived in a small town about 20 miles from the hospital. He had considerable residual motor difficulty while walking since he had had a stroke 6 months before with hemiplegia, but with significant improvement. His wife refused to consider home dialysis. She felt that she would be able to drive him back and forth for dialysis. This was started in April. The following August he and his wife had become increasingly frantic about the trips back and forth and his having to be on dialysis. His wife at one point insisted that we discontinue dialysis; we told her this was not her decision to make.

Finally the patient was taken off dialysis because he said he wanted this, although he would have continued dialysis if we had institutionalized him in our hospital or if we had been able to find a VA hospital available.

This brings up a matter which is going to be increasingly prevalent, namely the question of continuing dialysis in the elderly patient with comorbidity who has to be chronically institutionalized in a county hospital, a nursing home, and so forth.

This is an example of discontinuation because of psychosocial and comorbidity factors.

Case 008

A delightful 66-year-old meat packer, who had recently retired, was put on chronic dialysis and did extremely well. He had been twice widowed, the last time a year before he started on dialysis. He had only one family member, a son in his early thirties who lived some distance away and traveled around the country. He lived by himself in his old homestead with a housekeeper. A year after starting he became moderately depressed when his 70-year-old sister and only other relative died. This was a recapitulation of his previous wives' deaths. After being on dialysis for 5 years, he developed a cerebral thrombosis with a hemiplegia and coma and was admitted to the hospital. He was continued on dialysis for 3 weeks with no significant improvement and no recovery of significant consciousness. It was decided by a staff of three different physicians that this man's dialysis should be discontinued. He died quietly 10 days later.

This is an example of discontinuation because of severe comorbidity.

Chronic Dialysis with Severe Psychosocial Problems

Case 002

A 57-year-old former mechanic had diabetic nephropathy and Meniere's Disease with deafness in one ear and intermittent vertigo. He had retinopathy and was not able to read but could see differences between light and dark.

He had a devoted wife and a 15-year-old daughter in high school. He was started on dialysis after extended deliberation. At the time of considering hemodialysis, he said that he was so sick that he did not want to live like he was, but he was afraid to die and therefore would accept dialysis. At times, however, he would talk about wanting to kill himself and being angry because his wife had hidden his guns. A year and a half later, he had become increasingly irascible. It was a problem for his wife to get him into the car to transport him to dialysis, 40 miles away. His wife worked nights as a receptionist in a local hospital and at that time the now 16-year-old daughter tended to him. The wife tried to sleep and also take care of him during the day while the daughter was in school. He kept insisting that he wanted to stop dialysis, but he always came if his wife insisted enough. Frequently he appeared to act as though he was testing his wife. He became increasingly demented. After 2½ years he was brought into the hospital and given an extensive work-up regarding his irreversible mental and metabolic status. It was decided to discontinue dialysis as much for the sake of his wife and daughter as for the patient.

This is an example of discontinuation because of psychosocial problems.

Case 038

This 63-year-old man, who had moderately severe nephrosclerosis, had been an active farmer living some 50 miles from the hospital. He was started on hemodialysis and was considered to be a reasonably effective person who understood and could tolerate the procedure. At home he had a devoted wife. Two daughters lived in the vicinity in the same small town. After being on dialysis for approximately 1 year, he became progressively more demented with increasing difficulty in memory, particularly recent memory, and increasing difficulty integrating the stresses of dialysis. He became quite abusive of his wife and other members of the family. On dialysis he was generally quite docile and posed no particular problem. After about 2 years of dialysis, he began indicating that he did not want to come to dialysis anymore. It was an increasing problem for his wife to get him to make the 50-mile trip. This was more and more distressing for his wife, particularly during the northern New York State winters. It was obvious that the staff as well as the patient's wife and his grown children were in considerable conflict about whether or not to continue him on dialysis. It was felt that he was not able to comprehend the consequences of coming off dialysis. After deliberation for 2 or 3 months, it was finally decided by three physicians that we should no longer inflict the suffering entailed in dialysis on this patient who was becoming increasingly panicky about the procedure. This was done with the acquiescence of his family, but we emphasized that they in no way were making this decision.

This case is in the category of a patient whose dialysis was discontinued because of psychosocial problems.

Case 047

This 43-year-old large black man came to us acutely from a State Mental Hospital 100 miles away with end-stage renal disease. He had been chronically institutionalized for schizophrenia for 28 years. He had obvious thought-blocking, perseveration, delusions, and inappropriate affect. He was alternately combative and compliant on dialysis which was administered acutely because of severe fluid overload. He repeatedly indicated that he wanted no such treatment. There was, of course, the question of whether he appreciated the options available to him. Finally, he was taken off after 1 month and not put into the chronic dialysis category. As mentioned, he lived 100 miles away. It was evident that if he was dialyzed he would have to be institutionalized and this could only be done in a State Hospital. That was not feasible in the State Hospital where he had been for nearly three decades. This poses the problem of, are we or are we not going to dialyze those who do have severe irreversible psychotic mental illness and also persons with severe mental retardation requiring institutionalization?

CHRONIC DIALYSIS WITH PATIENT AND/OR FAMILY REQUEST TO STOP

Case 017

A 44-year-old black divorced mother of nine children started on dialysis because of renal failure due to nephrosclerosis. Throughout her course she had multiple complications including pericarditis requiring a pericardial window, repeated clotted shunts, and later a fistula which had to be revised many times using the upper and lower part of all four extremities.

A year later one of her daughters was considered as a possible donor. It was felt that the patient's prognosis and her multiple complications precluded the use of a live-related donor. She eventually had a cadaver kidney 2 years later, which was rejected completely after 4 months. Because of this she became quite depressed and paranoid and at times hallucinated.

She continued to have multiple access problems and increased difficulty eating and eventually became emaciated and unable to be out of the hospital for more than 2 weeks at a time. After 4 years of treatment it was eventually decided to discontinue dialysis.

This is an example of the patient who is eventually discontinued on dialysis, partly at her own request and partly due to the judgment of the staff as well as the conflict-ridden agreement of her many children. This type of problem can create many differences of opinion among the children and the professional staff.

Case 023

A delightful 67-year-old woman was initially put on acute dialysis for 3 to 4 weeks in view of her end-stage renal disease, the exact nature of which was not determined but which was probably acute glomerulonephritis. She had had rheumatoid arthritis for 27 years with a considerable deformity, but was able to get around with the assistance of a cane. She lived 80 miles from the hospital with her 66-year-old husband who was quite supportive and had retired a year before from his longstanding job as a mechanic. They had one child at home, a son, age 28, who had epilepsy and was retarded. A daughter, a nurse, was married and lived away from the household. The husband and the son were doing most of the housework. There was considerable question as to whether this woman should go on dialysis and she herself would not make the decision. She said this was a matter which she could not decide, whether she was going to die or not. This was something that should be decided only by God.

We finally started her on dialysis with the understanding that this was a 3-month trial. We would see, with her, how it worked out, particularly the problem of transportation back and forth. After a month of chronic therapy she herself said she didn't want to live like this. She felt that the problem was much too difficult for her. She also let us know that she felt it was too much of a burden to her family.

Therefore, we acceded to her wishes not to inflict the treatment any longer on her, much less on her family. Again, we let it be known emphatically that we were making the decision and it was not the family's decision.

This is an example of the patient deciding to terminate.

Case 005

A 60-year-old man had had multiple transfusions following an ileal femoral bypass and 3 months later developed serum hepatitis. With this he had severe hepatitis and hepatorenal syndrome and was dialyzed acutely. He became severely disabled, weak, and depressed and asked to be discontinued. His wife was 59 and he had two daughters in their thirties. He had always been an extremely active, outgoing man with an excavating business. It was felt by his wife and daughters that it would be too degrading for him to continue on the machine. The patient indicted that he wanted to stop dialysis and die. We acceded to his wishes.

This is an example of discontinuation at the patient's request.

CHRONIC DIALYSIS AND SUCCESSFUL RENAL TRANSPLANT WITH SEEMING PARADOXICAL DEPRESSION IN THE PATIENT

Case 012

A 47-year-old man was started on dialysis in May because of end-stage renal disease from interstitial nephritis due to methicillin. He had a long history of hypertension. He also had a history of mild recurrent asthma since age six, treated with steroids at times, but mainly with Isoprel. He claimed to be allergic to everything. He had one sister, who was married and had children. She lived in a distant city, had little to do with him, and refused to be a kidney donor. His mother and father had been divorced in his teens and he was much on his own. His father had remarried. Both his mother and father had died about 8 years before in their early sixties. He had been married once for 6 years, had no children, and was divorced 7 years before. He had a subsequent affiliation, living with a divorcee and her two children, which broke up 2 years before he began dialysis.

He had had multiple courses of psychotherapy and psychiatric hospitalizations over the previous 25 years with diagnoses of a severe obsessive–compulsive character with recurrent depression and at times had a diagnosis of schizophrenia.

He had been living by himself for 2 years with little or no social contacts except for the dialysis staff and patients and his psychotherapist, when he was called for a cadaver kidney transplant. This functioned quite well after a week of acute tubular necrosis. He was looking forward with apprehension to resuming his solitary life. The day before he was to be discharged home he became very anxious about going home and had a fulminating rejection which could not be reversed over the next 2 weeks. He went back on dialysis acutely and was discharged to his previous in-center dialysis status 3 weeks later.

This is an example of a patient with personality problems manifesting a severe anxiety and depressive reaction on being faced with discontinuation of dialysis due to transplantation. The anxiety is mainly due to separation from his main social relationships, the dialysis staff and patients.

CONCLUSION

These patients and their course have presented very agonizing problems for the physicians, the nurses, the technicians, and the social workers, all of whom knew well many of the patients and also their families. Perhaps fortunately, most of the dialysis staff did not have to care for these patients directly after the decision to discontinue dialysis was made. Most of the patients have died within 3 weeks of discontinuing dialysis.

It should be emphasized that the consideration and implementation of dialysis discontinuation is not a brief consolidated maneuver by any one individual. It involves an interacting process over time by several persons: the patient, his family, and the care-taking staff. The outcome is determined by the individual patients and their characteristics (MASS) and social resources (SPACE over TIME).

There are ethical problems here, such as what are the rights of patients, what are the rights of members of the family, and what are the responsibilities of physicians? In particular, there are problems concerning when a patient is competent to make a decision to continue dialysis. We have to take into consideration the problem of the effectiveness of dialysis and its continuation when patients become very disabled and the effect of this on family members, including spouses, children, and parents. To what extent may continuation be pathogenic for these other persons? These are matters which dialysis nurses, technicians, and social workers are often in a position to appraise for the individual and for other family members. They are matters which primary physicians in particular are going to have to consider as they care not only for patients on dialysis, but also for members of the family. The course of a few patients on dialysis and of the several patients who have successful transplants can make one enthusiastic about the treatment of end-stage renal disease. However, the course of some patients whose survival appears inflicted upon them against their will, causing turmoil in that smallest unit of society, the family, and the members thereof, at times makes one wonder about what we are accomplishing.

REFERENCE

1. REICHSMAN, F., and LEVY, N. B. Problems in adaptation to maintenance hemodialysis: A 4-year study of 25 patients. *Archives of Internal Medicine*, 1972, *130*, 359–365.

12

Modeling Home Hemodialysis Success
Finding the Obvious and Its Implications

JAMES C. ROMEIS, ROBERT W. HAMILTON, AND
CELIA A. SNAVELY

INTRODUCTION

Home hemodialysis refers to the place or social setting where a type of renal therapy is performed. It is contrasted with institution, hospital, or center settings. Depending on whether one's perspective is that of the physician, patient, patient's family or public program administrator, home and center settings have differing advantages and disadvantages. Under one set of circumstances, the home setting is preferred to a center setting. Under other circumstances, the center setting may be preferred. This study is designed to examine the effect of powerlessness on home dialysis outcome. Included is an overview of the relevant literature used to conceptualize the powerlessness relationship followed by results from the interviews. The data add to understanding factors which influence home dialysis outcome and have implications for emergent public policy designed to influence therapy setting selection.

BACKGROUND

In 1964, two small groups of patients in Seattle and London were among the first to undergo hemodialysis treatments in their homes. The selection of the patient's home as a setting for therapy was related in part to a more efficient use of scarce and costly institutional resources. Relative to an increasing number of patients needing hemodialysis, rap-

JAMES C. ROMEIS, PH.D. • Assistant Professor of Sociology, Department of Family and Community Medicine, Bowman Gray School of Medicine, Winston-Salem, North Carolina   ROBERT W. HAMILTON, M.D. • Associate Professor of Medicine, Department of Medicine; Medical Director, Artificial Kidney Clinic, Bowman Gray School of Medicine, Winston-Salem, North Carolina.   CELIA A. SNAVELY, A.C.S.W. • Instructor (Social Work), Department of Medicine, Social Worker, Artificial Kidney Clinic, Bowman Gray School of Medicine, Winston-Salem, North Carolina.

idly increasing public program costs, and a continuing need for optimal use of institutional facilities, research on factors which contribute to successful home hemodialysis therapy accumulates. Roberts et al.[1] estimated that finding ways to shift emphasis away from center dialysis to home dialysis or to cadaver donor transplantation would save $7000–$8000 per life year, or $284 million per year for the existing renal disease population.

Home hemodialysis is a pair or team event, but much of the research identifies factors associated with either the patient or the partner and how these factors influence outcome. Where psychosocial factors continue to be identified as problems for successful home therapy, our understanding of outcomes may improve by raising the level of abstraction and focusing on the social structure and social processes associated with the performance of the pair. We should uncover which attributes of the pair mitigate against success. To the extent that certain attributes interact and enhance success for the pair, it might be possible to develop more cost-efficient and efficacious screening mechanisms and training programs. Appropriate and well-timed social reinforcements tailored to the pair might result in more cumulative days at home and an improved quality of life for the pair.

The literature on psychosocial factors affecting home hemodialysis success or failure is extensive and may be categorized into three groups: (1) studies which focus on the patient, (2) studies which focus on the effect the patient has on others, such as spouse or children, and (3) studies of the patient–partner relationship. The stressful nature of the disease and the therapy for the patient are well documented. The suicide rate among patients has been estimated to be one hundred times greater than that of the general population.[2] Others[3-6] have identified the range and complexity of adjustment difficulties. Problems associated with adjustment and coping with the disease have been documented as an issue for the patient's family as well as for the patient himself.[7,8]

Powerlessness

Sociologically the expectations and the demands of the therapy may result in alienation. The patient and the partner may become estranged from the therapeutic process, its technology, one another, and finally themselves. The powerlessness variant of alienation[9,10] typifies the dilemma. By powerlessness we mean the extent to which individuals perceive they are in control of their lives versus the extent to which they perceive that their lives are controlled by fate, chance, or other powers beyond themselves. From a social learning theory perspective, powerlessness is conceptually parallel to Rotter's locus of control.[11,12] For a recent review and critique of this literature see Strickland.[13]

A sociological vantage of powerlessness may add to identifying correlates of home success when the level of abstraction is raised to the pair. For example, if we follow the implications of powerlessness within the patient–partner dyad, we might theoretically expect successful home pairs to perceive they were in control of their lives and their health (low powerlessness) compared to center patients who would not be as likely to perceive themselves to be in control of their lives and health (high powerlessness). Parenthetically, it is instructive to note how a center setting is sometimes referred to as passive care. A pair characterized by high powerlessness might not be defined as suitable home candidates, might have a great deal of difficulty mastering the home-training program, and may ultimately require numerous back-up treatments in-center. Accordingly, the center begins preparing for the failure. A pair characterized by low powerlessness might be more likely to pursue home dialysis options, master the home training program quickly, have fewer back-up days, and generally have a better home experience.

This hypothetical relationship is presented in Table 1. The probability of success is greater for patients and partners characterized by low powerlessness. Patients and partners who are characterized by high powerlessness would have a higher probability of "failure."

We do not know what to predict when one member of the pair is low on powerlessness and the other is high on powerlessness. Mock et al.[14] suggest our expectations are generally on track and give some clues about what to expect from discrepant pairs. Table 2 indicates how a sample of VA patients and their wives scored on a general locus of control measure and thus how powerlessness between the pair may relate to setting performance.

Their data indicate that center patients perceive themselves to be more powerless than home patients (8.3 versus 5.8). Wives of center and home patients arrive at a score similar to that of their husbands (9.9

TABLE 1
Hypothetical Relationship between Patient–Partner
Powerlessness and Probability of Home
Hemodialysis Outcome

	Partner powerlessness	
Patient powerlessness	Low	High
Low	"Success"	?
High	?	"Failure"

TABLE 2
Mean Numbers of Questions
Answered in the External Direction
on Locus of Control ($N = 32$)[a]

Setting	Patients	Wives
Home	5.8	7.5
Ex-home	6.3	11.2
In-center	8.3	9.9

[a]Reconstructed from Mock and Kopel.

versus 7.5). Ex-home patients, those who attempted a home setting but returned permanently to a center setting, scored closer to the home patients (6.3), but their wives had the highest powerlessness scale scores (11.2). These data do not show if the perceptions of the ex-home patients' wives were produced by the home failure or if their perceptions of powerlessness contributed to the home failure. We would, nevertheless, be inclined to ask if powerlessness contributes to setting selection and setting success or failure.

METHOD

During the spring and summer of 1979, adult (18 and over) home patients and their partners were interviewed regarding setting expectations, what influenced their setting selection, problems they anticipated, problems they experienced, and the perceived advantages and disadvantages associated with the setting. A comparable interview was completed with adult center patients except it reflected their center experiences.

In addition, Wallston and Wallston's[15,16] 32-item Multiple Health Locus of Control Scale (MHLC) was given to center patients, home patients, and the partners of the home patients. The MHLC is a 6-point Likert-type attitude scale designed to measure beliefs about control or powerlessness over general life- and health-specific events. The MHLC has five subscales: Internal (I), Chance (C), Internal Health Locus of Control (IHLC), Chance Health Locus of Control (CHLC), and Powerful-Others Health Locus of Control (PHLC).

A typical item reflecting the generalized Internal (I) subscale is: "When I make plans, I am almost certain to make them work." An Internal Health Locus of Control (IHLC) item is: "If I get sick, it is my own behavior which determines how soon I get well again." An example of the generalized Chance (C) subscale is: "To a great extent my life is controlled by accidental happenings." An example of a Chance Health

Locus of Control (CHLC) item is: "No matter what I do, if I am going to get sick, I will get sick." Finally, an example of the Powerful-Others Health Locus of Control (PHLC) is: "Having regular contact with my physician is the best way for me to avoid illness."

For this report, responses were collapsed and dichotomized into agree–disagree categories. Scoring thus reflects the Mock et al.[14] approach. The I and C subscale scores range from 0 to 7. The health-specific (IHLC, CHLC, PHLC) subscale scores range from 0 to 6. High powerlessness is reflected by high scale scores.

RESULTS

Table 3 describes the social and demographic characteristics of the study population.

There are no major differences between the average age of the center and home patients. Center patients' average age was 47.44 years and home patients' average age was 48.92 years. There is a slightly higher percentage of younger patients in the center (24.1%) compared to younger patients (19.2%) at home. This difference reflects marital status differences, with center patients more likely to be unmarried. There are no important differences between the sex distribution of center or home patients, but there are slightly more females dialyzing in-center than males.

When health status is defined as the number of the months on hemodialysis both groups are essentially equal. The center hemodialysis patients had been dialyzing for an average of 20.6 months. None of the center patients had been on home hemodialysis. The home patients had been dialyzing at home for an average of 17.9 months. Four patients had dialyzed in-center for over a year before going home. Seventy-three percent of the home partners were spouses, two were daughters, three were paid assistants, and two were friends. Two center patients were omitted because of illness and inability to comprehend the interview questions.

Important differences between the two patient groups are related to home eligibility. Marital status and thus the functional requirement for a partner affects home eligibility. Racial characteristics appear important because nonwhite center patients were more likely to be single and live in home situations not physically adaptable. More nonwhite patients also said their homes were socially unsuitable. For example, one center patient complained of an "alcoholic brother" who often and unexpectably would "come busting into the house" for impromptu parties. When such factors are coupled with occupational status, educational attainment, and gross household income differences, a social class

TABLE 3
Frequency Distribution of Group Characteristics

	Center patients ($N = 29$)	Home patients ($N = 26$)	Home partners ($N = 26$)
Age (in %)			
19–39	24.1	19.2	38.5
40–60	56.2	61.7	45.1
61 +	19.7	19.1	16.4
Average	47.44	48.92	45.73
Sex (in %)			
Male	48.3	53.8	30.8
Female	51.7	46.2	69.2
Marital status			
% Married	51.7	88.5	96
Race			
White	49.3	84.6	80.8
Non-white	51.7	15.4	19.2
Current/former occupational status (in %)			
Blue collar	69	38.1	26.9
White collar	31	57.1	50.0
Self-employed	—	4.8	7.7
Education (in %)			
< 7	13.8	19.2	3.8
7–12	48.3	26.9	23.1
High school	24.1	23.1	19.2
Some college	10.3	26.9	50.0
College	3.4	3.8	3.8
Household size (in %)			
1	20.7	8	
2	27.6	52	
3	20.7	16	
4 +	31.0	24	
Group household income (in %)			
< $3000	17.9	12	
$3001–$5000	32.1	16	
$5001–$8000	32.1	12	
$8001–$11,000	7.1	8	
$11,001–$15,000	7.1	24	
$15,001–$20,000	3.6	12	
< $20,001	0	16	

factor appears related to setting selection. These data suggest the lower the patient's social class, the greater the likelihood the patient will end up in a center setting.

Looking at class-related factors to understand differences between settings, one sees that 69% of the center patients had blue-collar jobs while 61.9% of the home patients had white-collar jobs or were self-employed. Even though formal education may not relate to ability to perform home therapy, only 13.7% of the center patients had above a high school education, compared to 30.7% for the home patients. Finally, gross household income is lower for center patients than home patients. Eighty-two percent of the home patients have annual gross household incomes of $11,000 or less. The home patient's income distribution is bimodal, with 40% having $8,000 a year gross household income or less and 52% having annual gross household incomes above $11,000. Thus, in general, social class factors appear related to setting selection. However, there are clearly patients and partners who have little education and income but who are quite successful in the home setting.

Table 4 indicates how the MHLC subscale scores correlate between home patients and home partners. A moderate–strong relationship between the pair was expected. As Table 4 indicates, there are no statistically significant relationships (< 0.05) between the home patients and the home partners for any of the MHLC subscales. The data in Table 4 are thus contrary to our expectations.

The first three columns in Table 5 compare the mean number of responses in the powerlessness direction for the MHLC subscales. The

TABLE 4
Spearman Correlations between Home Patients
and Home Partners

	Home partners				
Home patients	I	IHLC	C	CHLC	PHLC
I	0.321	0.285	0.073	0.258	0.061
IHLC	−0.118	0.077	0.187	0.088	−0.012
C	0.119	0.164	0.076	0.199	−0.112
CHLC	0.065	0.145	0.024	0.321	−0.145
PHLC	0.340	0.168	0.168	0.082	0.239

TABLE 5
Mean Number of Responses in Powerlessness Direction and Group Differences

	1	2	3	4		5	
Scale	Center patients	Home patients	Home partners	t 1:2	p	t 2:3	p
I	4.679	5.160	5.077	1.115	—	0.188	—
IHLC	3.536	3.346	3.462	−0.408	—	−0.263	—
C	3.750	2.038	2.538	−3.479	0.001	−1.157	—
CHLC	3.310	2.346	2.423	−2.046	0.05	−0.199	—
PHLC	4.241	3.769	2.385	−1.244	—	3.188	0.001

t-test differences between center and home patients are in Column 4. T-test differences between home patients and their partners are in Column 5. Contrary to expectations, Table 5 does not indicate there are important differences in powerlessness between center and home patients and between home patients and their partners.

We expected home patients to have lower I subscale scores than center patients. These data show all groups scored on the high end of the I subscale. The home patients scored the highest on the I subscale of the three groups, and there are no statistically significant differences between the groups. For the I subscale, these data suggest an interpretation opposite to the one suggested by the Mock et al. data.[14] The other subscale scores are in the expected direction, except the scores decrease to the middle values of the subscales. The C and CHLC subscales scores for the center and home patients are statistically different and suggest that center patients perceive the general and health-specific effects of luck, fate, and chance more than home patients. However, all groups scored in the middle range of the subscales.

Column 5 also indicates results contrary to our expectations. Home partners arrived at a score similar to that of home patients but only the PHLC subscale is statistically different. However, again, average scores are in the middle range of the scale. Patients may have reasonably accurate perceptions of their powerlessness relative to their partner's because a patient's success in the home setting is functionally tied to partner assistance. Center patients' PHLC scores increased relative to the other health-specific subscale scores and may indicate an accurate perception of control over their health by center staff.

Because of these unanticipated findings and as a way of extending this analysis, five cases were reexamined. Three cases will become part of an ex-home category when the population is reinterviewed. One case involves a paid assistant who failed and was reinterviewed with her new partner. The fifth case involves a patient who was apprehensive about her partner's reliability. Because the partner had small children, the patient believed their care could interfere with the therapy schedule. The only interesting finding in the case analysis was that the paid assistant's MHLC scores increased slightly after the first failure. The other cases resemble the tabular data and do not help isolate why these results are contrary to expectations.

DISCUSSION

This research was designed to examine the complementarity of perceptions among home hemodialysis patients and their partners with the intent of enlarging the context for understanding the determinants of home dialysis success or failure. The literature suggests that perceptions of control or powerlessness are psychosocial factors which interact within the dyad and thus relate to setting selection and its concomitant success or failure.

Identical MHLC scale measures were obtained from center patients, home patients, and home partners. It was expected that center patients would have significantly higher powerlessness scores than home patients. Also, it was expected that home patients and their partners' scores would be positively correlated and similar in strength. The results were contrary to expectations and forced a reexamination of the basis for these expectations. Because these are initial findings, the following interpretations of the results are possible.

One interpretation is methodological. The population is small and does not allow for sufficient quasi-experimental or statistical controls to examine relationships conclusively. There are no measures on potential partners (spouses) of center patients but 50% of this group do not have family partners and many of the rest indicate a family member is unwilling to assist them. Our coding method reduced MHLC variation and thus true differences may not have been detected. However, nondichotomized scale scores for the home patients and partners were analyzed and the results did not differ appreciably. The data are cross-sectional and from one patient pool making clear statements about the relationships tenuous. It is anticipated that as the number of observations increase and when follow-up interviews are completed, the effects of many of these limitations will become known.

Another interpretation is that these are negative findings and powerlessness is not directly related to hemodialysis setting or success. Center patients, home patients, and home partners all scored moderately high on the general powerlessness subscale and scores were not statistically different. There were statistical differences between the C and CHLC subscales for the two patient groups but the scale values were not high. No correlation was found between home patients' and home partners' perceptions of powerlessness. Only one subscale was found to be statistically significant between home patients and their partners but it was based on moderate scale values. The negative results interpretation also suggests that powerlessness specifically and psychosocial factors generally are exaggerated as predictors of setting success or failure. Instead social class and lifestyle-related factors may better explain outcome differences. It is important to separate sociological from psychological factors when examining the relative importance of determinants of home dialysis success.

A final interpretation argues that rather than negative findings, these are sociological findings related to the obvious—behavior is best understood when it is related to the social context in which it occurs. Instead of negating the importance of powerlessness and the importance of raising the level of abstraction to the pair, the level of abstraction requires an additional boost. These data suggest we need to systematically examine the complementarity of the pair as their complementarity is organized by the home-care program's structure, philosophy, and requirements. The importance of program organization, structure, and staff beliefs for treatment modality and therapy setting has been noted but research has yet to identify relationships.[3,17,18] Fox observes that when crucial developments in therapy research are subjected to historical analysis, treatment modality preferences reflect the commitments of certain medical scientists and by extension the programs they directed.[18] To what extent future breakthroughs are developed by the emerging second generation of dialysis specialists remains to be seen but reinforces the importance of understanding program structure when analyzing outcome statistics.

For example, this program emphasizes patient independence, patient control, and self-care. The partner functions as a "third hand" when needed and an aide in the event of emergency. Organizationally, the partner provides emotional and other psychosocial supports but these are tailored to reinforce patient independence. In other programs the responsibilities for the pair are organized differently. Partners play major roles and patients play passive roles. A program philosophy may also diffuse to center patients. Differently structured home-care programs may produce patients and partners with high scale scores which in turn relate to setting selection and performance in the home setting. This program, however, may have "produced" scale scores consistent with stated and unstated preferences for patient control.

THE MODEL

This latter interpretation led to development of the following model. In Figure 1, home dialysis success or failure is conceptualized as a function of five generalized patient resource variables which are filtered through the organizational structure of the home-care program or intervening variable. The outcome variable is separated into three sequentially related subvariables: home setting eligibility, home-training performance, and the eventual home therapy experience. "Success" refers to satisfactory performance in an outcome as defined by the program. "Failure" is the unsatisfactory performance of an outcome which is also determined by the program and may occur during any sequence but usually results in a destabilizing influence on the therapy and thus the patient returns to a center setting. Failure does not preclude future

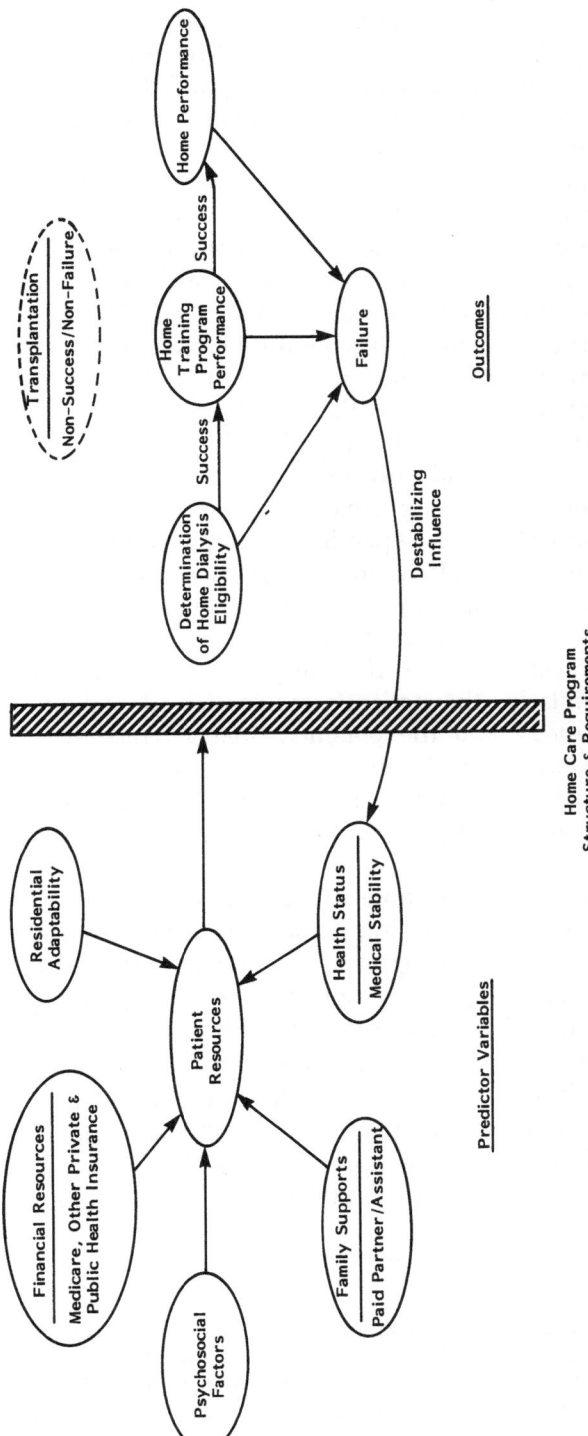

FIG. 1. The home dialysis model: Variables influencing success or failure.

home setting selection, reentry into the home training program and eventual long-term success. In the context of this model, transplantation, change to other treatment modalities, and death may occur at any time but should be carefully considered before a relationship to either success or failure is established.

This sequential ordering of outcome variables is intended to better understand success and failure statistics because too often published program data do not report the total patient population, the number of patients entering a program, the number of patients who attempted home training, the number of patients dialyzing at home, and the number who return to centers permanently because of problems (medical and/or extramedical) with the home therapy. When total population data are reported, success and failure statistics will be better understood as well as the reasons why home dialysis accounted for 40% of hemodialysis in 1972 and only 13% in 1976.[19,20]

The patient resource variables, or predictor variables, are factors which are conceptually independent but empirically interrelated, and the magnitude of their relative importance on outcomes is not known. In this model each resource variable is considered to be equal in weight, although there is an implied weighting. Clearly, the patient's health status and medical stability will affect the program's determination of home eligibility. Similarly, the patient's residential adaptability to the machine's technology and the patient's financial resources are factors. Finally, the extent to which the patient is able to rely on family supports or nonfamily assistance plus a multiplicity of psychosocial factors will affect the patient's ability to meet the performance expectations of the home program.

Knowledge about variations in the organizational structure of home care is crucial to understanding home dialysis success and failure. Existing knowledge about program structures is indirect and difficult to compare. Published reports do not describe in enough detail the structure of programs, their philosophy, their leadership, and so forth. As organizational structure information is added, processes and relationships will be shown to be more complex. However, until this information is added, models demonstrating the relative importance of variables will be quite limited. Moreover public policy designed to influence setting opportunities and success rates will be equally limited.

REFERENCES

1. ROBERTS, S. D., MAXWELL, D. R., and GROSS. T. L. Cost effective care of end-stage renal disease: A billion dollar question. *Annals of Internal Medicine*, 1980, 92, 243–248.
2. ABRAM, H. S., MOORE, G. P., and WESTERVELT, F. B., Jr. Suicidal behavior in chronic dialysis patients. *American Journal of Psychology*, 1972, 127, 1199.

3. FRIEDMAN, E. A., GOODWIN, N. J., and CHAUDRY, L. Psychosocial adjustment of family maintenance hemodialysis. *New York State Journal of Medicine*, 1970, *70*, 768–774.
4. LEVY, N. B. (Ed.), *Living or dying: Adaptation to hemodialysis*. Springfield, Illinois: Charles C. Thomas, 1974.
5. LEVY, N. B. Psychosocial factors in rehabilitation of the patient undergoing maintenance hemodialysis. In B. Chyatte (Ed.), *Rehabilitation in chronic renal failure*. Baltimore: Williams and Wilkins, 1979, pp. 46–64.
6. CZACZKES, J. W., and KAPLAN DE-NOUR,A. *Chronic hemodialysis as a way of life*. New York: Brunner/Mazel, 1978.
7. TSALTAS, M. O. Children of home dialysis patients. *Journal of American Medical Association*, 1976, *236*, 2764–2766.
8. BEARD, M. P. Changing family relationships. *Dialysis and Transplantation*, 1975, *4*, 34–41.
9. SEEMAN, M. S. The meaning of alienation. *American Sociological Review*, 1959, *24*, 783–791.
10. SEEMAN, M. S. Alienation and engagement. In A. Campbell and P. Converse (Eds.), *The human meaning of social change*. New York: Russell Sage, 1972, pp. 467–527.
11. ROTTER, J. B. Generalized expectancies for internal versus external control of reinforcement. *Psychological Monograph*, 1966, *80*, 609.
12. ROTTER, J. B. Some problems and misconceptions related to the contruct of internal versus external control of reinforcement. *Journal of Consulting and Clinical Psychology*, 1979, *43*, 56–67.
13. STRICKLAND, B. R. Internal–external expectancies and health related behaviors. *Journal of Consulting and Clinical Psychology*, 1978, *46*(6), 1192–1211.
14. MOCK, L., TODD, A., and KOPEL, K. Psychosocial aspects of home and in-center dialysis. *Dialysis and Transplantation*, 1977, *56*, 32–43.
15. WALLSTON, B. S., WALLSTON, K. A., KAPLAN, G. D., and MAIDES, S. A. Development and validation of the health locus of control (HLC) scale. *Journal of Consulting and Clinical Psychology*, 1976, *44*, 580–585.
16. WALLSTON, K. A., and WALLSTON, B. S. (Eds.), *Health locus of control*. Health Education Monographs, *6*(2), 1978, 160–170.
17. BLAGG, C. R. Home hemodialysis. *American Journal of Medical Scientists*, 1972, *264*, 168.
18. FOX, R. C. *Essays in medical sociology*. New York: John Wiley and Sons, 1979.
19. DHEW, Facility Report No. 2: End stage renal disease, medical information system. Series 1-The National Reported by Network. Washington, D.C.: Health Care Finance Administration, 1976.
20. BLAGG, C. R. Incidence and prevalence of home dialysis. *Journal of Dialysis*, 1977, *1*, 475–493.

13

Life without the Machine
A Look at Psychological Determinants for Successful Adaptation of Patients on CAPD

HOWARD J. BURTON, LINO CANZONA, LOKKY WAI, RONALD R. HOLDEN, JOHN CONLEY, AND ROBERT M. LINDSAY

INTRODUCTION

Although peritoneal dialysis for the treatment of renal failure became a reality earlier in this century, the advent of the more efficient and convenient hemodialysis retarded the progress of peritoneal procedures. After a slow start, peritoneal dialysis now appears to be gaining acceptability. It is seen by Gutman[1] as at least an equally satisfactory alternative to hemodialysis, and by Fenton et al. as a major advance in promoting home dialysis.[2]

This renewed enthusiasm undoubtedly can be traced to two major events. The first was the introduction of a permanent and safe silastic catheter which overcame high infection rates and inconvenient access devices.[3] The second event was the development of continuous ambulatory peritoneal dialysis (CAPD) by Popovitch et al.[4] and its refinement by Oreopoulos et al. at Toronto Western Hospital in Canada.[5]

HOWARD J. BURTON, M.S.W., M.SC. (Hig.) • Assistant Professor, Faculty of Nursing, University of Western Ontario, London, Ontario, Canada.   LINO CANZONA, B.S.W., M.S.W., D.S.W. • Associate Professor, Social Work Department, King's College, University of Western Ontario, London, Ontario, Canada.   LOKKY WAI, M.A., PH.D. • Staff, Health Care Research Unit, University of Western Ontario, London, Ontario, Canada.   RONALD R. HOLDEN, M.A., PH.D. • Researcher, Health Care Research Unit, University of Western Ontario, London, Ontario, Canada.   JOHN CONLEY, B.P.E., M., PH.D. • Health Promotion Directorate, Department of Health and Welfare, Ottawa, Canada.   ROBERT M. LINDSAY, M.D., F.R.C.P.(C.), M.R.C.P. (Edin.) • Director of Renal Unit, Victoria Hospital, Faculty of Medicine, University of Western Ontario, London, Ontario, Canada. This research was supported by Grant Number DM338, "Adaptation to Home Dialysis," awarded by the Ontario Ministry of Health.

In the last several years, the widespread publicity given to CAPD has gained the attention of many previous skeptics. Currently it is being used in an appreciable number of centers in Canada and the United States. In fact, approximately 55% of all patients placed on home dialysis in Ontario (Canada) are being treated by this therapy mode.[6]

The efficacy of CAPD is well documented. Already there are several publications describing its physiological and procedural advantages. These include "steady-state" biochemical stabilization of chemistries,[7] control of blood pressure without antihypertensive medicine,[8] decreased or absent need for phosphate binding agents,[7] and improved clearance per week of retention products in the "middle molecular" weight range (500–3000 daltons).[8] It is believed by most to be cost effective,[9] requires no partner,[8] has a shorter training period,[7] results in minimum cardiovascular stress[10] and minimal dietary restrictions,[7] and does not require anticoagulants.[8]

Information on the psychosocial well-being of patients on CAPD, especially on their psychological functioning, is just beginning to appear. This paper presents additional information to that already presented to the First International Symposium on CAPD (Paris),[11] to the CAPD International Symposium II (Austin, Texas),[12] and to the Pan Pacific Symposium on Peritoneal Dialysis (Melbourne, Australia).[13] It focuses on determining the level of a patient's psychological adjustment using objective measures of personality traits and subjective judgements of how well the patient is doing psychologically. It concludes with the presentation of regression models that suggest the relative relevancy of the personality determinants of psychological adjustment.

Technique

As a new method of peritoneal treatment, CAPD is a safe and simple technique. It is believed by many to be a revolutionary approach to the treatment of renal failure. It is a process wherein the patient dialyzes continuously over a 24-hour period without being dependent on a dialysis machine. The technique consists of connecting a 2-liter collapsible plastic bag containing a commercially available dialysate to a permanent catheter in the abdominal area following a rigorous sterilizing regimen.[8] The bag is hung on a special portable stand and the solution emptied into the abdomen. The plastic container and the infusion tubing is rolled up and placed in a cloth pocket suspended from the patient's waist during the prolonged dwell time. To remove the fluid, the bag is placed below the abdomen to permit drainage by gravity. The exchange of fluid takes an average of 40 minutes and is usually carried out four times per day, 7 days a week. The time the dialysate remains in the abdomen can be varied up to 8 hours to accommodate the patient's activity.

STUDY DESIGN

This research paper is part of a major study whose objectives are:

1. To evaluate the influence that physiological, psychological, social, and economic functioning and the training and support received by the dialysis patients have on their ability to adapt to a program of home dialysis.
2. To analyze those factors that facilitate the adaptation of patients to home dialysis so that more accurate predictions in patient selection may be made.
3. To analyze the influence of treatment methods employed on the adaptation of the dialysis patient.

The realization of these objectives hopefully may lead to successful home dialysis adjustment in a higher percentage of patients with chronic renal disease.

The study design incorporates two stages: a retrospective phase to explore adaptation in persons who commenced a home dialysis training program between June 1, 1975, and June 1, 1978, and a prospective phase to follow patients from commencement of home dialysis training through their first and second years of adjustment to a home program.

Patient Population

The data was obtained from patients in 16 dialysis centers in Ontario, Canada, who participated in the retrospective phase. From a sample of 260 patients of mixed modalities, a subsample of 54 CAPD patients was generated who had no previous home experience and had not changed modalities during the study. The sample consisted of 29 males and 25 females with a mean age of 50.17 years (range 19–74 years), mean education of 10.28 years, and who had been, on the average, at home for 6.89 months (range of 3–31 months and median of 5.64 months).

DATA COLLECTION AND INSTRUMENTATION

Three instruments were utilized to collect the data. First, the dialysis unit staff were asked to fill out a clinical evaluation form, which attempted to ascertain how each clinician in an independent judgement felt the patient adapted physically, psychologically, socially, and economically, as well as in terms of supportive systems available to them and their ability to meet their total dialysis responsibility.

Secondly, patients' hospital records were reviewed to obtain relevant medical and physiological data. Finally, a home interview averaging 2 hours in duration was given by trained interviewers to obtain personal demographic, social, physical, psychological, economic, vocational, sexual, and support systems data. These three data collection activities occurred concurrently.

TABLE 1
Basic Personality Inventory—Scale Descriptions

Depression	Reports a usual feeling of confidence, cheerfulness and persistence, even when experiencing disappointment. Has an optimistic attitude about his future.	Inclined to be downhearted and show extreme despondency; considers himself to be inadequate; may be listless, remote, and preoccupied; looks at his future pessimistically.

Sample item: My present situation is hopeless.

Denial	Accepts his feelings as part of himself; not afraid to discuss unpleasant topics. Can answer questions about himself frankly; avoids impression management. Shows normal affect.	Lacks insight into his feelings and the causes of his behavior. Avoids unpleasant, exciting, or violent topics. Relatively unresponsive emotionally.

Sample item: I care about what other people think of me.

Anxiety	Remains calm and unruffled even when confronted by unexpected occurrences. Takes things as they come without fear or apprehension. Maintains self-control even in a crisis situation.	Easily scared. Little things, even an idea, can throw him into a frenzy of anxiety. Afraid of novelty and of the possibility of physical or interpersonal danger.

Sample item: I feel frightened when I have to go out alone.

Social introversion	Enjoys company. Likes to talk and knows many people. Spends much of his time with others.	Avoids people generally. Has few friends and doesn't say much to those he has. Seems to be uncomfortable when around other. Prefers asocial activities.

Sample item: I enjoy being with people.

Self-depreciation	Manifests a high degree of self-assurance in dealings with others. Not afraid to meet strangers; speak with confidence about a variety of topics; believes in his own ability to accomplish things.	Degrades himself as being worthless, unpleasant, and undeserving. Generally expresses a low opinion of himself and refuses credit for any accomplishment.

Sample item: I have given up hope of ever amounting to anything.

Basic Personality Inventory Instrument

From the home interview schedule, the Basic Personality Inventory,[14] developed out of the work of Hoffmann et al.[15] was selected as the objective measure of psychological adjustment. The BPI is a 12-scale, 240-item, true/false inventory devised using modern principles of test construction for item writing and selection procedures.[16,17] The 12 scales of the BPI measure the constructs of hypochondriasis, depression, denial, interpersonal problems, alienation, persecutory ideas, anxiety, thinking disorder, impulse expression, social introversion, self-depreciation, and deviation. These scales are based on a multimethod factor analysis of the Differential Personality Inventory[18] and the Minnesota Multiphasic Personality Inventory (MMPI). These constructs represent relatively independent aspects of traditional dimensions of psychological dysfunctioning.[15] Although the BPI is still in the process of being validated and normal ranges for each scale are being established, initial research has shown it has suitable psychometric properties.[15,19-22] For example, Reddon[21] reports coefficient alphas ranging from 0.57 for "anxiety" to 0.80 for "depression" with a sample of 1444 university students. Holden, Holmes, Fekken, and Jackson,[19] using 123 university students report stability coefficients ranging from 0.63 for "denial" to 0.85 for "depression" using a 1 month test–retest interval. Due to the BPI's superior internal consistencies, relative orthogonality of scales, and the test's short length, it could be regarded as a more efficient instrument than other multiscale inventories.

For the retrospective study, five of the BPI scales were used: depression, denial, anxiety, social introversion, and self-depreciation. Descriptions of high and low scorers on these scales, as well as sample items, are contained in Table 1.

Clinical/Self-Report Evaluation Instrument

Subjective psychological adjustment outcome measures were obtained separately from the patient during the home interview, and from the nephrologist and other members of the medical team as part of their clinical evaluation. Each was asked to respond independently to the question of how they felt the patient was doing psychologically. The question response was scaled 1–5, where 1 indicated "very well," and 5 "very poorly." Evaluation scores of the medical team were the average of the individual clinical judgements. The number obtained was used as the psychological adjustment score (PAS).

RESULTS

Personality Differences between Selected Groups

One of the first sets of analyses which was conducted was to ascertain whether there were personality trait differences between:

1. The general population norm and the CAPD sample
2. CAPD patients who succeeded in the home program and those who failed
3. CAPD patients who transplanted and those who remained on CAPD

Table 2 shows the difference in BPI scores between the general population and the CAPD patients. General population norms were obtained from a random sample of 196 adults selected and stratified for sex and domicility in Tillsonburg, a small Ontario community (6700 pop.) located in southwestern Ontario. As can be seen from the table, CAPD patients tend to have higher levels of depression, denial, anxiety, self-depreciation, and social introversion than the general population. Such differences are statistically significant at the 0.05 level for all BPI variables with the exception of social introversion. This latter finding was contrary to what was expected and may reflect the conservative nature of small communities to be somewhat insular in their responses to outside inquisitors.

Differences in personality traits between CAPD patients who succeeded and those who failed their home dialysis program are presented in Table 3. Persons who succeeded were those patients, interviewed between June 1, 1978, and April 30, 1979, who were still on home dialysis as of May 30, 1980. Failures were those individuals who returned to center for reasons other than transplant and were being dialyzed in hospital, or had died as of May 30, 1980. The t-tests performed on the avail-

TABLE 2
Personality Trait Differences between CAPD
Patients and a General Population Norm

BPI	CAPD (N=54)	Tillsonburg (N=196)
Depression[a]	5.11	2.84
Denial[a]	9.45	7.95
Anxiety[a]	7.43	6.32
Self-depreciation[a]	33.16	2.49
Social introversion	5.08	4.67

[a] $p < 0.05$.

TABLE 3
Difference in Personality Traits between CAPD Patients Who Succeed
and Those Who Fail a Home Program

BPI	Success (N=25)	Failure (N=11)	t	Significance
Depression	4.9867	6.4322	−0.90	0.376
Denial	9.5368	9.9904	−0.45	0.654
Anxiety	7.8526	7.6364	0.11	0.912
Self-depreciation	3.0926	3.4407	−0.31	0.762
Social introversion	5.9326	3.9091	1.30	0.204

TABLE 4
Personality Trait Differences between Transplanted and Success Groups of
CADP Patients

BPI	Success (N=25)	Transplant (N=5)	t	Significance
Depression	4.9867	2.8316	1.09	0.287
Denial	9.5368	7.8632	1.17	0.253
Anxiety	7.8526	4.8526	1.23	0.228
Self-depreciation	3.0926	2.8500	0.17	0.869
Social introversion	5.9326	3.4316	1.19	0.243

able data show that there is no statistical significant difference of personality traits between the two groups.

Personality trait differences between patients who transplanted and those who remained on CAPD are reported in Table 4. It indicates that, although patients who were transplanted exhibited consistently lower scores on basic personality traits than those who remained on CAPD, such differences between the two groups are not statistically significant at the 0.05 level.

Objective versus Subjective Evaluations

Correlation analysis was carried out to examine the relationships between the objective assessment of psychological well-being (BPI) and the evaluation on psychological adjustment as judged by (1) the patients themselves, (2) the nephrologists, and (3) the medical team. The medical team's evaluation is a composite score of independent clinical judgements of the patient by members of the medical team including the nephrologist. The results of the analysis are summarized in Table 5.

It can be seen from Table 5 that "depression" correlates positively with the patient's, the medical team's and the nephrologist's eval-

TABLE 5
Correlations of Evaluations on Levels of Psychological Adjustment
with Basic Personality Inventory Variables

BPI	Medical teams' evaluation	Patients' evaluation	Nephrologists' evaluation
Depression	0.5002	0.6296	0.3471
	($p < 0.001$)	($p < 0.001$)	($p < 0.026$)
Denial	−0.1144	−0.1800	−0.2175
	($p < 0.238$)	($p < 0.130$)	($p < 0.116$)
Anxiety	0.2595	0.3144	0.4743
	($p < 0.051$)	($p < 0.023$)	($p < 0.003$)
Self-depreciation	0.3378	0.4986	0.5244
	($p < 0.015$)	($p < 0.001$)	($p < 0.001$)
Social introversion	0.0116	0.3132	0.1725
	($p < 0.471$)	($p < 0.023$)	($p < 0.173$)

uations. This suggests that a lower or higher evaluation score provided by the patient, the medical team, or the nephrologist corresponds with a lower or higher level of depression in the patient, as computed from the scores obtained through the administration of the BPI. The table also shows that the correlations are significant at the 0.05 level. However, it must be noted that the strongest correlation exists between the patients' own evaluation of their level of psychological adjustment and their level of depression. The weakest correlation exists between the nephrologists' evaluation of the patients' psychological adjustment and the patients' own depression score on the BPI.

In the analyses of the construct "denial," the association between the objective measure (BPI Denial Score) and the psychological adjustment as judged separately by the patient, the nephrologist, and the medical team is weak and not statistically significant.

The associations between the patient's "anxiety" score and the clinical evaluation of the medical team, the patient, and the nephrologist were all significant. The strongest correlation, however, exists between the nephrologist's evaluations and the level of "anxiety," with the weakest relationship showing between the medical team's evaluation and the patient's BPI "anxiety" score.

Correlations between the patient's "self-depreciation" score and the evaluation by the medical team, the patient, and the nephrologist were all found to be significant. The strongest relationship existed between the nephrologist's clinical evaluation and the BPI scores of "self-depreciation." The weakest relationship exists between the medical team's evaluation and the BPI "self-depreciation" scores.

Analyses of the association between the BPI "social introversion" scores and the clinical and patient self-report evaluations of level of

TABLE 6
Correlations between the Clinical/Self-Report Evaluations

Clinical self-report	Medical teams' evaluation	Patients' evaluation	Nephrologists' evaluation
Medical teams' evaluation	1.0000		
Patients' evaluation	0.3667	1.0000	
	($p < 0.004$)		
Nephrologists' evaluation	0.7406	0.3056	1.0000
	($p < 0.001$)	($p < 0.023$)	

psychological adjustment were found to be statistically significant only for the patient's evaluation and his BPI score.

Subjective Evaluations: Clinical versus Patient Self-Report

Table 6 shows the correlation coefficients between the three subjective evaluations of the nephrologist, the patient, and the medical team. They are all significant ($p < 0.03$), but with the exception of the correlation between the medical team and the nephrologist, the relationships are weak. It should be noted that the nephrologist's rating is also incorporated in the medical team's composite score and the strength of the relationship could be somewhat spurious.

Regression Models

The final set of analyses addressed the question of whether or not meaningful statistical models could be built to predict the levels of psychological adjustment of CAPD patients based on the assessment of judgements made by the medical team, the patient, and the nephrologist using the objective scores obtained from the five BPI personality variables, "depression," "denial," "anxiety," "self-depreciation," and "social introversion." By subjecting the data to multiple regression analysis, three statistical models were developed. All beta coefficients in the models are standardized regression coefficients. The interpreting code for all models is as follows:

PAS = Psychological adjustment score
DEP = Depression raw score
 SD = Self-depreciation raw score
DEN = Denial raw score
  A = Anxiety raw score
 SI = Social introversion raw score

Based upon a sample of 32 CAPD patients, a statistically significant predictive model ($R = 0.62$; $p < 0.02$) was constructed using the nephrologist's evaluations. The model accounts for 38% of the variation within PAS scores. This model, referred to as Model A, is:

$$PAS = 0.67(SD) + 0.387(A) - 0.289(DEP) - 0.175(SI) + 0.126(DEN)$$

Utilizing a sample of 41 CAPD patients, a statistically significant predictive model ($R = 0.64$; $p < 0.001$) was developed using patient self-report evaluations. This model, accounts for 41% of the variation within PAS scores. The model, referred to as Model B, is:

$$PAS = 0.56(DEP) + 0.13(SD) - 0.07(DEN) - 0.07(A)$$

With a sample of 40 CAPD patients another statistically significant predictive model ($R = 0.57$; $p < 0.003$) was built. This model using medical team evaluations, accounts for 32% of the variation within PAS scores. The model, referred to as Model C, is:

$$PAS = 0.55(DEP) - 0.30(SI) + 0.13(SD)$$

Differences in sample sizes used in the models are a function of excluding evaluations which are not complete; that is, individual evaluations with missing data were not considered for analysis.

CONCLUSIONS

Based upon the above analyses, the following conclusions can be made:

1. While depression, anxiety, self-depreciation, and social introversion manifest themselves to a greater degree in the CAPD dialysis group than in the general population, the differences between patients who remain on CAPD and those who do not are not significant. This is equally as true for the success and transplant group comparisons.

2. In general, CAPD patients are better in assessing their levels of depression and social introversion than either the nephrologists or the medical team. The nephrologist is better in assessing patients' levels of anxiety and self-depreciation than either the patients themselves or the medical team. CAPD patients are better in assessing their overall levels of psychological well-being as defined by the five basic personality traits of the BPI than are either the nephrologist or the medical team. However, the subjective evaluations of patients, nephrologists, and medical teams give unreliable indications of the level of patient denial which is best determined by an objective assessment tool.

3. The weak–moderate (although significant; $p < 0.05$) relationships between the clinical or patient self-rating evaluations and the objective assessment (BPI) indicate that other variables have to be examined.

4. The regression equations developed show trends only. The trend, at present, indicates that depression shows the strongest influence upon the PAS as defined by the medical team, and that the factor most related to the patient's own adjustment score is self-depreciation.

5. Contrary to expectations, denial seems to have little influence on any of the PAS values. The change in signs from positive in Model A, to negative in Model B, and the disappearance of denial in Model C altogether suggests further study of denial is needed to better assess its influence on the PAS. The weights for denial in Model A and B do not differ significantly from zero and the sign change may be attributable to measurement error.

6. Statistically speaking, the best regression model so far in terms of predictability of psychological well-being is that which is based on the patient's own psychological adaptation scores (Model B).

DISCUSSION

In the last 15 years research on the psychosocial aspects of an individual's reaction to his chronic renal disease has been preoccupied with the many stresses that this disease precipitates and has been directed to the psychological dynamics activated by the array of crises and stresses.

This preoccupation with the psychological aspects of dialysis is not surprising considering the magnitude of problems that the disease inflicts on the patients and their families. Nor should it be surprising that researchers are currently expending a great deal of effort at establishing which personality traits are good predictors of successful psychological adjustment and which clinical assessment instruments offer the best hope in patient selection for the various treatment options. The results from this research address both of these issues.

While it was not unexpected that dialysis patients manifest greater personality dysfunctioning than individuals from the general population, it was confounding that personality profiles did not differ significantly between those who succeed on a home program and those who failed. Whether prolonged patient experience on CAPD will alter this finding remains to be seen. Analysis of data on patients with lengthy exposure to home hemodialysis using identical BPI scales revealed significant personality profile differences between success and failure groups.[23] The question is whether differences are attributable to length of time on a home program, treatment modality, or some other antecedant variable, for instance, age.

The study also illustrates the individual merits of three subjective methods of determining the quality of a patient's psychological well-being. The belief that a relationship exists between a person's perception of health and how that individual functions and the correlation between self- and physician-rated health has been the subject of a number of investigations.[24-28] It is generally agreed that some degree of positive association is present between self- and physician-rated health and that self-rated health is reliable over short terms.

Findings from this study corroborate the positive association between the subjective evaluations of the patient and the professionals and the reliability of patient self-assessment. In general, the data and analyses tends to support our contention that statistical models based on multiple regression offer the best hope for predicting levels of psychological adjustment of a CAPD dialysis population.

SUMMARY

In summary, based on a sample of 54 patients from 16 home dialysis programs in Ontario, Canada, who were on continuous ambulatory peritoneal dialysis for a limited time, it can be concluded that psychological determinants for successful adaptation may be predicted through the use of a regression model involving the determinants of the Basic Personality Inventory (BPI). The psychological adjustment scores obtained from the regression models and applied to an Index of Psychological Well-Being should assist health professionals not only in the selection of individuals who will psychologically do better on this modality, but should also assist in monitoring patient psychological adjustment when on the CAPD program. Further development of regression models is underway by including other psychological variables believed to have an influence on psychological well-being. These will be reported upon subsequently.

ACKNOWLEDGMENTS. The principal and co-investigators in this study are Professor Howard Burton, Dr. Lino Canzona, Dr. Robert Lindsay, and Professor Sally Palmer. The participating nephrologists are listed herewith and their help is acknowledged: Drs. C. J. Barnes, C. Cameron, W. Cameron, D. C. Cattran, P. E. Cordy, R. Couture, W. P. Fay, S. S. A. Fenton, B. Haberstroh, B. Hall, R. W. Johnson, E. Kinsey Smith, J. Lien, T. Liu, R. Manning, P. Morrin, D. Oreopoulos, D. Page, G. Posen, C. S. P. Saiphoo, A. G. Shimizu, R. Uldall, and C. C. Williams.

REFERENCES

1. GUTMAN, A. Toward enhancement of peritoneal clearance. *Dialysis and Transplantation*, 1979, *8*, 1075.

2. FENTON, S. S. A., CATTRAN, D. C., BARNES, N. M., and WAUGH, K. J. Home peritoneal dialysis. A major advance in promoting home dialysis. *Transactions of American Society for Artificial Internal Organs*, 1977, *23*, 194–202.

3. TENCHKHOFF, H., and SCHECHTER, H. J. A bacteriologically safe peritoneal access device. *Transactions of American Society for Artificial Internal Organs*, 1968, *14*, 181.

4. POPOVICH, R. P., MONCRIEF, J., DECHARD, J. B., BOMER, J. B., and PYLE, W. K. The definition of a novel portable/wearable equilibrium peritoneal dialysis technique. *Abstracts, Transactions of American Society for Artificial Internal Organs*, 1976, *5*, 181–183.

5. OREOPOULOS, D. G., ROBSON, M., and IPETT, S. A simple and safe technique for continuous ambulatory peritoneal dialysis (CAPD). *Transactions of American Society for Artificial Internal Organs*, 1978, *24*, 484–489.

6. BURTON, H. J., CANZONA, L., LINDSAY, R. M., and PALMER, S. *Adaptation to home dialysis*. The Health Care Research Unit Report, The University of Western Ontario, 1980.

7. OREOPOULOS, D. G., CLAYTON, S., DOMBROS, N., ZELLERMAN, G., and KATIRTZOGLOU, A. Experience with continuous ambulatory peritoneal dialysis (CAPD). *Transactions of American Society for Artificial Internal Organs*, 1979, *25*, 95–97.

8. MONCRIEF, J. W., NOLPH, K. D., RUBIN, J., and POPOVICH, R. P. Additional experience with continuous ambulatory peritoneal dialysis (CAPD). *Transactions of American Society for Artificial Internal Organs*, 1978, *24*, 476–483.

9. FENTON, S. S. A., CATTRAN, D. C., ALLEN, A., RUTLEDGE, P., AMPIL, M., DADSON, J., LOCKING, H., SMITH, A., and WILSON, D. Initial experiences with continuous ambulatory peritoneal dialysis. *Artificial Organs*, 1979, *3*, 206–209.

10. MONCRIEF, J. W. Continuous ambulatory peritoneal dialysis. *Dialysis and Transplantation*, 1979, *8*, 1077–1081.

11. LINDSAY, R. M., OREOPOULOS, D. G., BURTON, H. J., CONLEY, J., WELLS, G., and FENTON, S. S. A. Adaptation to home dialysis: A comparison of CAPD and hemodialysis. *Proceedings of the 1st International Congress CAPD*, Paris, 1980, 120–130.

12. LINDSAY, R. M., OREOPOULOS, D. G., BURTON, H. J., CONLEY, J., and WELLS, G. A comparison of CAPD and hemodialysis in adaptation to home dialysis. In J. W. Moncrief, R. P. Popovitch (Eds.), CAPD Update. New York: Masson Publishing, 1981, 171–179.

13. LINDSAY, R. M., OREOPOULOS, D., BURTON, H. J., CONLEY, J., RICHMOND, J., and WELLS, G. The effect of treatment modality (CAPD vs. Hemodialysis) in adaptation to home dialysis. *Proceedings of the Pan Pacific Symposium on peritoneal dialysis*, Melbourne, 1980.

14. JACKSON D. N. *The basic personality inventory*. London, Canada: Research Psychologists Press, 1980.

15. HOFFMAN, H., JACKSON, D. N., and SKINNER, H. A. Dimensions of psychopathology among alcoholic patients. *Journal of Studies on Alcohol*, 1975, *36*, 825–837.

16. JACKSON, D. N. A sequential system for personality scale development. In C. D. Spielberger (Ed.), *Current topics in clinical and community psychology*. Vol. 2. New York: Academic Press, 1970, pp. 61–96.

17. JACKSON, D. N. The dynamics of structured personality tests. *Psychological Review*, 1971, *78*, 229–248.

18. JACKSON, D. N., and MESSICK, S. *The differential personality inventory*, London, Canada: Research Psychologists Press, 1971.
19. HOLDEN, R. R., HELMES, E., FEKKEN, G. C., and JACKSON, D. N. Person reliability and psychopathology (manuscript in preparation), 1982.
20. KILDUFF, R. A. *Reliability and faking susceptibility of the basic personality inventory*. Unpublished Master's thesis, Department of Psychology, The University of Rhode Island, 1979.
21. REDDON, J. R. *Rural–urban personality and adjustment among Alberta high school youth*. Unpublished Master's thesis, Department of Rural Economy, The University of Alberta.
22. SMILEY, W. C. *Multivariate Classification of Male and Female Delinquent Personality Types*. Unpublished Doctoral dissertation, Department of Psychology, The University of Western Ontario, 1977.
23. CONLEY, J., BURTON, H. J., and LINDSAY, R. M. Home dialysis won't work if—: A psychological perspective. *Proceedings of the Fifth Annual Symposium of The Canadian Society of Dialysis Perfusionists*, Ottawa, Canada, 1980.
24. TISSUE, T. Another look at self-rated health among the elderly. *Journal of Gerontology*, 1972, *27*, 91.
25. PALMORE, E., and LUIKART, C. Health and social factors related to life satisfaction. *Journal of Health and Social Behavior*, 1972, *68*, 68.
26. SUCHMAN, E., PHILLIPS, B., and STREIB G. An analysis of the validity of health questionnaires. *Social Forces*, 1958, *36*, 223.
27. FRIEDSAM, H. J., and MARTIN, H. W. A comparison of self and physicians' health ratings in an older population. *Journal of Health and Social Behavior*, 1963, *4*, 179.
28. LINN, M. W., HUNTER, K. I., and LINN, B. Self-assessed health impairment and disability on Anglo, Black and Cuban Elderly. *Medical Care*, 1980, *18*, 282–288.

II

Dialysis and Renal Transplantation

14
Psychonephrology
Reminiscence and Review

JOHN P. MERRILL

In 1913 Dr. Abel and his colleagues at Johns Hopkins University Medical School published a paper on the use of an "artificial kidney"[1] for the treatment of poisoning with aspirin, then a common method of attempting suicide. Their experimental subjects were dogs who had been fed or given intravenously large amounts of aspirin. The apparatus they employed was a series of tubes made of the membrane collodion, very much like some of the cellophane membranes which are used today, except that it had to be extruded by hand and all the connections made by the investigators. In 1913 heparin was unknown, so Abel used hirudin, the anticoagulant injected by the leech to prevent coagulation in the process of sucking blood. In spite of the primitive apparatus, it was the best available at the time and Abel recorded the removal of large amounts of aspirin from dogs. In his discussion he also mentioned that this apparatus perhaps when perfected might be used to sustain human patients with acute kidney failure until their own kidneys had recovered enough function to sustain them. This was indeed prophetic because in the early 1950s it became a reality.

Since that time a good many investigators attempted the use of semipermeable membrane to remove toxins, or even to isolate hormones from animal and human blood. Between 1913 and 1946 one of the most interesting attempts was that of Necheles,[2] a gastroenterologist, who used guinea pig peritoneum as semipermeable membrane to study whether or not there was a substance in the blood which caused increased gastric secretion. In view of the fact that Necheles was probably one of the first to discover the value of the peritoneal membrane as a dialyzing surface, that he was a gastroenterologist, and his work was done in the capital of China at the Peking University Medical School, we cannot but take pause. However, in 1945 and 1946 Dr. Willem Kolff, well

JOHN P. MERRILL, M. D. • Professor of Medicine, Harvard Medical School, Director, Renal Division, Peter Bent Brigham Hospital, Boston, Massachusetts.

known to most of you, made one of the great leaps forward. Kolff then worked in the little Dutch town of Kampen under the conditions of German occupation. He devised an apparatus made of rubber tubing, crude wooden slats, and cellophane which has now been marketed. This "artificial kidney" proved to be an efficient method for treating renal failure.[3] When one remembers that Kolff did this, with German soldiers looking over his shoulder, and that it succeeded beyond the expectations of anyone who had knowledge in the field, one must admire the psychologic trauma that both Kolff and his patients surmounted.

Shortly following World War II Dr. Kolff visited the Peter Bent Brigham Hospital and talked about his device and his results. Dr. George Thorn, then the Chairman of the Department of Medicine at the Peter Bent Brigham Hospital and the Hersey Professor at Harvard Medical School, became interested. He persuaded Dr. Carl Walter, a skilled surgeon and engineer, to devise an apparatus built from the blueprints kindly lent to them by Dr. Kolff. With these they constructed a new artificial kidney—this one built of stainless steel instead of wood, plastic instead of rubber, and with many other accessories to which Kolff could not possibly have had access during the German occupation of Holland. With this new apparatus I, and a fourth year Medical Student named Lloyd H. Smith, currently the Chairman of the Department of Medicine at the University of California at San Francisco, added the final touches which we believed would make it totally safe, at least technically, for use in humans.[4,5] This was in the late 1940s. The term nephrology had not yet been invented, nor had human subjects committees which today have so much to do with any new techniques or drugs that are applied to human treatment. Needless to say, for those interested in the moral, ethical, social, and psychologic problems of advances in medical therapy vis-à-vis human experimentation, these committees have great importance. However, in 1949, there was virtually nothing in the way of treatment for people with terminal renal failure. An artificial kidney did have something to offer. We therefore felt justified in applying such therapy to people who without it would be dead in a week; we had good reason to believe we could keep them alive for months.

Today we have many excellent journals edited and contributed to by dialysis patients and conferences which stress the important psychologic, socioeconomic, and ethical problems of dialysis. In those days, however, all of those problems belonged to the physician and not to the comatose patient. We felt, however, that since there was no recourse we were justified in attempting this form of therapy. Our first treatment of a patient with chronic renal failure was done in 1948. Because of technical difficulties which we had not foreseen, the duration of the dialysis was only 3½ hours. We were all extremely disappointed. The following morning I arrived to see the patient and he certainly was no better. I went home that evening, having done everything I could, extremely discouraged. Again, you can imagine the psychic trauma to the physician. However, on Sunday, the second day after dialysis, I arrived in the hospital to see the patient eating a hearty breakfast and reading the Sunday newspaper. This was a lesson it took us a long while to learn. Because of the short dialysis period we had not markedly corrected imbalances that had occurred in a patient with chronic renal failure over the years and therefore we had not produced what we now know as "dialysis dysequilibrium." Several weeks later when we had corrected the technical problems, we were able to dialyze such patients for a period of 6 hours with an apparatus that had a urea-dialysate of some 180 ml/hr. All of these patients with chronic renal failure did very badly and for at least 4 years after our first use of the artificial kidney I was to write that it had no use in the treatment of chronic renal failure. Nevertheless, in the treatment of acute renal failure when the disease and the chemical disorganization had come on suddenly it was a miraculous tool.

About this time, in the early 1950s, Dr. David Hume and I were experimenting with kidney transplantation. In those days we had no ready method for suppressing the immune response and the dogs with transplanted kidneys did not do well. Nevertheless, because of a report from Chicago (which later proved to be incorrect) recording long-term survival of a transplanted kidney, Hume and I decided to go ahead. Our reasons were these: Our patients were terminal patients with renal failure and without some form of substantive therapy would be dead in weeks. We had available a good source of cadaver kidneys which would not necessitate removing a kidney from a healthy donor for what was then really an unproved form of therapy. Hume then transplanted 9 kidneys into patients, using a technique which did not involve entering the abdomen and the retroperitoneal space. To our great amazement, 4 of these patients survived long beyond the expected time.[6]

I think it takes no imagination to visualize the problems with which the surgeons and medical people wrestled at that time. As an afterthought I must tell you that prior to our efforts the French had attempted kidney transplantation. Their donors were patients who had been executed by the guillotine. A surgeon was on hand to promptly remove the kidney from the newly decapitated donor and transplant it into the chronically ill recipient. One can appreciate the soul-searching that went on in this kind of operation. Nevertheless, the end was for human good and patient survival.

In 1954 we were presented with a young man with terminal renal failure. A brilliant young internist at the Brighton Public Health Hospital had recognized that the patient had an identical twin and he reasoned that if the twin were indeed identical then there should be no rejection response between them. He telephoned me, and the patient was admitted to the hospital and kept alive on the artificial kidney for some weeks. Skin was transplanted between him and his brother; it survived. We felt that this was positive evidence that other tissues would survive and on December 28, 1954, Dr. Joseph Murray and Dr. J. Hartwell Harrison transplanted a kidney from Ronald to his sick brother Richard Herrick.[7] The kidney functioned immediately and well and the recipient lived with normal kidney function for a good many years. Eventually he developed recurrent glomerulonephritis in his kidney, but died of a massive myocardial infarction with a BUN of only 60.

Again, it is not hard to imagine the psychic, ethical, and even legal problems which confronted us in removing a normal kidney from a normal individual when it was not for his benefit, and transplanting it into his sick brother. All of us were temendously concerned, searching our souls and the law. Eventually it was the law which decided that the healthy twin would be so traumatized by the fact that he had not been allowed to save his brother's life that it would injure his psyche. I do not ask my readers to question the logic of this decision because it obviously was successful, but again let me remind you that the physicians involved at this point had more psychologic trauma than the patient and certainly as much as the donor who is to be much admired for his choice.

Transplantation of kidneys between identical twins was a technically proven device for the saving of the life of an otherwise terminally ill patient, but there were a limited number of identical twins. How to treat patients who were not identical twins?

In 1959 we had an opportunity to explore this when two male twins, born on the same day, were sent to us. Skin grafts had been exchanged between them before they came to us and at 15 days (normal time being 10–13 days) the grafts looked quite intact. However, as we dialyzed the sick twin and watched the healthy one it became apparent that the graft on the healthy one was beginning to fail. We then transplanted a second skin graft from the sick twin to the healthy twin and that was rejected in an accelerated response (5 days), positive proof that he and his twin were not identical.

How then to suppress the immune response between these twins whose tissues were obviously close but not identical? Other investigators had shown that it was possible to suppress the immune response by total body irradiation in which all of the antibody cells were destroyed. In order to allow the animal to survive, however, bone marrow had to be transplanted and this represented major problems. We had tried this approach in humans but bone marrow never survived. However, since the two nonidentical twins were so closely related it occurred to us that one might use sublethal irradiation, that is enough irradiation to destroy all but the basic stem cells of bone marrow and yet allow the patient to receive a transplant. With transplant in place the regrowing marrow from very immature cells would then "learn" to recognize the transplanted tissue as "self," an experiment for which Peter Medawar and Burnett had received a Nobel Prize.

How did one know what sublethal irradiation was? How much irradiation could be given to a patient without killing him? Here again the psychologic problem was enormous. How could a doctor possibly decide this? Fortunately, or unfortunately, as you choose to view it, Dr. Shields Warren, one of our greatest radiopathologists, and I had both been participants in the atomic bomb drop. We met at Bikini; he then went on to Hiroshima and Nagasaki and had some idea of what represented lethal and sublethal irradiation. From these data we decided upon a dose of 400 rads. as sublethal. For those of you interested in psychonephrology, imagine what it meant to the physicians involved to decide even on the basis of the best evidence they had whether or not the treatment they were giving to the patient was going to kill him or allow him to survive. To make a long story short, our approach did work and our patient survived and did well,[8] becoming Chairman of the Department of Philosophy at Indiana University.

In the early 1960s two things occurred which changed nephrology drastically. One was the invention of the shunt by Quinton and Scribner which made chronic dialysis possible and the other was the appreciation of the fact that immunosuppressive drugs developed by Dr. Joseph Murray and Dr. Roy Calne would drastically suppress the immune attack against transplanted organs. Into this era was born chronic dialysis and transplantation.

Nevertheless, there remained one predominant decision which caused deep concern to the physician; that was the definition of "brain death." When can one remove a kidney from a patient who is still breathing with artificial apparatus, whose heart is still working with artificial apparatus, but whose brain is totally dead and not revivable? This problem occupied hours of our time and a good deal of agony, but it eventually became soluble, and thus began an era of greater psychic trauma for the patient and somewhat less for the physician.

What of the present? Most of the patients, nurses, and social workers know better than I about the present. The nurses, technicians, and patients have taken over much of the responsibility for patients on chronic dialysis and transplantation. The federal government has taken over much of the responsibility for the economic support of such individuals. Nevertheless there remain problems of which you are all aware. Is the cost of all of this worth it? Should we be treating terminally ill diabetics? Older patients? Compare the experience in the United States with that in England where poor-risk patients are denied therapy for economic reasons. Compare the problems between the dialysis nephrologists and the transplant patients. Are people sequestered in dialysis units because their care is paid for by the federal government? Should they be on home dialysis or on transplantation programs? I don't pretend to know the answer to these questions in every case. What I do know is that there is no simple answer. Those who espouse a holistic answer for every area of the country do not understand the problem. Home dialysis, in which we were the first to publish a paper[9], seemed to me at the time to be the answer to the problem: freedom of choice, much less expensive. To my great disappointment this has not proven to be true. You are all well aware of the arguments, pro and con. Dialysis has certainly become the practical method for many people for maintaining healthy lives. People can travel around the world and if they are affluent enough can maintain the dialysis establishments in various homes. New apparatus is available to make it simple and more effective. Whether or not various forms of hemodialysis versus chronic ambulatory peritoneal dialysis, for example, are to be preferred, I am convinced remains a problem of individual preference.

As far as transplantation goes, we now have realized the *summum bonum* in animal work; that is, we have achieved specific immunologic unresponsiveness. What this means is that we are able now to make an animal unresponsive to a specific organ from a specific donor strain but still remain responsive to other antigens, that is to reject infection by viruses, fungi, and protozoa. As yet we have no proof that we can apply this to the human, but it looks most promising.

One thing we do need to remember is that there is no question but that the mortality rate of patients from transplantation of cadaver kidneys is no greater than that to be expected in a long-term program of chronic dialysis. In my opinion, therefore, any patient in a dialysis center should be properly screened as a potential cadaver transplant recipient. One of the recent unsolved problems which is being attacked is whether this is being done.

In conclusion, I must say that I have stressed some of the technical advances in dialysis and transplantation. However, I must tell you that some of the greatest progress that has been made in this area is the concern and contributions of the patients' organizations, the nurses, technicians, social workers, and others. What we saw as simply a technical and scientific project has grown into a broad economic, psychologic program to which psychologists, psychiatrists, nurses, social workers, and so many others have greatly contributed and into which we feel ourselves fortunate to welcome them as colleagues.

REFERENCES

1. ABEL, J. J., ROWNTREE, L. G., and TURNER, B. B. On removal of diffusible substances from circulating blood by means of dialysis. *Transactions of the Association of American Physicians*, 1913, *28*, 51–54.
2. NECHELES, H. Method of vivi-dialysis. *Chinese Journal of Physiology*, 1927, *1*, 69–80.
3. KOLFF, W. J., and BERK, H. T. J. Artificial kidney, dialyzer with great area. *Geneesk, gids.*, 1943, *5*, 21.
4. MERRILL, J. P., THORN, G. W., WALTER, C. W., CALLAHAN, E. J., III, and SMITH, L. H., Jr. The use of an artificial kidney. I. Technique. *Journal of Clinical Investigation*, 1950, *29*, 412.
5. MERRILL, J. P., SMITH, S., III, CALLAHAN, E. J., III, and THORN, G. W. The use of an artificial kidney. II. Clinical experience. *Journal of Clinical Investigation*, 1950, *29*, 425.
6. HUME, D. M., MERRILL, J. P., MILLER, B. F., and THORN, G. W. Experience with renal homotransplantation in the human. Report of 9 cases. *Journal of Clinical Investigation*, 1955, *34*, 327.
7. MERRILL, J. P., MURRAY, J. E., HARRISON, J. H., and GUILD, W. R. Successful homotransplantation of the human kidney between identical twins. *Journal of the American Medical Association*, 1956, *160*, 277.
8. MERRILL, J. P., MURRY, J. E., HARRISON, J. H., FRIEDMAN, E. A., DEALY, J. B., Jr., and DAMMIN, G. J. Successful homotransplantation of the kidney between nonidentical twins. *New England Journal of Medicine*, 1960, *262*, 1251.
9. MERRILL, J. P., SCHUPAK, E., and HAMPERS, C. L. Hemodialysis in the home. *Journal of the American Medical Association*, 1964, *190*, 468.

15

Cultural Aspects of Adjustment to End-Stage Renal Disease

Jon Streltzer

INTRODUCTION

From the beginning of the availability of chronic hemodialysis as a treatment for end-stage renal disease (ESRD), it has been recognized that major adjustments in life style are imposed on most patients. The inevitability of psychological distress and social disruption has led to the great interest in factors associated with psychosocial adjustment to ESRD. The impact of cultural background on such adjustment has been studied very little, however. Culture is known to affect symptom choice and beliefs about illness and its treatment. The importance of cultural background on adjustment to chronic illness is not well understood, however.

A "classic" study with clear-cut findings was that of Zborowski, who studied chronic pain patients.[1] He found that cultural background greatly influenced reactions to pain and its treatment. "Old Americans" were stoic in their response to their pain in contrast to Jews and Italians who were likely to complain. The Jews tended to resist medications, however, in contrast to the Italians. These observations were made without statistical analysis and potentially confounding variables such as age, sex, economic status, chronicity of pain, and type and amount of medication were not examined. Nevertheless, this study demonstrates that cultural background potentially has a significant impact on response to a chronic illness with implications for treatment approaches.

Hawaii's multiethnic society is in many ways an excellent population for the study of cross-cultural differences in response to end-stage renal disease. The ethnic distribution of civilian population is approximately as follows: Japanese—27.6%, Caucasian—25.8%, Hawaiian (part Hawaiian)—18.3%, Filipino—10.3%, mixed (non-Hawaiian)—9.4%,

Jon Streltzer, M.D. • Associate Professor of Psychiatry, University of Hawaii at Manoa, John A. Burns School of Medicine, Honolulu, Hawaii.

TABLE 1
Approximate Ethnic Distribution of Dialysis Patients

Hawaiian	25.0%
Japanese	21.0%
Caucasian	16.0%
Filipino	14.0%
Micronesian and Guamanian	12.0%
Chinese	7.0%
Caucasian–Oriental	2.5%
Samoan	1.3%
Korean	0.8%
Black	0.4%

Chinese—4.5%, Korean—1.3%, black—0.7%, Samoan—0.5%, and other—1.5%.[2]

Hawaii is known for its tolerance and appreciation of different cultures and the many ethnic groups are able to live harmoniously side by side. Evidence that these ethnic groups respond differently is present in a recent study of ethnic differences in the treatment of postoperative pain.[3] Caucasians received significantly more parenteral narcotic analgesics following elective cholecystectomy than the Oriental groups. Multivariate analysis revealed, however, that racial group accounted for only 6% of the variance.

The observations and studies to be presented here involve patients treated at the Institute of Renal Diseases, St. Francis Hospital, Honolulu, Hawaii. As of June 30, 1980, the Institute of Renal Diseases was treating 268 hemodialysis patients. This included patients from all the major Hawaiian Islands, Guam, Micronesia, Samoa, and Tahiti. The approximate ethnic breakdown of these patients is seen in Table 1. Compared to the general population in Hawaii, the Hawaiian and Filipino groups were somewhat overrepresented and the Caucasians underrepresented.

THE ETHNIC GROUPS OF HAWAII

Some background information about the different ethnic groups will help to provide a framework for the observations to follow. The Hawaiians, of course, are the native population of Hawaii. Hawaiians have not been dominant politically or economically during the entire twentieth century. Pure Hawaiians are quite rare as are those who can speak the Hawaiian language. Nevertheless, the Hawaiian cultural heritage—the music, food, dance, crafts, and friendliness—is extremely highly valued by the general population. The Hawaiians were quite accepting of immigrant groups to their islands, particularly the Caucasians, and intermarried readily, something that is ordinarily taboo in dominant cultures. Popular stereotypes associated with Hawaiians include laziness and lack of motivation, and on the positive side, being easy-going, loving, and generous—the aloha spirit.[4] Expectations based on this stereotype might be that Hawaiians would be friendly patients but likely to be noncompliant to diet and fluid restrictions.

The Caucasians were the first immigrant group to Hawaii and for many years they were dominant politically and economically. Many Caucasians at present are relatively recent arrivals from the mainland. Stereotypes associated with the Caucasians are that they are aggressive, successful, independent, and boastful. Family ties seem to play a much smaller role in the life of the Caucasians than with Orientals and Polynesians.[5] One might predict that Caucasians would have more difficulty adjusting to chronic dialysis than other groups because of less family support and less ability to accept a dependent role.

The Japanese immigrated in great numbers to Hawaii between 1868 and 1924, mostly as cheap labor for the sugar cane plantations. Since statehood in 1959, they have come to be the dominant political group in the Islands. Popular stereotypes of the Japanese are that they are orderly, stoic, and loyal, with family ties superseding all others. Negative stereotypes are that they are stubborn, clannish, quiet, and inarticulate.[6]

The Chinese of Hawaii, for the most part, immigrated during the last half of the nineteenth century to work on the sugar plantations. Despite representing only about 5% of the population of Hawaii, the Chinese have reached positions of prominence in business, politics, and the professions. The stereotypic image of the Chinese in Hawaii is shrewd, frugal, hard-working, cold, and stoic.[7]

The Filipinos, the fourth largest ethnic group in Hawaii, began to arrive in large numbers after 1910. Many in the Filipino population are still first-generation immigrants. Stereotypic images associated with Filipinos include lazy, hot-tempered, hard-working, stoic, and having great respect for authority.[8] Expectations based on stereotypes for Japanese, Chinese, and Filipinos with regard to adjustment to ESRD might be that they would be compliant patients, respecting the authority of the doctors and nurses. They might also be stoic patients preferring to please the doctor rather than reveal their physical symptoms.

CLINICAL EXPERIENCES WITH DIFFERENT CULTURAL GROUPS

In general, experience with this patient population based on 5 years of work as liaison psychiatrist and discussions with staff members, reveal that expectations based on stereotypes are difficult to substantiate. In only a few cases have cultural issues seemed to dominate the clinical picture.

Case Example

An elderly Hawaiian woman developed ESRD and had multiple other medical complications. She chose not to be treated with chronic dialysis, accepting the fact that she would die otherwise. Family sessions were required for the members of the immediate family to understand and accept the patient's decision. When this was done, however, the family began a celebration of the patient's life during her last few days. Her room was constantly filled with members of the extended family, reminiscing about the past. Guitars played Hawaiian music, women danced the hula, and little children played around the bedside. The patient was never left alone, and after several days she died peacefully.

The phenomena of large numbers of extended family members being present in a hospital when a relative is critically ill is often seen in the Hawaiian group; in this case the family response was particularly beautiful and created a good feeling in the staff also.

Case Example

A 40-year-old married Samoan woman seemed unable to learn self-dialysis and a psychiatric consultation was requested. The patient reported that she would completely forget what was told her during teaching for self-dialysis. In fact, she could not remember why she needed to be on the kidney machine. She said she sat at home for hours at a time with her mind a complete blank and her husband had to manage the household chores for her. She seemed totally mystified by this experience. She demonstrated no sign of organic brain syndrome and was diagnosed as having a dissociative reaction with hysterical amnesic episodes secondary to extreme anxiety associated with the onset of kidney failure. She responded rapidly to psychotherapeutic support and was able to learn self-dialysis. She has done well for several years now.

It is not uncommon for Samoan patients in Hawaii to present with hysterical states, including "classic" conversion reactions. It would appear that this patient's cultural background influenced her symptom choice and perhaps also the fact that her anxiety was unrecognized until she failed to learn during self-dialysis training.

Frequently, however, there is great difficulty evaluating the impact of cultural background on patient response.

Case Example

A 26-year-old college-educated Japanese (Okinawan) male from an outer island complained of severe bone pain. He was very difficult to evaluate because of his minimal verbalizations and neutral affect. It was thought that his inability or unwillingness to describe his feelings, perceptions, desires, and beliefs reflected cultural background. However, when his mother flew over to visit him in the hospital, she complained how she could never get this son to open up and express what was on his mind in contrast to everyone else in the family.

PSYCHOLOGICAL TEST DATA

Psychological test data is available on 95 patients, including the majority of those living on the major island of Oahu. This data in combination with clinical observations can be used to evaluate some of the hypotheses generated by the ethnic stereotypes. Table 2 shows scores on the Beck Depression Inventory.[9] This is a simple self-report questionnaire where high scores are indicative of a high level of depression. Overall, the scores are not much higher than that of the general population and the difference can be accounted for by the somatically oriented questions on the inventory. Our results are similar to those seen in cancer patients tested in this same inventory[10]; that is, depression scores measured by this scale are not particularly high. There are no significant differences among ethnic groups. Thus far, this scale does not provide evidence of a differential in coping abilities among ethnic groups.

Table 3 shows scores on the Nowicki–Strickland Scale, which is a measure of locus of control.[11] The highest possible score is 40, and higher scores indicate more externality, that is, a greater belief that what happens is not subject to one's personal control. The stereotype of Caucasians being more independent- and achievement-minded than other

TABLE 2
Mean Score on Depression Scale (BDI) by Ethnic Group

Hawaiian (n = 26)	10.5 ± 7.5
Caucasian (n = 20)	12.9 ± 8.7
Japanese (n = 18)	11.5 ± 6.7
Filipino (n = 13)	15.8 ± 16.7
Chinese (n = 11)	11.3 ± 10.7

TABLE 3
Mean Score on Locus of Control Scale (NSS) by Ethnic Group

Hawaiian (n = 26)	15.3 ± 5.1
Caucasian (n = 20)	15.4 ± 4.8
Japanese (n = 18)	16.8 ± 7.8
Filipino (n = 13)	17.0 ± 5.3
Chinese (n = 11)	13.5 ± 5.1

TABLE 4
Mean Score on Social Desirability Scale (MCSDS) by Ethnic Group

Hawaiian ($n = 26$)	22.0 ± 5.9
Caucasian ($n = 20$)	17.7 ± 6.4
Japanese ($n = 18$)	19.4 ± 7.2
Filipino ($n = 13$)	20.0 ± 4.7
Chinese ($n = 11$)	22.5 ± 5.2

groups would lead one to expect that they might score lower on this scale than the other groups. In fact, once again, there are no significant differences among any of the groups on this scale.

Table 4 shows scores on the Marlowe–Crowne Social Desirability Scale.[12] This is a scale that measures tendency to give socially desirable responses and can also be considered a measure of tendency to use denial. We have found that mean scores on this scale are quite high for our dialysis population in comparison to other populations and we have interpreted this as reflecting a greater tendency of dialysis patients to use denial.[13] All of the means seen here are quite high. The differences between the Caucasian and Hawaiian group and the Caucasian and Chinese group are both statistically significant at the 0.05 level. Higher scores on this scale correlate with lower scores on the depression scale indicating that denial probably is a protective mechanism against depression in dialysis patients.[13] On the other hand, lower scores occur in patients more responsive to psychotherapy.

TRANSPLANT FAILURE

We have found some support for this possible finding that Hawaiians have a higher tendency to use denial. In a study of patients' reactions to transplant failure, we found that 24 out of 25 patients had good psychological adjustment upon returning to chronic hemodialysis. However, their coping styles fell into two distinctly different groups: those who went through a grief process with resolution and those who used a great deal of denial without evidencing other than minimal grief and depression throughout the whole process. The ethnic breakdown for these two groups is seen in Table 5. Hawaiians were overrepresented among the deniers although this finding does not quite reach significance.

Thus, we have data that suggests Hawaiians may be more likely to use denial and Caucasians less. Whether this has any clinical significance is not clear. A potential area of clinical impact is that of compliance. The demands of diet and fluid restrictions can be difficult for dialysis patients, yet compliance is crucial to their well-being.

TABLE 5
Response to Transplant Failure

	Grief[a]	Denial[a]
Hawaiian	2	7
Caucasian	5	2
Japanese	3	0
Filipino	2	1
Chinese	1	0

[a]$\chi^2 = 8.14$, $df = 4$, $p < 0.10$.

TABLE 6
Fluid Compliance among Ethnic Groups

	Compliers	Borderline	Noncompliers
Hawaiian	5	5	4
Caucasian	4	2	3
Japanese	1	4	1
Filipino	2	1	2
Chinese	3	1	4

Compliance

Table 6 shows the ethnic breakdown of patients who were classified according to fluid compliance.[13] We studied 46 patients in depth from which three groups were defined. Noncompliers were patients who gained excessive weight (>2.5 kilograms) the majority of the time between dialyses. Compliers were those who gained 2 kilograms or less weight between dialysis at least 75% of the time. The rest of the patients fell into a borderline group in between. As can be seen, strikingly similar results were found for all ethnic groups. Despite the lack of ethnic differences with regard to compliance, it may be that staff reacts differently to noncompliance in Hawaiians as opposed to the other groups. Psychiatric consultation seems more likely to be requested for an Oriental who repeatedly gains too much weight than it is for a Hawaiian.

Home Hemodialysis

Another area in which culture might have a potential impact is home hemodialysis. Home dialysis allows the patient increased freedom and flexibility in terms of time and mobility, but it requires collaboration with a dialysis partner. Usually the partner is the patient's spouse. Some couples do very well with home dialysis; others are unable to manage and the patient must be dialyzed in a facility. The type of relationship a patient has with the spouse has been shown to correlate with success in home dialysis.[14]

We have found no difference in success in home hemodialysis training among couples from different ethnic groups as can be seen in Table 7.[15] In addition, at the time of the study, there were 14 mixed-marriage couples who had been home trained. Table 8 demonstrates the variety of combinations of ethnic groups in these couples.[15] Table 9 demonstrates the interesting finding that the intercultural marriages were significantly more successful in home training and home hemodialysis.[15] It should be noted that mixed marriages are readily accepted in Hawaii and indeed are the statistical norm at present.[16]

Table 7
Homocultural Home Hemodialysis Couples

Ethnic background	No. of couples	No. of failures
Japanese	12	2
Caucasian	8	3
Hawaiian[a]	8	2
Filipino	6	1
Chinese	3	1
Total	37	9

[a]Includes part Hawaiian.

Table 8
Interethnic Home Hemodialysis Couples

Patient		Spouse	
Sex	Ethnic background	Sex	Ethnic background
M	Caucasian	F	Hawaiian[a]
M	Filipino–Hawaiian	F	Portuguese
M	Portuguese	F	Japanese—local
F	Filipino	M	Caucasian
F	Filipino–Puerto Rican	M	Hawaiian[a]
M	Hawaiian–Caucasian	F	Japanese
M	Chinese	F	Caucasian
F	Japanese	M	Hawaiian[a]
F	Japanese	M	Filipino
F	Filipino	M	Japanese
F	Korean	M	Caucasian
F	Hawaiian[a]	M	Japanese
F	Japanese	M	Filipino
F	Hawaiian[a]	M	Caucasian

[a]Includes part Hawaiian.

TABLE 9
Success in Home Hemodialysis Related to
Cultural Composition of Marriage

	Success	Failure
Intercultural	14	0
Homocultural	28	9
$\chi^2 = 4.133,\ df = 1,\ p < 0.05$		

Cultural issues have clearly been important in home training in some individual cases.

Case Example

A 60-year-old Samoan man with diabetes and blindness developed ESRD. He immediately decided on home dialysis with his two daughters ages 22 and 14 being the partners who would learn the procedure. The 22-year-old daughter was married with a small child, yet the patient insisted that she live with him and help take care of him rather than live with her husband. He also insisted that the 14-year-old come home immediately from school and not participate in any extracurricular school activities in order that she may help care for him. Both daughters felt obligated to go along with the father's wishes although they both privately expressed their unhappiness at the disruption of their lives. The patient was confronted about the impact of his decision on his daughters' lives and he became tearful. Nevertheless, he insisted that it was an important part of the way of life of his people that children must place the needs of the parents above all else. The children did learn home dialysis, but shortly thereafter the patient died of medical complications.

Case Example

An elderly Filipino couple was referred for psychiatric consultation because of failure to learn during home training. The couple revealed that they felt that their young Caucasian nurse–teacher was too talkative, too loud, and too critical, and treated them in a manner they felt was disrespectful. They felt angry and anxious and were unable to concentrate on what the teacher was telling them. They were unable to express any of this to their teacher. As a result of this interview with the couple, the consulting psychiatrist was able to explain the problem to the teaching nurse in terms of cultural expectations of behavior and resulting implications for teaching approach. This led to a change in the relationship between the nurse and the couple and home dialysis training then proceeded smoothly. The couple has done very well with home dialysis.

PREJUDICE

Another area in which cultural differences potentially have an impact on adjustment to ESRD has to do with relationships among patients and staff. Racial harmony would seem necessary for proper patient care; prejudice is an issue worth examining.

Case Example

A 29-year-old single, Caucasian male, had great difficulty adjusting to chronic hemodialysis. Among other things, he frequently came into conflict with the treating staff. He often felt that his dialysis was not being run properly and would sometimes miss dialysis sessions. He stated that he did not like Orientals and he felt that he was being discriminated against because he was a blonde Caucasian who had recently arrived from the mainland. It was observed, however, that the two nurses who had the most conflict with this patient were both Caucasian.

Case Example

A 55-year-old married, Japanese man was known for his outbursts of temper, occasionally yelling and swearing during dialysis. Many times he would complain about the "damn haoles" (Caucasians). Nevertheless, he was able to develop a close relationship with the Caucasian psychiatric liaison nurse. This ultimately led to great improvements in the patient's behavior.

Despite the above examples, overt expressions of racial prejudice seem to be quite uncommon. Furthermore, the multiracial staff does not seem to take racial epithets seriously. Staff members tend to act as if racial insults are merely a surface manifestation of deeper emotional conflicts and clinically this does appear to be the case.

"DIALYSIS CULTURE"

From another perspective, ESRD programs could be viewed as having a culture of its own, with unique traditions, customs, rituals, beliefs, and expectations. Dialysis patients must make significant accommodations in their life style in order to be treated with maintenance hemodialysis. A great deal of their time is involved in this treatment. They often must make significant changes in their dietary habits. They are dependent upon the machines and the treating staff for their lives yet they are encouraged to function as independently as possible. This can create a "double-bind" situation leading to adjustment difficulties.[17]

Dialysis patients who are treated in the facility get to know the treating staff extremely well and they become very sensitive to nuances in interpersonal relationships.[18] For some patients the human contacts in the dialysis unit are the most significant ones in their lives. Nurse–patient interactions can have profound effects on patients' mood and sense of well-being. Dialysis patients can become exquisitely sensitive to such seemingly trivial matters as who gets put on the dialysis machine first and how much time a nurse spends talking to another patient.

Likewise, staff can develop intensely strong feelings toward the patients. Staff members will attend patients' funerals and weddings. There is a fairly high incidence of social contact with patients outside the unit. Occasionally a staff member develops a sexual relationship with a patient and may even marry one.[19] These and other special aspects of the hemodialysis milieu create what could be called a "dialysis culture." Dynamics associated with the dialysis culture can often override factors associated with individual cultural background in determining adjustment to ESRD.

Case Example

A young Caucasian nurse with a thick southern accent developed a seemingly improbable, close relationship with an older first-generation Korean–American woman patient who worked as a bar hostess. The nurse provided transportation for the patient to and from dialysis and also included the patient in her family's social activities. When the nurse planned to return to her native state in the deep South, the patient induced a great deal of guilt in the nurse for leaving, implying that dialysis would be intolerable without the nurse present. Indeed, the nurse invited the patient to move to the mainland with her and live with her family. The patient, feeling she would be very much out of place in a Southern state, declined.

CONCLUSIONS

We have not found significant differences in the adjustment of different cultural groups to ESRD. There may be a tendency for Hawaiians to use denial more than other groups; however, the clinical implications of this are not clear. We have not found good evidence substantiating hypotheses generated by popular racial stereotypes. In individual cases, however, cultural background may be the crucial factor in determining response to aspects of ESRD or its treatment. Viewing the hemodialysis milieu as having its own special culture may prove to be the most fruitful way of understanding issues associated with adjustment to ESRD.

REFERENCES

1. ZBOROWSKI, M. Cultural components in responses to pain. *Journal of Social Issues*, 1952, *8*, 16–30.
2. RESEARCH and STATISTICS OFFICE, HAWAII DEPARTMENT OF HEALTH. *Population report, issue no. 9*, October 1977, Honolulu, Hawaii.
3. STRELTZER, J., and WADE, T. C. The influence of cultural group on the undertreatment of postoperative pain. *Psychosomatic Medicine*, 1981, *43*, 397–403.

4. YOUNG, B. B. C. The Hawaiians. In J. F. McDermott, W. S. Tseng, and T. W. Maretzki (Eds.), *People and cultures of Hawaii, a psychocultural profile*. Honolulu: The University Press of Hawaii, 1980, 5–24.

5. MARETZKI, T. W., and McDERMOTT, J. F. The Caucasians. In J. F. McDermott, W. S. Tseng, and T. W. Maretzki (Eds.), *People and cultures of Hawaii, a psychocultural profile*. Honolulu: The University Press of Hawaii, 1980, 25–52.

6. ROGERS, T. A., and IZUTSU, S. The Japanese. In J. F. McDermott, W. S. Tseng, and T. W. Maretzki (Eds.), *People and cultures of Hawaii, a psychocultural profile*. Honolulu: The University Press of Hawaii, 1980, 73–99.

7. CHAR, W. F., TSENG, W. S., LUM, K. Y., and HSU, J. The Chinese. In J. F. McDermott, W. S. Tseng, T. W. Maretzki (Eds.), *People and cultures of Hawaii, a psychocultural profile*. Honolulu: The University Press of Hawaii, 1980, 53–72.

8. PONCE, D. E., and FORMAN, S. The Filipinos. In J. F. McDermott, W. S. Tseng, and T. W. Maretzki (Eds.), *People and cultures of Hawaii, a psychocultural profile*. Honolulu: The University Press of Hawaii, 1980, 155–183.

9. BECK, A., WARD, C., MENDELSON, M., MOCK, J., and ERBAUGH, J. An inventory for measuring depression. *Archives of General Psychiatry*, 1961, 4, 561–571.

10. PLUMB, M. N., and HOLLAND, J. Comparative studies of psychological function in patients with advanced cancer. I. Self-reported depressive symptoms. *Psychosomatic Medicine*, 1977, 39, 264–275.

11. NOWICKI, S., and DUKE, M. P. A locus of control scale for noncollege as well as college students. *Journal of Personality Assessment*, 1974, 38, 136–137.

12. CROWNE, D. P., and MARLOWE, D. *The approval motive: Studies in evaluative dependence*. New York: John Wiley and Sons, 1964.

13. YANAGIDA, E. H., STRELTZER, J., and SIEMSEN, A. Denial in dialysis patients: Relationship to compliance and other variables. Unpublished manuscript.

14. STRELTZER, J., FINKELSTEIN, F., FEIGENBAUM, H., KITSEN, J., and COHN, G. L. The spouse's role in home hemodialysis. *Archives of General Psychiatry*, 1976, 33, 55–58.

15. STRELTZER, J. Intercultural marriages under stress: The effect of chronic illness. In W. S. Tseng, J. F. McDermott, and T. W. Maretzki (Eds.), *Adjustment in intercultural marriage*. Honolulu: The University Press of Hawaii, 1977, 113–120.

16. McDERMOTT, J. F. Toward an interethnic society. In J. F. McDermott, W. S. Tseng, and T. W. Maretzki (Eds.), *People and cultures of Hawaii, a psychocultural profile*. Honolulu: The University Press of Hawaii, 1980, 225–232.

17. ALEXANDER, L. The double-bind theory and hemodialysis. *Archives of General Psychiatry*, 1976, 33, 1355–1356.

18. STRELTZER, J. Psychiatric problems in chronically-ill patients: hemodialysis, diabetes, and cancer. In H. Leigh (Ed.), *Psychiatry in primary care medicine*. Addison-Wesley Publishing Company, In press.

19. MOE, M., and STRELTZER, J. Implications of patient's sexuality for nursing staff. *Dialysis and Transplantation*, 1981, 10, 912.

16

Growing Up with Renal Failure
Problems and Perspectives

MARY ANN GANOFSKY, DENNIS DROTAR, AND
SUDESH MAKKER

For the past 10 years, we have been caring for children and adolescents with renal failure (RF) and their families in an evolving program of comprehensive pediatric care that features attention to psychosocial development, involvement of child and family in treatment decisions, and family-oriented intervention concerning psychological crises which arise in the course of physical treatment.[1-3]

Our relatively small patient group and strong emphasis on continuity of care throughout all stages of treatment have provided a context for clinical experiences which suggest realistic principles for the psychosocial management of adolescents with ESRD, enhancing their maturity and independence, adaptation to life with a chronic illness, and compliance with medical regimens.

MEDICAL AND PSYCHOSOCIAL OUTCOME OF OUR PATIENT POPULATION

Pediatric and adolescent transplantation began in our facility in 1970. As of this writing, there have been 47 transplants, both live–related (L/R) and cadaveric, in 37 patients ranging in age from 5 through 20 at the time of transplant.

This paper describes our clinical experiences with 21 adolescent and young adults with RF (ages 15–24). In this group, there have been 24 kidneys transplanted into 18 patients. Fifteen patients have functioning

MARY ANN GANOFSKY, A.C.S.W. • Pediatric Social Service, Rainbow Babies and Children's Hospital, Cleveland, Ohio.   DENNIS DROTAR, PH.D. • Division of Pediatric Psychology, Associate Professor in Psychiatry and Pediatrics, Case Western Reserve University, School of Medicine, Cleveland, Ohio.   SUDESH MAKKER M.D. • Associate Professor, Case Western Reserve University, School of Medicine, Division of Pediatric Nephrology, Rainbow Babies and Children's Hospital, Cleveland Ohio.

transplants. Six others, who are on dialysis, include four on the cadaver list, one who is presently opting for chronic dialysis, and one who is a chronic dialysis patient following two failed transplants. These adolescents have a varied race and sex distribution which includes 70% male, 30% female; 80% white, 20% black. They have been recipients of both cadaveric (75%) and L/R transplants (25%). The group's intellectual abilities range from mildly retarded through above-average intelligence. The varied economic composition of the families ranges from welfare recipients to middle class and includes a few families in which the fathers are executives in their companies. The patients are from urban, suburban, and rural homes.

These adolescents' adaptation to living with chronic renal failure and its treatment as measured by functioning in life situations such as school and with peers has generally been good. Although none of the group is as yet totally financially independent or living on their own, a majority (13 of 21) are still in school. Of the 21, 11 are high school graduates. Six are presently in college, including one who is in medical school and another who is due to graduate from college this winter. Eight of the younger patients are still in high school. Only two, ages 20 and 21 respectively, dropped out of high school without receiving a diploma. This rate of school attendance is especially impressive because almost all of the patients missed considerable time in school with every-other-day dialysis and repeated hospitalizations. Many (14 of 21) have had or currently have some type of employment. However, most report that they have faced discrimination in securing jobs because of their chronic illness. Six of the group is presently neither working nor attending school. Four of these six have been referred to the Bureau of Vocational Rehabilitation (BVR). These adolescents' social adaptation in peer group and heterosexual relationships has been delayed. Yet 17 of 21 patients have age-appropriate contacts with peers involving a wide range of activities. Of 17 young adults who are age 17 or older, 11 have normal dating patterns including one, age 21, who plans to marry soon. Our findings coincide with the good potential for long-term rehabilitation of children and adolescents with RF noted by others.[4-6]

In all programs that treat adolescents with RF the question of compliance with the medical regimen is an important one. Our experience has yielded some interesting and unanticipated results: With adolescents on dialysis, we have had rather unremarkable success in securing their cooperation with fluid, dietary, and medication requirements. However, in the posttransplant phase of treatment, we have had exceptionally good compliance from patients in the taking of steroids. There have been *no* kidneys lost due to patients stopping their medication. Given our patients' noncompliance with treatment regimens while on dialysis and the serious and distressing compliance problems that adolescents and adults have had with steroid therapy at other centers,[6] we were both surprised and pleased by this finding.

EARLY WORK WITH ADOLESCENTS IN PSYCHOSOCIAL CRISIS

Our clinical approach to adolescents and their families has changed dramatically over a 10-year period as we have gained experience. Our trial-and-error encounters with adolescents, particularly those patients in the midst of severe psychosocial crises, gradually led to the development of a comprehensive care approach which differs dramatically from the way psychosocial issues were addressed in the early phases of our work.

In 1971, dialysis and transplant selection committees were set up at our hospital to determine who should be offered the treatments for the disease. By 1973, the increasing number of pediatric patients and our experiences with two patients, including one adolescent with renal failure referred for a severe psychological crisis,[7] led us to gradually restructure our case-by-case involvement so that we could contribute to the total care of the children adolescents and their families. The newness of dialysis and transplantation in a pediatric population precluded hard and fast guidelines for psychosocial intervention with adolescents. In fact, a number of professionals at our hospital felt that many adolescents and families could not cope with the stresses and setbacks that are associated with dialysis and transplantation. In the interest of developing a more humane focus of total care, we became closely involved with each and every RF patient and family; this involvement has since taught us much about how adolescents confront this stressful disease and its constraining treatment regimens.

Our difficult, and at times, overwhelming initial confrontations with adolescent problems will be all too familiar to those who work with such patients. Perhaps the most difficult problem for any treatment staff is the out-of-control, screaming patient. We have seen a good number, including several in our adolescent population, such as C., a 14-year-old girl from a very deprived and chaotic family, who was referred to our facility when she was comatose from uremia with a pathological fracture of the femur secondary to renal failure. When she awoke, she struck out, hit staff, threw things, refused medications, and got out of bed with the leg cast and refractured her hip. She was hospitalized for 9 months, mostly for management of the fracture. The first 4 months of that hospitalization were a nightmare. She refused contact with any helping person. She withdrew and was silent and frequently verbally abusive. Her behavior, which included agonizing screaming while being dialyzed, is still remembered very clearly, not only by C. herself, but by other patients dialyzed with her 6 years ago.

Another very common problem presented to treatment staffs is the withdrawn, depressed, or totally uncommunicative adolescent. T., a 16-year-old girl, was under our care for several years prior to the onset of dialysis at age 16. In that period, a wide variety of staff members were unable to effectively establish any kind of relationship for even the most elementary of purposes: education regarding the disease and the treatment courses. After she had begun dialysis and was transplanted 6 months later her withdrawal continued despite ongoing efforts on our part to interact with her.

Children and adolescents who seem emotionally intact when they begin treatment for renal failure can deteriorate under the stress of complications, particularly a failed transplant. We have seen this kind of problem on several occasions: A., a 15-year-old girl, received her sister's kidney after a transplant rejected 5 years ago. In the ensuing period she was relegated to chronic dialysis because of high antibody titers which made locating a cadaver transplant difficult. Unfortunately, this transplant also was rejected and the posttransplant nephrectomy course (a 2-month hospitalization) involved numerous complications including: significantly low platelets (due to the immunosuppressive therapy), chronic fever due to a CMV infection, a massively enlarged right leg due to edema, and loss of hair probably due to uremia, medication, and poor nutrition. This 15-year-old, who had maintained quite adequate school attendance while on dialysis and who had good peer relationships, was now behaving like an infant. She retreated to sleep (partially due to uremia, but also due to depression), refused to eat, and was unwilling to get out of bed. When forced to do so, she would shake and crumble to the floor unless physically supported by others. She described hallucinations and cried out fearfully that people were trying to kill her.

There are also the patients, like B., who present as argumentative and challenge every medical decision. B. is a 19-year-old man who had lived his entire adolescence knowing he would eventually receive dialysis and transplantation. His older brother was transplanted twice in 1972 at age 16, when B. was 12. His brother was a remarkably compliant, accepting patient who was well liked by the dialysis staff. B.'s mother feared that he would not be so well liked by the staff because he questioned everything in an argumentative way, precluding any resolution of an issue. Her observations proved to be correct. Because B. required chronic dialysis longer than was initially anticipated, the considerable frustrations engendered by his protracted time on dialysis and his difficult temperament provided an arena for conflicts between B., the dialysis technicians, and the physicians.

COMPREHENSIVE CARE FOR ADOLESCENTS

These patients and many others like them have provided us much grief, anxiety, and ultimately some enjoyment as we have weaved a path through their adolescence altered by chronic illness. Their resiliency and response to our support as well as our mistakes have suggested principles of comprehensive care for adolescents that are geared to their unique developmental needs.

Continuity of Relationship

The hallmark and most essential component of our treatment program has been the continuity of care provided by physicians and mental health professionals. It is from this continuity that all else follows. Our persistent contacts with adolescents and their families over protracted periods of time and through the various phases of physical treatment have provided the best opportunity to form meaningful relationships with them. Yet even with the provision of continuity of care it has not been easy to establish and maintain relationships with adolescents in crisis. For example, C.'s hospitalization was highlighted by our efforts to make contact with her on a human level. To that end, a psychology intern, the attending nephrologists, renal fellows, and I visited daily for very short periods making no demands other than to express our interest in her. Slowly, but surely, she responded to these contacts. However, her behavior was so difficult as to require considerable work on our part with the nursing staff who had to put up with her on a daily basis. In 6 years we have cared for her through two courses of maintenance dialysis, two cadaveric transplants, orthopedic surgery for removal of the femoral head, a total hip replacement, and multiple attempts at fistula placements. Many of her hospital admissions have been fraught with disasters—some of her making and some of ours. Yet each succeeding admission has revealed a surprising maturation and development toward independence, which stands in stark contrast to her initial upset. She now understands her disease and its treatments, hates it, yet accommodates as best she can to its demands. With each treatment setback, she continues to be difficult. For example, as recently as 2 months ago when she was readmitted for another fistula placement preparatory to a possible third course of dialysis, she adamantly refused the surgery. As before, her physician spoke quietly with her and when he concluded she agreed to the procedure. When she described this episode, she said, "Dr. M. uses black magic; he always gets me to change my mind!" When we suggested to her that no black magic was involved but rather that he conveyed that he cared what happened to her, and she accepted his caring attitude, C. smiled in agreement. She has grown emotionally in a way that we would not have predicted at the outset. We have provided her with the reliable presence of adults who would not desert her in the midst of a treatment crisis or of her anger but would continue to support her. In many ways, we believe we have served as a kind of surrogate family which has aided her development by providing an emotional experience that contrasted sharply with her early experiences of abandonment and separation.

Enhancing Adolescents' Control of and Partnership in Treatment

With many adolescents, a battle of monumental proportions can develop over the next phase of physical treatment, particularly a new surgery. Often, the adolescent's refusal to "be cut on again," is not directly related to a desire to die, but rather to a wish to control more of what is happening to him or her. When this is understood by the treatment team and when the adolescent is given a chance to state it, a surprisingly amicable solution to what initially appears to be an intractable problem can ensue.

Adolescents with ESRD are forced to accept one of the most controlling physical treatments ever devised at a time in their development when issues of autonomy and independence from adults, and sensitivity to restrictions in their activities are at their zenith.[8] In our early work, we tried numerous methods to encourage adolescents' compliance with the fluid, dietary, and medication requirements of dialysis. Efforts at education and discussion by a variety of staff often deteriorated into sessions of nagging and only produced alienation on both sides. We have learned from our patients that as much as possible the management of their own bodies should be left to them. We attempt to be a supportive guide by providing information that relates to their individual condition. Our adolescents are given very complete information and then told, "You know what's expected and you know the consequences." In the manner of patient parents, we provide a relationship in which the adolescent feels safe enough to share their struggles with compliance. For example, J., a 19-year-old man, who suffered two failed transplants within 5 months last year and is currently awaiting a third try, described his struggles with dietary compliance: "I know what I'm supposed to do, but it's sure hard when you go out with your friends on Saturday night and not eat and drink what they do." We responded to J. by not preaching about compliance, but by letting his body be his teacher. J. has, until recently, been one of the lucky ones who could transgress dietary restrictions without complications. Now he's facing problems with decreased urinary output and rising blood pressure. He has the ability and the information to make the connections between these facts and what he needs to do to maintain his previous state of well-being while on dialysis. Knowing him, we expect that in time he will make the necessary adaptations.

We strive to develop a sense of mutual respect and dialogue in which the adolescent is seen as an active partner in, rather than a passive recipient of, treatment. Our continuous support during crises provides ample opportunities for staff and patient to have an open and honest exchange about the treatment, its restrictions, and its complications. Right from the outset and at each critical juncture of treatment, we outline for patients what we know about their care and prepare them for the good as well as the bad that can occur. Within this context, we always emphasize our unfailing expectation that they will eventually have a successful transplant.

Supporting Adolescents during Periods of Regression versus Independence

When patients are in the midst of a severe medical crisis, we have found that the most useful tool we have to offer is ourselves. Being with them for both physical support and empathic listening during these periods has paid significant dividends. With young children, the form that physical support can take is often easy to perceive. With adolescents, it may not be so clear. Yet if the care-giver is patient and listens hard enough, the adolescent will very often tell the staff member what he needs. For example, J. invited the senior author, rather off-handedly, to be present at a meeting he had scheduled with the doctor to discuss prospects for his third transplant. He and I had previously discussed these matters and my role in the meeting turned out to be that of advocate; he needed to ask someone questions he was afraid to raise with his physician. Another kind of support was given to F., a 19-year-old woman who on the day of her cadaver transplant insisted that I stay at the hospital and accompany her to the operating room for moral support as I had done 6 years earlier when her twin sister received a transplant.

There are many times when adolescents need support and understanding during crises of physical treatment. The regressed or dependent state that many patients fall into is often a response to the severe stresses of physical treatment and cannot be turned around rapidly. Such regressions are often understandable (rather than pathological) reactions to the extreme stress and enforced dependency of physical treatment. Rather than viewing very dependent behavior as a problem that always requires modification, we often attempt to accept the behavior, understand the reasons for it, and provide support and close follow-up of psychological progress. The same meticulous attention that is paid to adolescents' medical and surgical recovery is also necessary for their psychological state. Severely regressed behavior may require a management plan that takes months to achieve rather than days or weeks. For this reason, the mental health consultant's "long view" of the situation can provide reassurance to the staff and family that the adolescent will improve emotionally as they improve physically. Extensive contact with the patient and family by the treatment team is critical to facilitate psychological recovery from severe regression. For example, the severe regression experienced by A., the 15-year-old girl described earlier, required frequent contacts with her and her family. During recovery from the transplant nephrectomy, A.'s family (parents, siblings, aunts) were seen very frequently by both the social worker and the nephrologist to apprise them of A.'s medical condition, reassure them that physical health would return, and support them in their efforts to encourage A. toward recovery.

Over the course of time, we have developed an increased tolerance of regression because our experience has taught us that when children and adolescents are physically healthy, that is, with normal or near-normal renal function, they are generally well-adjusted, adequately functioning human beings. Good physical health and the adolescent's striving for maturity allow the care-giver to accept and even foster regression in a sick adolescent. Severe dependency is not a normal state and will often be altered as soon as the patient can physically do so. The potential resilience of adolescents should never be overlooked or underestimated.

Despite our tolerance for adolescent dependence when it is understandable, a major thrust of our comprehensive care program is toward enhancing maturation and independence. To accomplish this, we provide close follow-up on each adolescent's functioning in life situations and of their general state of well-being. A brief description of the life adjustment of disturbed adolescents described earlier illustrates their resiliency. For example, T., now 21, with a 5-year functioning cadaver kidney is about to be married; B., after a second transplant 9 months ago, started working amost immediately after discharge and will begin his sophomore year for the third time this fall; A., amongst the 'most seriously disturbed of our patients, after 5 months of arduous recovering from the transplant failure is accepting the need for chronic dialysis, returning to high school, and joining the volunteers who speak for Organ Recovery Inc., on the importance of transplantation. C., at the age of 20, without a high school diploma, has decided to accept a referral to the Bureau of Vocational Rehabilitation (BVR). F. is working full time and attending college (as she did while she was dialyzed for a year) and J., a high school graduate who cannot find a job because of the chronic dialysis, has been referred to BVR. As a dialysis patient, he is exceedingly well liked by the staff for his humor, charm, and adaptive acceptance of the demands of his disease.

Offering Hope Tempered by Reality

Our treatment team has tried to be inventive in the ways we offer hope for adolescent patients for whom another transplant is impossible. Perhaps the most important element of this hope is our persistent caring for the patient, in spite of the withdrawal, irritability, and depression that can accompany dialysis. When we convey to adolescents that we perceive their return to chronic dialysis as good and as a way to help them get ''back on their feet,'' we communicate a powerful message of hope and expectation that the adolescent's life will return to the previous level of adaptation. To implement this expectation, a great deal of time must be provided to parents whose disappointment over the failed transplant and fears in seeing their child very sick with kidney rejection or infection can be overwhelming. In addition to directly supporting parents, we have found that it is necessary to help them begin to set realistic and achievable goals as to when the child should be expected to do more for themselves, return to school, and begin coming to the outpatient dialysis treatments by themselves. This approach unifies the work of both staff and parents and provides the adolescent with a supportive network of concerned care-givers who share similar expectations for their independence.

The adolescents themselves can provide important models to other patients as they share experiences. In our setting, children and adolescents are given ample opportunity to talk to each other before they begin dialysis. Even more important, when an adolescent is newly transplanted, we encourage them to visit the dialysis unit to afford the staff the chance to discuss with those still on dialysis their prospective transplants. This can be an opportune time to discuss the posttransplant course and its complications, for example, rejection, steroid therapy, weight gain, and the eventuality of a good functioning kidney that will ultimately lead to low-dose immunosuppressive therapy. As in all our discussions, hope, the unifying theme, is balanced with a straightforward message about the negative effects of steroids following transplantation. Our communications about this painful reality are accompanied by statements that the symptoms of cushingnoid appearance and increased appetite will diminish as the steroid dosages are decreased. Adolescents are encouraged to meet patients who are at various posttransplant stages, that is, at 3 months, 6 months, 1 year, and more, so that they can experience the effects of the medication firsthand. Our impression is that adolescents' compliance with steroids following transplantation is enhanced by our honest presentation of the prospects for side effects in ways that also communicate that they are expectable but short-term burdens. Our clinical impressions are supported by reports which link patients' perceptions of physicians' understanding and concern[9] and explicit, honest explanation[10] with patient compliance.

IMPLICATIONS

Many unanswered questions remain about the physical survival and long-term psychological adaptation of these young persons. Our retrospective view, which is supported by others,[5,11] suggests that with a long-term commitment by a treatment staff to a continuous and available relationship, adolescents can understand, accept, and make the necessary adjustments to living with kidney failure and its treatments. We recognize that our experience is colored by the impact of our particular setting and may not generalize to settings such as community-based dialysis units or very large university-based transplantation centers.

There is a critical need for various centers to gather comprehensive outcome data concerning adolescent psychosocial adjustment, including compliance with medical regimens. The gathering of such data will provide an important first step toward the eventual identification of the specific features of comprehensive medical care that are associated with positive versus negative psychosocial outcomes. Our experience strongly suggests that variables such as continuity of patient–physician relationship, honesty of explanation, degree to which the patients' concerns are listened to and considered, and the provision of special support during times of stress may well be associated with ESRD adolescents' ability to successfully negotiate a stressful treatment regimen and maintain independent care following transplantation.

REFERENCES

1. DROTAR D., and GANOFSKY, M. A. Mental health intervention with children and adolescents with end-stage renal failure. *International Journal of Psychiatry in Medicine,* 1976, 7, 181–194.
2. DROTAR, D., GANOFSKY, M. A.,and MAKKER, S. Comprehensive pediatric management of severe emotional reactions of children to dialysis and transplantation. *Dialysis and Transplantation,* 1979, 8, 983–986.
3. DROTAR, D., GANOFSKY, M. A., MAKKER, S., and DEMAIO, D. A supportive approach to renal transplantation in children. In N. B. Levy, (Ed.), *Psychonephrology I: Psychological factors in hemodialysis and transplantation.* New York: Plenum Publishing, 1981.

4. KORSCH, B. M., NEGRETE, V. F., GARDNER, J. E., WEINSTOCK, C. L., MERCER, A. S., GRUSHKIN, C. M., and FINE, R. N. Kidney transplantation in children: Psychosocial follow-up study on child and family. *Journal of Pediatrics*, 1973, *83*, 399–408.
5. GRUSHKIN, C. M., KORSCH, B. M., and FINE, R. N. The outlook for adolescents with chronic renal failure. *Pediatric Clinics of North America*, 1973, *20*, 953–963.
6. FINE, R. N., MALEKZADEH, M. H., PENNISI, A. J., ETTENGER, R. B., VITTENBOGAART, C. H., NEGRETE, V. J., and KORSCH, B. M. Long term results of renal transplantation in children. *Pediatrics*, 1978, *61*, 641–650.
7. DROTAR, D. The treatment of a severe anxiety reaction in an adolescent boy following renal transplantation. *Journal of the American Academy of Child Psychiatry*, 1975, *14*, 451–461.
8. SCHOWALTER, J. E. Psychological reactions to physical illness and hospitalization in adolescence. *Journal of the American Academy of Child Psychiatry*, 1977, *16*, 500–516.
9. FALVO, D., WOEHLKE, P, and DEICHMANN, J. Physician behavior and its relationship to patient compliance. Paper presented at the Annual Meeting of the American Psychological Association, New York, N.Y., 1979.
10. SCHMITT, D. Patient compliance: The effect of the doctor as the therapeutic agent. *Journal of Family Practice*, 1977, *4*, 853–856.
11. KORSCH, B., FINE, R. N., GRUSHKIN, C. M., and NEGRETE, V. F. Experiences with children and their families during extended hemodialysis and kidney transplantation. *Pediatric Clinics of North America*, 1973, *18*, 399–408.

17

Habilitation of the Child with Chronic Renal Failure

ANNETTE C. FRAUMAN

In the not-too-distant past, habilitation of the child with chronic renal failure was not an issue; all children with chronic renal failure died or were severely impaired. When dialysis and transplantation for children became technically possible, the techniques leading to physical survival were of consuming interest. Devising clinically feasible methods of hemodialysis for a 5-kg child was a sufficiently demanding task. Developing surgical techniques and immunosuppressive regimens making possible transplantation for children was equally challenging.

A paper published in 1964 by Riley[1] presented the view that the multitude of stresses and problems experienced by children in renal failure were so severe as to raise serious questions as to the advisability of dialysis and transplantation. He believed that the quality of life obtained by dialysis and transplantation was so poor as to very often not be worth the time, effort, and money involved. In addition, the increased life span was minimal. Dr. Barbara Korsch was among the first to be interested in the social, psychological, and developmental care of children in renal failure, and the interventions necessary to improve their quality of life. She began to demonstrate that children with renal failure and their families require a great deal of support beyond the medical and pharmacological regimen.[2]

We now have a rapidly growing population of children either on dialysis or posttransplantation who need carefully planned care in order to become functional adults, coping with their physical disorder but continuing to live maximally satisfying and useful lives. We are beginning to acquire some information about the problems these children and their families face and how we can go about helping them.[3] It is difficult, however, to devise and implement effective psychosocial studies of children with chronic renal failure. The population is small and only in se-

ANNETTE C. FRAUMAN, R.N., M.S.N. • Assistant Professor, College of Nursing, University of Florida, Gainesville, Florida.

lected types of studies can one compare children of varying development levels. Much of the information in this paper is based on detailed clinical observation and interviews with parents and children for that reason.

I have used the term *habilitation* in the title of this paper as opposed to *rehabilitation* as a more appropriate term for the care of a child who has not reached his developmental potential and has not yet entered society as a fully productive member. *Habilitation* also implies not re-ability but ability to perform a task for the first time. In addition, *habilitation* reflects the vital necessity of considering the child's physical, emotional, and intellectual development. The goal of care for the child with chronic renal failure is physical survival along with the child's development into a happy, useful adult.

Children in renal failure may present the health care team with a multitude of behavioral problems including acting-out, noncompliance, withdrawal, and school phobias. They frequently exhibit apathy and a sense of powerlessness in dealing with their illness. These behaviors can be very frustrating to those providing health care. This complex of behaviors and their accompanying consequences can be termed the "poor little thing" syndrome.

Frequently when children with any long-term problem are discussed we hear the expression "the poor little thing!" While this view is certainly understandable, it is not a helpful or therapeutic attitude. To a great extent, children and their families pattern their attitudes about the child's illness from the attitudes of health care providers. While the empathic viewpoint is necessary, care must be taken to operationalize that attitude in appropriate therapeutic ways. The child who is told, verbally or nonverbally, that he is a "poor thing" will soon come to believe it, and act upon his belief. Helping children and their families to have normal attitudes and expectations will greatly facilitate the child's normal development into a happy productive adult.

FAMILY

The family is a crucial element in dealing with the child with renal failure. The family becomes the patient: a multi-individual patient unit. The family can include parents and siblings (older and younger) as well as grandparents and other extended family members. The significant constellation of family members may change over time, influenced by the stage of development of the family itself, as well as its members.[4] In many families, pets are considered to be an integral part of the family unit. For adolescents, the kinship group may assume diminished importance, with peers, employers, and teachers assuming some functions previously served by the family.

The developmental level of the family and its members should be considered. This developmental level may range from that of a newly married couple with a first child, to a couple in their sixties whose child was born in their middle years. Each of these families' level of development has its own implications for the care-giver. For example, a very young couple will depend heavily on their own parents for support, regressing from previously achieved independence. While an older family may have fewer financial problems because of maximal career achievement, they may resent their heavy burden of parental responsibilities at this stage of life. In addition, consider the developmental level of individual family members. It is unrealistic to expect mature parenting behaviors from a 17-year-old mother, especially with the added stress of a child on dialysis.

Although children with renal failure and those in a posttransplant state have a great deal of direct contact with the health care system, the vast majority of their lives is spent with their families and in their communities. Therefore it is essential to involve the family in the care of the child, assisting them to care for their child rather than having the major responsibility for care rest with the health care system. In addition, family members will require care from the health care team. If a family member is a transplant donor, both concentrated physiological and psychosocial intervention is necessary. However, other family members will also need support to maintain their effective coping strategies.

The illness trajectories of renal failure can vary widely, depending on treatment modality and the success of interventions. Children in renal failure may gradually worsen, may stabilize on dialysis, or be successfully transplanted and assume an essentially normal life style. Children in all of these situations require continued psychosocial as well as physical care. This care must be a unified team approach involving not only the staff of the nephrology unit, but the in-patient pediatric units and those providing care for the child in the community. All of those involved should see the child's problem realistically, but realize that this child has the potential to lead a normal life in many ways. The child and his family need assistance from knowledgeable care-givers in order to achieve maximal normalization.

Specific Developmental Considerations

In order to help the child and family, health care providers must consider the individual child, with his unique cognitive, emotional, and physical developmental levels. Each child also, no matter how young, exhibits individual preferences, coping mechanisms, and temperament which should be considered in planning his care.

Parents who have an infant with renal failure need support and assistance in accepting this imperfect infant. While both parents may—during the pregnancy—idealize their expected child, an infant with renal failure certainly does not resemble the "Gerber baby." In addition, parents may have experienced great anxiety about their coming baby, an emotion which is now confirmed.[5] One very important way new parents can be helped is to involve them in the care of their infant; after all, it is their baby. While assisting them to feel confident in providing normal care for their child, they can learn much from health care workers about the child's illness and the special care which it necesitates, thereby gaining a feeling of confidence. Feeling comfortable in caring for their infant will facilitate their incorporation of the child into the family.

A sick toddler is almost a contradiction in terms. Toddlers normally are growing rapidly, moving rapidly, and asserting their independence. Toddlers in renal failure grow poorly and typically look much younger than they actually are. This is the ideal time to intervene in order to prevent the "poor little thing" syndrome. Again, expectations can dictate behavior, and small size may lead to infantile behavior. Engaging the toddler in normal activities including active play, interactions with other children, and simple but honest explanations of the illness can help the child to view himself realistically.

Preschool children go further in achieving independence. This is a good time to begin to involve the child in activities outside the home. Not only does this give the care-giver, usually the mother, some much-needed relief from constant care, but the child begins to achieve a degree of independence in a gradual manner as he copes with the added responsibilities. If the child is currently receiving in-center dialysis, school schedules and his treatment schedules will need to be coordinated. Waiting until first grade or age 6 to expose the child with renal failure to the world outside his home may produce severe stresses in the child and his family, resulting in a reluctance to attend school.

School-age children with renal failure or those in a posttransplant state should be considered as individuals functioning within a family and community. In the past, all too frequently, these children remained at home, going out only for dialysis or for clinic visits. More recently, these children have become or remained involved in church groups and activities, including physical education and clubs. This facilitates normal development and enables the school-age child to see himself as a capable individual, involved in his community and with peers.

Adolescents can be among the most frustrating pediatric patients because of their inconsistencies and egocentricity. However, adolescence is a crucial developmental stage for the child with renal problems. Body image is very important to the adolescent. Renal failure causes many obvious physical changes including pallor, wasting, and delayed puberty. Posttransplant steroids may cause acne, a cushingnoid facial appearance, increased hair growth, and continued growth failure. It can require much ingenuity and creativity from families and care-givers to help the adolescent to have a positive self-image.

An additional consideration is the developing sexuality of the adolescent with chronic renal failure. Sexuality is a normal part of development, but one which is too often ignored. When dealing with adolescent sexuality, the focus is frequently problematic rather than developmental, concentrating on venereal disease, unwanted pregnancy, and abortion. Adolescents with chronic disease need assistance with sexual development. Achieving intimate relationships with peers influences the achievement of independence and the promotion of a normal life style.[6]

Achieving independence is one of the major tasks of adolescence and young adulthood. This can be very difficult for the adolescent and the family, particularly if there has been little preparation in previous years. Parents may recognize the need for the adolescent to achieve independence but can not quite bring themselves to trust anyone, even the adolescent himself, with the care they have given for many years.

COMMON PROBLEMS

Discipline

One of the problems families frequently have questions about is that of discipline. Discipline can help a child to feel secure within the limits of his world and also will make his behavior much more sociably acceptable. Discipline is a normal part of a child's life and development. Most often when parents ask the members of the health care team about disciplining their child, they get one of the two answers. Either, "Discipline him just as you do your other children" or they are given a personal philosophy of discipline. Neither is helpful.

In order to discipline an ill child, families have first to deal with their guilt about this child's illness. This makes it almost impossible to "discipline as you do the others." In addition, a family's normal method of discipline may be to spank, and it is virtually impossible to safely spank a child with three drainage tubes and an external shunt. In this case, the family may need assistance in modifying methods of discipline.

Guiding parents to see the necessity of setting limits for the child's security and development usually helps. It also helps to point out that allowing the child free rein may lead to intolerable testing by the child, an explosion of anger from the parent, and subsequent severe punishment or even child abuse. In addition, parents should be helped to set priorities for discipline since their "guilt tolerance" may make it impossible to set limits in all areas.

Fear of Death

An ever-present concern of the families of children with renal failure is the fear of imminent death, no matter how remote this possibility may seem to an objective observer. The child and his family will need support when another child with the same condition dies. Families of children with any chronic illness come to know others through hospitalization, clinics, and support groups. It is better to deal honestly and factually with the death while considering the privacy of both families. An additional consideration is that families need continuing support from health care providers known to them after the death of a child. Particularly if the illness has been severe and lengthy, as is usually the case with renal failure, the initial reaction may be relief, followed by guilt and sorrow as a reaction to the relief felt initially. Family members need to have the opportunity to express these feelings to someone with whom they have established a trusting relationship.

While the care of children in renal failure is complex, these children can be helped to become satisfied, productive members of society. There is little, if any, point in the physical survival of a child if he remains dependent and unable to function. Through the use of thoughtful assessment of the child and family, planning of creative, individualized intervention and thoughtful, long-term follow-up, these children and their families can achieve a relatively normal life as well as one which is satisfying and productive.

REFERENCES

1. RILEY, C. M. Thoughts about kidney homotransplantation in children. *Journal of Pediatrics*, 1964, *65*, 797–800.
2. KORSCH, B. M., FINE, R. N., GRUSHKIN, C. M., and NEGRETE, V. F. Experiences with children and their families during extended hemodialysis and kidney transplantation. *Pediatric Clinics of North America*, 1971, *18*, 625–637.
3. SIMMONS, R. G., KLEIN, S. D., and SIMMONS, R. L. *Gift of life.* New York: John Wiley and Sons, 1977.
4. DUVALL, E. M. *Family development.* 4th Ed. New York: J. B. Lippincott, 1971.
5. CAPLAN, G. *Principles of preventive psychiatry.* New York: Basic Books, 1964.
6. FRAUMAN, A. C., and SYPERT, N. S. Sexuality in adolescents with chronic illness. *The American Journal of Maternal Child Nursing*, 1979, *4*, 371–375.

18
Children and Adolescents on Hemodialysis and Transplantation Programs

STEPHEN ARMSTRONG

I try not to sound like Woody Allen when I say this, because while the point is made more tolerable by humor, we tend to forget the pain of it also. The thesis is that we forget the universal fact of death, we who are pledged to treat illness; we forget and repress the pain of death and the psychological demands that death makes upon us as an inevitable fact of our lives. We tend to do this more with children and adolescents than with adults, because a child's death strikes us as untimely and cruel, a life cut short, an event worse than tragic because children and adolescents are innocent and we, as adults, partake of their spotlessness and assumed longevity. In treating children and adolescents, therefore, we must attend not only to their growth, habilitation, and promise in life, but also to our capacities to remember and tolerate untimely death, loss, or grief.

THE CHILD OR ADOLESCENT'S GROWTH

All psychological develoment occurs in the context of biologi-cal–physiological–medical parameters.[1] Over the course of childhood a disabled child learns to understand and appreciate the unique aspects of his physical disability, in as best a way as possible. A 6-year-old on a mixed child–adult dialysis unit wondered whether Mr. B's machine "got angry" when it beeped. The thought certainly is age-appropriate and was expressed clearly to the treatment staff. (The moon, after all, "rests" when it goes down; the sun is "sad" on cloudy days, and dreams are "like a movie in my head when I sleep.")

Because the patient has to invest so much energy to understand the circumstances of the illness and treatment, however, the understand-

STEPHEN ARMSTRONG, PH.D. • Associate Clinical Professor, Tufts University School of Medicine; Pediatric Psychology, Baystate Medical Center, Springfield, Massachusetts.

ings may not parallel chronological development; they may not develop properly; or objective meanings may fuse with specific emotional meanings.

An 18-year-old on the same unit withdrew into sleep, under a sheet, during all dialysis treatments. His reason? He said that "people and the machines remind me of angry things going off that I can't stop." (This reasoning is also animistic.)

I find there are three "loaded" understandings that children and adolescents need help with, merely as a part of their development. First is the notion of the iatrogenicity of treatments,[2] second is the sick role,[3] and, third, the developmental notion of independence and separation from the family of origin.[4]

First, iatrogenicity: I find that most children and adolescents are smart and can spot a "con" pretty accurately. They know that "sticks" can hurt, people can and do get sick as a result of the treatment, and nobody gives away unmixed blessings. Adolescents in particular will not tolerate a lie in regard to problems of treatment "making me feel worse." For one thing, adolescents think that a lie is directed at them personally (as opposed to an adult's conception of an impersonal "professional lie")—and, looked at from an age-normative point of view, the adolescent is justified in thinking so; certainly many of his peers think so.

"Did that hurt?" asked the nurse.

"Yes," replied the 15-year-old.

"Shouldn't have," the nurse replied (a professional lie, since the procedure hurts most people most of the time). The nurse has now undermined her treatment alliance with the adolescent, and he will now spend the next 4 hours testing her veracity. Does she have a boyfriend? Does she smoke dope? Does she remember to take him off the machine at noon? All because she does not want to say that she missed the stick, or that the pills taste lousy, or that the treatment does, on occasion, make one feel badly.

Second, the "sick role": Assuming that the transplantation program or hemodialysis program works routinely, the ill child is returned to "healthy" society (family or school) with notions of doing what healthy kids do—yet not quite. And when things do not go well, the child must signal, one way or another, reentry into the sick position. To the extent that the child, parents, teachers, nurses, and physicians have confused views about how many "normal standards" are not required when the child is "sick," the "sick" and "well" roles also are confused, and the child withdraws farther (from the adults around) and must rely on "special" or "private" communication channels through selected persons. These private channels are often misunderstood, which is when the psychiatric consultant gets called in.

Third, independence and separation: We tend to assume that adolescents become separate, independent adults who live away from their families. Yet they come from childhoods stratified by sick roles, tight bonding to parental and medical figures, and the mortification of illness. An ill child would be crazy to separate from the family of origin, and would likely die. A number of adolescents think the same way and would do almost anything, including destroy a healthy transplant, rather than separate completely from their families of origin.[4]

THE FAMILY CONTEXT

Not too many recommendations are available routinely to siblings of sick children, since (the sib feels that) nearly everyone focuses on the sick child. How is the sib to handle jealousy, or guilt, or "survivor guilt," or support his or her parents through stress? How are parents to get on with the problems of developing the family's life, when there may be a periodically empty seat at the table, or the meal has to be specially prepared anyway?

I have found it useful to classify families on three dimensions[7] because it helps me think through exactly where I need to put some therapeutic energy:

1. The family's developmental age. Is this a young family, just starting out, or an older couple with a last child? What do they imagine doing with each other in 10 or 15 years; where will they be living? And what did they expect when they began having children years ago?

2. Subsystem relationships[8]. Family therapists like to think of the marital dyad and children as "subsystems" in the family, and each subsystem relates to all others in characteristic ways[9]. Is one child isolated from, or in conflict with, the others? Do the parents support one another, or are they "split" (as to how they see the "sick role")?

3. Emotional structure. Children are fanatically loyal to parents when they think the parents are under stress or that the family may fall apart. Yet who sets the tone for loyalty in the family? Are the children responsible for this, or can the parents provide loyalty to the children, to help the kids work out competition, jealousy, or guilt with the ill child? Who has authority, who disciplines, and who cares?

THE CONTEXT OF TREATMENT

I usually find some professionals on the dialysis or transplant unit who are upset with the physicians, for one reason or another, some of which may be valid. Yet we must underline also the stringent ethical standards[10] that physicians must adhere to, as well as the personal standard of risking failure in attempting to improve the child's or adolescent's treatment.[11] These standards imply an unusual amount of character on the physician's part, which is why alleged "lapses" tend to be seen in such overcast light. In close proximity to a threatened death, this light can be terribly oppressive; at such moments we must try to remember our fears about death also.

The treatment for chronic renal failure comes in four types for children and adolescents. A number of results provide psychologically descriptive commentaries, which I mention briefly; but I have found no single report to be truly "integrative" of the psychology of each treatment, and I suspect that many readers would find some of these reports antiquated or below their own level of clinical experience.

Transplant Alone[12–16]

The central concerns with children are surgical risk, rejection risk, and the psychological response to a relatively large, palpable organ donated by someone else, perhaps through that person's own death.

Transplant Donation[17–20]

Child or adolescent donors are subject to "higher" donation criteria than are adult donors. Their legal, medical, and ethical rights require very careful inspection.

Combined Dialysis and Transplant Programs[21,22]

Combined programs tend to be more acceptable from the treatment staff's point of view than unitary dialysis-alone programs; but the long-term psychological differences are not clear yet.

Dialysis Alone

The central questions in these programs involve: what age to begin treatment[23]; the cumulative deficits in development in children[21,24–26] or pre-adolescents[27]; and the handling of a child's or adolescent's anxiety reactions to dialysis.[28,30] There is one case report[31] of severe psychological deterioration on dialysis, linked to a child's feelings of being psychologically abandoned by parents to a hopeless treatment.

STAFF REACTIONS

I mentioned before our universal pledge to health and intense ambivalence about death. These are hardly new observations,[32,33], but they are amplified with children, as the note of Salisbury[31] demonstrates. I would like to make a point of a negative case example and a second example, positive, to underline how strong the staff feelings can run.

An 11-year-old girl was admitted to the hospital with acute and chronic renal failure. She was edematous, hypertensive, anuric, and in congestive heart failure. Her acute problems were managed apropriately, and 2 months later she was accepted for the chronic hemodialysis protocol, which calls for kidney transplantation as soon as possible.

The psychiatric consultant who evaluated her then found her to be immature, depressed about her illness, and mourning the hospital separation from her parents. The social worker found the parents' cooperation deficient. The physicians felt a powerful ethical commitment to treat her, even though her prognosis was guarded. Because of the parents' poor engagement in the treatment, physicians were nonplussed and made no effort to clarify treatment responsibilities, risks, liabilities, or priorities with the parents.

The patient was dialyzed three times per week, and underwent a bilateral nephrectomy after 7 months. Histological sections revealed chronic pyelonephritis. She received a cadaveric transplant 9 months post onset, but the graft rejected and had to be removed. Medical complications required hospitalization for 5 months further.

Throughout that period the patient's mother refused to visit her. The nursing notes mentioned the patient's "wish to die, and get out of this world," or noticed her crying, wanting her mother, refusing to eat, or sleeping most of the day.

After leaving the hospital, blood potassium levels, never having been higher than 5.5 mEq/liter, rose slowly to toxic levels. At this time, unknown to her physicians, the girl began eating noxious substances when unsupervised at home. She received out-patient hemodialysis for another 8 months, but her condition deteriorated. The staff noted her excessive appetite at the clinic and suspected that the girl was not being fed well at home.

At the clinic it was noted that she kept pulling out some of her hair, that she rarely had been bathed, and that her clothes were filthy. New clothes were given to her by the nurses but never were worn, and the mother did not respond to the staff's questions about them. Another psychiatric consultant found the patient in genuine despair. The parents refused to meet with the consultant.

The patient was readmitted to the hospital because of seizures at 23 months post onset. The blood potassium level was then 6.9 mEq/liter and the pH was 6.95. For the first time the child acknowledged eating noxious substances such as wooden match heads, cigarette paper, and brick mortar. She ate at least one book of matches 2 days prior to admission and four wooden match heads about 18 hours prior to admission. Her parents reported finding a whole box of wooden matches with the heads chewed off. Shortly after admission the potassium concentrated in her blood reached 8.8 mEq/liter. (The toxic component in matches is potassium chlorate. Sixty wooden matches or

90 book matches contain 1 gm of potassium chlorate, a lethal dose for children.)

On psychiatric consultation the girl would not communicate at all. She was disoriented, unable to concentrate or to express any feelings. She picked scabs on her hands apparently without pain. After improving with hospital dialysis, she was returned home.

Two weeks later, when she was brought again to the emergency room, she was dead, having died almost 2 years to the day since she first came to the hospital for kidney disease. Blood studies indicated a potassium level of 8.0 mEq/liter and autopsy showed stomach contents consistent with ingestion of a large number of matches.

Her parents again found several books of headless matches at home. I think it is fair to say that the physicians and nurses went through agony with the child and that everyone was disappointed that their treatments, which offer such life-sustaining promises, proved so ineffective in the face of the child's psychological abandonment. The staff itself had to confront the temptation to abandon her in the midst of her awful difficulties.

As much as physicians and nurses can give and help children in treatment, they must have channels for their concerns away from the day-to-day, sometimes morbid, aspects of their work. Thus, readers will understand how salutory have been the following experiences for the nurses, technicians, and physicians who started a summer camp for children and young adolescents on dialysis.

Camp Okawehna (a Seneca Word Meaning "Kidney")

The idea started one Friday afternoon, at a "happy hour," when we were musing over some of the youngsters we knew who had returned, unhappily, from an Easter Seals camp. The clinic's head nurse contacted the only other camp we had heard of, a 4-bed unit in northern New York, for information. We decided that we did not want to build a "clinic in the woods," so some volunteer nurses started looking for camps that we could rent within easy driving distance of the home clinic. By now the idea had taken off, and one nurse found some church leaders who had a church camp about 40 miles out of town. The primary nephrologist found a pediatric nephrologist who would come to the camp with his family, and a number of other people started thinking of financial and program support.

The first year has 27 children from the southeast United States for one week, and subsequent years have enrolled more children; other clinics' staff have donated their time in planning both the program and the financing. The activities are designed to treat these youngsters much as other children, and include such things as nature hikes, vollyball games, relay races, crafts, swimming, movies, flag-raisings, mail calls, softball games, singing, campfires, and awards ceremonies—and, of course, meals. There have been all-week scavenger hunts, talent shows, and flag-making for individual cabins.

The talent shows have been what one might expect from kids who know a lot about medicine and who need to poke fun at it. One was titled

"M*U*S*H—Medicine Undergoes Severe Harassment," with a plot line about transplantation, looking for a missing organ in a nurse.

One transplanted girl was surprised to find that one of the "normal" looking adults was herself a transplant recipient. She found this out while they were walking together and the girl tripped. She reached out for the adult's arm and felt the buzz of a fistula, and it dawned on the youngster that the adult was one of "them."

An obvious benefit of the camp is that the children had new reference points for their lives; instead of being a "child on dialysis," they were members of cabins, teams, or groups, wherein identity derived from the group, not a medical treatment.

Many of the clinics had sent notes to the home clinic saying that such-and-such a child was "whiny, crying," or depressed. To be sure, there were some homesick pangs, but we have found little evidence for childhood depression or estrangement from the camp.

The Camp Okawehna experience underlines six aspects of child and adolescent development:

1. The camp reduces the child's world to a microcosm that is handleable, masterable.
2. The camp creates a social microcosm with other children, a spirit and life that is communicable, expressive, and expansive.
3. The inevitable conflicts that do arise between children, or between children and adults, are played out in a medium that does not require elaborate cognitive or verbal skills, in action, with symbolic representation made concrete; this is in contrast to conflicts that arise on dialysis or transplant units, those that do require elaborate emotional and cognitive development.
4. The camp has the quality of playfulness and transience, as light does on water, delightful and fluid.
5. For the staff, the camp is a safe sublimation and extroversion of the fear of death; it is creative, fully invested, and reduces guilt for having hurt a child in treatment.
6. The camp creates its own history for the staff, a history that forestalls time and creates a group cohesion; pain, and death, are less readily apparent.

These two examples indicate how much we need "normal" developmental experiences—being "held tight," warmly, in a strong family, and going to camp—to bring up children and adolescents on dialysis and transplant programs. These examples point out how important it is that we remember how to play, to run, to jump, to dance lightly in life, how we can temporarily anaesthetize the pain of loss and the treatments themselves, and how many different ways we and the children each walk along our own life's path. Thus, there can be no single best collection of precepts for bringing children and adolescents into adulthood on dialysis and transplantation regimes. We merely have to be aware of our own sense of death and to provide what health we can, normally.*

ACKNOWLEDGMENTS. The case history of the 11-year-old girl is taken from an article published in the *Journal of the Tennessee Medical Association*. Some of the material on Camp Okawehna was published in an article in *Dialysis and Transplantation*.

REFERENCES

1. HARDING, R. K., HELLER, J. R., and KESLER, R. W. The chronically ill child in the primary care setting. *Primary Care*, 1979, 6, 311–324.
2. CALLAND, C. H. Iatrogenic problems in end-stage renal failure. *New England Journal of Medicine*, 1972, 287, 334–336.
3. CALLAHAN, E. M., CARROLL, S., and REVIER, S. P. The "sick role" in chronic illness: Some reactions. *Journal of Chronic Diseases*, 1966, 19, 883–897.
4. ARMSTRONG, S., JOHNSON, K., and HOPKINS, J. Stopping immunosuppressant therapy following successful kidney transplantation: Two year follow-up. In N. Levy (Ed.), *Psychonephrology I: Psychological factors in hemodialysis and transplantation*. New York: Plenum, 1981, pp. 247–254.
5. DE-NOUR, A. Adolescents' adjustment to chronic hemodialysis. *American Journal of Psychiatry*, 1979, 136, 430–433.
6. GRUSHKIN, C. M., KORSCH, B. M., and FINE, R. N. The outlook for adolescents with chronic renal failure. *Pediatric Clinics of North America*, 1973, 20, 953–963.
7. TSENG, W. S., and McDERMOTT, J. F. Triaxial family classification: A proposal. *American Academy of Child Psychiatry Journal*, 1979, 18, 22–43.
8. DROTAR, D., GANOFSKY, M. A., MAKKER, S., and DeMAIO, D. A family-oriented supportive approach to dialysis and renal transplantation in children. In N. B. Levy (Ed.), *Psychonephrology I. Psychological factors in hemodialysis and transplantation*. New York: Plenum, 1981, pp. 79–92.
9. KOSSORIS, P. Family therapy, an adjunct to hemodialysis and transplantation. *American Journal of Nursing*, 1970, 70, 1730–1733.
10. CURRAN, W. J., and BEECHER, H. K. Experimentation in children. *Journal of the American Medical Association*, 1969, 210, 77.
11. FOX, R. C., and SWAZEY, J. P. *The courage to fail: A social view of organ transplant and dialysis*. Chicago: University of Chicago Press, 1974.
12. BERNSTEIN, D. M. After transplantation—the child's emotional reactions. *American Journal of Psychiatry*, 1971, 127, 1189–1193.
13. FINE, R. N., EDELBROCK, H. H., RIDDELL, H., MALEKZADEH, M. H., PENNIST, A. J., ETTENGER, R. B., VITTENBOGAART, C. H., and KORSCH, B. M. Renal transplantation in children. *Urology*, 1977, 9, 61–71.
14. FINE, R. N., KORSCH, B. M., STILES, Q., RIDDELL, H., EDELBROCK, H. H., BRENNA, L. P., GRUSHKIN, C. M., and LIEBERMAN, E. Renal homotransplantation in children. *Journal of Pediatrics*, 1970, 76, 347–357.

*For more information on Camp Okawehna, contact Jeanne Hopkins, R.N., The Dialysis Clinics, Inc., 1714 Hayes Street, Nashville, Tennessee, 37212.

15. KORSCH, B. M., NEGRETE, V. F., GARDNER, J. E., WEINSTOCK, C. L., MERCER, A. S., GRUSHKIN, C. M., and FINE, R. N. Kidney transplantation in children. Psychosocial follow-up study on child and family. *Journal of Pediatrics*, 1973, *83*, 339–408.

16. MALEKZADEH, M. H., PENNIST, A. J., UITTENBOGAART, C. H., KORSCH, B. M., FINE R. N., and MAIN, M. E. Current issues in pediatric renal transplantation. *Pediatric Clinics of North America*, 1976, *23*, 857–872.

17. BERNSTEIN D. M., and SIMMONS, R. G. The adolescent kidney donor: The right to give. *American Journal of Psychiatry*, 1974, *131*, 1338–1343.

18. FOST, N. Children as renal donors. *New England Journal of Medicine*, 1977, *296*, 363.

19. LEWIS, M. Kidney donation by a 7 year-old identical twin child: Psychological, legal, and ethical considerations. *American Academy of Child Psychiatry Journal*, 1974, *13*, 221–245.

20. SWENSON, O., GIVEN, G., KING, L. R., INDRISS, F. S., and HARRIS, N. L. Kidney transplants in children. *Journal of Pediatric Surgery*, 1971, *6*, 245.

21. KHAN, A., HERNDON, C. H., and AHMADIAN, S. Social and emotional adaptation of children with transplanted kidneys and chronic hemodialysis. *American Journal of Psychiatry*, 1971, *127*, 1194–1198.

22. SAMPSON, T. F. The child in renal failure: Emotional impact of the treatment on the child and his family. *American Academy of Child Psychiatry Journal*, 1975, *14*, 462–476.

23. RAIMBAULT, G., and ROYER, P. L'enfant et son image de la maladie. *Archives Francaise Pediatrique*, 1967, *24*, 445–462.

24. FINE, R. N., KORSCH, B. M., GRUSHKIN, C. M., and LIEBERMAN, E. Hemodialysis in children. *American Journal of Diseases of Children*, 1970, *119*, 498–504.

25. FINE, R. N., DePALMA, J. R., LIEBERMAN, E., DONNLL, G. N., GORDON, A., and MAXWELL, M.H. Extended hemodialysis in children with chronic renal failure. *Journal of Pediatrics*, 1968, *73*, 706–713.

26. GRUSHKIN, C. M., KORSCH, B., and FINE, R. N. Hemodialysis in small children. *Journal of the American Medical Association*, 1972, *221*, 869–873.

27. HUTCHINGS, R. H., HICKMAN, R., and SCRIBNER, B. H. Chronic hemodialysis in a pre-adolescent. *Pediatrics*, 1966, *37*, 68–73.

28. KALLEN, R. J., ZALTZMAN, S., COE, F. L., and METCOFF, J. Hemodialysis in children. *Medicine*, 1966, *45*, 1–50.

29. DROTAR, D. The treatment of a severe anxiety reaction in an adolescent boy following renal transplantation. *American Academy of Child Psychiatry Journal*, 1975, *14*, 451–462.

30. SAMPSON, T. F. Use of fantasy for conflict resolution in the pediatric hemodialysis patient. In N. B. Levy (Ed.), *Psychonephrology I: Psychological factors in hemodialysis and transplantation.* New York: Plenum, 1981, pp. 177–184.

31. SALISBURY, R. E. Behavioral responses of a nine year-old child on chronic dialysis. *American Academy of Child Psychiatry Journal*, 1968, *7*, 282–295.

32. EISENDRATH, R. M. The role of grief and fear in the death of kidney transplant patients. *American Journal of Psychiatry*, 1969, *126*, 381–387. ·

33. GELFMAN, M., and WILSON, E. S. Emotional reactions in a renal unit. *Comprehensive Psychiatry*, 1972, *13*, 283–290.

19

Biopsychosocial Evaluation of Sexual Function in End-Stage Renal Disease

KATHLEEN DEGEN, JAMES J. STRAIN, AND BARNETT ZUMOFF

INTRODUCTION

This paper discusses the prevalence of sexual dysfunction in end-stage renal disease (ESRD); the biologic, psychologic, and social aspects of sexual dysfunction; and finally, the evaluation process itself.

PREVALENCE

The prevalance of sexual dysfunction in end-stage renal disease is quite remarkable, as high as 100% according to some studies.[1,2] In uremic men, 28–88%[3-5] have partial or total impotence and/or difficulty in ejaculating and 44–100%[6,2] report decrease in frequency of intercourse and/or decrease in libido. Some studies indicate that sexual functioning may improve on dialysis[5]; others report a decline. Levy found that 49% of 202 men reported their sexual problem to be worse on dialysis, 12% reported improvement, and 39% reported no change.[6] These studies were based on unstructured or structured interviews or self-administered questionnaires. Karacan's study of five uremic men using nocturnal penile tumescence measured by Strain Gauge Manometer during REM sleep reported in 1978[7] indicated a considerable reduction in total tumescence time during sleep in patients with end-stage renal

KATHLEEN DEGEN, M.D. • Assistant Clinical Professor of Psychiatry, Columbia University College of Physicians and Surgeons; Assistant Attending Psychiatrist, Consultation–Liaison Service, St. Luke's-Roosevelt Hospital Center, St. Luke's Site, New York, New York. JAMES J. STRAIN, M.D. • Professor of Clinical Psychiatry, Director, Psychiatry Consultation–Liaison Service, Mt. Sinai School of Medicine, City University of New York, New York. BARNETT ZUMOFF, M.D. • Chief, Division of Endocrinology and Metabolism, Department of Medicine, Beth Israel Medical Center, New York, New York.

disease, despite comparable total sleep duration relative to age-matched, randomly selected, normal population controls. The decrease persists in both the night before and night after dialysis. He also found a significant decrease in the number of tumescence episodes on the night preceding dialysis.

In summary, the types of sexual dysfunction encountered by ESRD patients are:

1. Inhibited sexual desire (decrease or loss of libido) in men and women[8]
2. Partial or total impotence (erectile dysfunction)
3. Difficulty in ejaculating in males; insufficient or absent lubrication in females[8]

Very little is known about impairment of the orgastic phase in females. One would expect orgastic phase dysfunction in females also, paralleling male ejaculatory difficulty, just on a purely physiologic basis. In fact, Golden and Milne in their study reported 6 out of 11 women had less frequent orgasms or loss of orgasmic response.[8]

Biologic dysfunction in male and female ESRD patients can be due to any of the following:

1. Drugs: Antihypertensives such as methyl dopa (an alpha blocker) or reserpine interfere with the orgasmic phase; anticholinergics given to control itching, for example, periactin or benedryl, interfere with the excitement phase
2. Autonomic neuropathy: giving hypo- or hyper-esthesia, which interferes with sensation and muscle contraction (the orgasmic phase)
3. Vascular disease (adequate engorgement of genitals in men and women and lubrication in women can't take place)
4. Hemotologic—low hematocrit (some patients experience a return of desire and sexual capacity after blood transfusion)
5. Endocrine abnormality.

Vascular disease is often the sequela of long-standing hypertension and/or diabetes mellitis and is connected in many patients with their renal failure. Common endocrine abnormalities reported in uremic men are as follows:

Subnormal plasma levels of triiodothyroine[9,10,11] and testosterone[9,12,13]; elevated prolactin[9,14,15] and cortisol[9,16,17]; and increased lutenizing hormone in about 50%.[18-20] There has been one report concerning the plasma level of adrenal androgens.[9]

In our study at the Steroid Institute at Montefiore Hospital and Medical Center we found decreased 24-hour mean plasma levels of

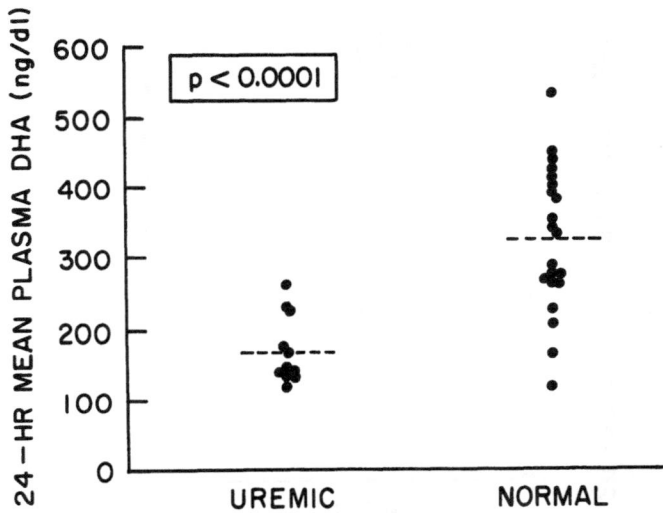

FIG. 1.   Twenty-four-hour mean plasma DHA in normal and uremic men (age-matched).

dehydroisoandrosterone (DHA) and dehydroisoandrosterone sulphate
(DHAS), and high cortisol. Eleven ESRD men were studied.

Figure 1 shows the 24-hour mean plasma dehydroisonandrosterone
in normal and uremic men. The average for uremic men was 164 mg/dl.
The average for 22 age-matched controls was 330 mg/dl with significance
at the 0.0001 level.

Figure 2 shows the 24-hour mean plasma DHAS in normal and uremic men. Uremic men had an average plasma concentration of 40 μg/dl
compared with 21 age-matched normals' concentration of 74 μg/dl. This
is significant at the 0.0005 level.

The biologic effects of DHA and DHAS are not known. There have
been no clinical or animal experimental virilizing effects. Whether they
have any effect on sexual or reproductive functions despite their lack of
virilizing effects remains an open question. What is known is that DHA
and/or DHAS is a major, probably obligatory intermediate in the
biosynthesis of testosterone in the testes (Figure 3). As you can see, cho-
lesterol goes to hydroxipregnenolone which forms either DHA, found to
be low in uremic men, or cortisol, which is high, indicating a probable
defect at the level of activity of the enzyme 17,20 desmolase. A decreased activity of 17,20 desmolase would give a high level of cortisol
and a low level of DHA and testosterone. It has seemed logical to relate
the frequently observed subnormal plasma testosterone levels to the frequently observed erectile dysfunction, but there has not been any clear-
cut demonstration of definite correlation in individual patients, nor has

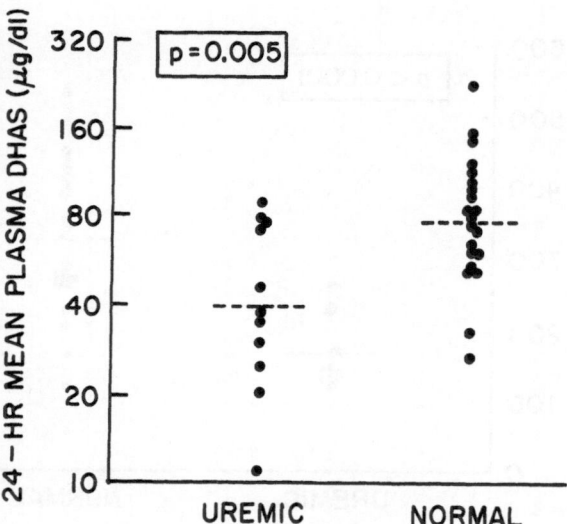

FIG. 2. Twenty-four-hour mean plasma dehydroisoandrosterone sulfate in normal and uremic men (age-matched).

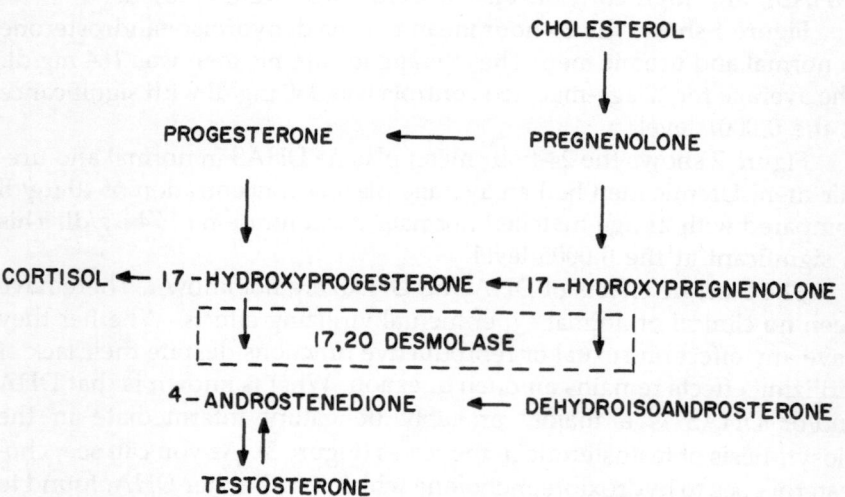

FIG. 3. The low levels of DHA and testosterone and the elevated levels of cortisol in
the uremics clearly imply decreased activity of 17,20-desmolase.

it been shown that testosterone therapy favorably effects the erectile
dysfunction.

Some researchers hypothesize that other abnormalities such as zinc
deficiency are related to erectile dysfunction. In one study zinc was

shown to increase potency in more than half of the patients studied.[21] In 1977 Antoniou et al. conducted a study of eight impotent uremic men in whom no organic or psychological causes could be found. Four patients were treated with zinc, four with a placebo. All four treated with zinc had improved potency and experienced worsening of sexual functioning 4 weeks after zinc was discontinued. This was associated with reduced levels of plasma testosterone. The placebo did not improve sexual functioning or raise testosterone levels in any of the controls, according to this study. However, this was not a blind study. Another abnormality noted is parathyroid hormone increase.[21,23] One study done by Loew et al. in 1975[23] found a significant correlation between the degree of impotence and the magnitude of secondary hyperparathyroidism. Two dialysis patients who were impotent for several years became potent after subtotal parathyroidectomy.

Fischer[24] and Karacan[7,25] and Jovanovic[26] documented that in adult males at least 80% of REM periods of sleep are associated with NPT. A penile circumference increase of 16–20 mm at the tip is a common indicator of normal tumescence. In our study at Montefiore of five uremic patients complaining of erectile dysfunction, only one reached a level of tumescence of 20 mm in one episode.[9] This is below normal for his age. Testimony of the five patients in our study about their erectile difficulties proved to be accurate when assessed by Strain Gauge Manometer measurement of penile tumescence during REM sleep.

Psychologic Aspects

ESRD patients have a number of major psychological stresses to deal with

1. They may experience a loss of function of major organ systems. This may include:

- Loss of erection in males and engorgement and lubrication in females
- Loss of ejaculation in males, of orgasmic capacity in females
- Loss of intercourse
- Loss of procreation[8,27,28]
- Loss of urination[29]

Kaplan De-Nour believes that the loss of or threat of loss of urination causes regression to pregenital stages of development and renewed hypercathexis of urination. She speculates that potency troubles in male uremics may also be due to regression to pregenital stages of development caused by loss of urination.

2. Hemodialysis patients experience loss of what Strain calls "narcissistic integrity,"[30] that is, the loss of the fantasy we all have that we

are invulnerable and omnipotent. These patients have the potential to live very fearful lives in not being able to deny their vulnerability and mortality.

3. They often experience fear or concerns about punishment, that is, illness is viewed as a punishment for some wrongdoing or past sin. Also, the machine for some patients may represent an omnipotent, castrating parent who is punishing them for some wrongdoing. One patient, when asked what he felt was responsible for his sexual dysfunction, said angrily, "the machine did it." He was unable to elaborate how or why the machine had done it.[31]

4. Some patients may become concerned about their loss of control. Certainly they have to submit to a great deal of care-taking by the technicians, nurses, and physicians. Their skin has to be cleaned; needles have to be put in; the pressure of the dialysis machine, their blood pressure and electrolyte balance must be constantly monitored; and so forth. Some patients may actually experience a very strong activation of dependency wishes—feelings of helplessness and the wish to return to an infantile state—and this could conceivably interfere with their sexual performance.

5. Many express intense fear about the possible loss of erectile capacity (males) and orgasmic capacity (females), and that this will lead to other losses, for example loss of a spouse, self-esteem, loss of value to others. For males, erectile capacity seems tied to their sense of themselves as men to the extent that decreased or absent erectile capacity means they are no longer men, either in their own eyes or those of others. Sexual capacity in women does not seem to be so important in stabilizing a feminine identity, and most can still regard themselves as female when they experience diminished or absent sexual function. This speculation, however, warrants further study.

SOCIAL ASPECTS

Social stress in ESRD includes:

1. Arousal of stranger anxiety. ESRD patients have to deal with a large number of health care providers, nurses, technicians, social workers, and physicians. Turnover of staff, at least at the Bronx Dialysis Unit, was great, so that the patients often have to get used to unfamiliar people, which is stressful.

2. Fear of unfamiliar places is also aroused. Given the wide variety of complications of their illness, ESRD patients frequently have to receive care in a number of different facilities, for example, the dialysis unit, blood bank or transfusion unit, in-patient service, neurologist's of-

fice, endocrinologist's office, cardiologist's office, dermatologist's office, and so forth. They have a disease which eventually involves virtually every other system in their bodies, and fear about unfamiliar places and situations is a social stress of considerable dimension.

3. Most of the patients talk openly about their fear of loss of love and approval. That is, as a sick person they fear they will no longer be loved by their friends and family. This fear often becomes a reality.[31-33] Separation and divorce, and the frequency of infidelity of spouses are very explicit parameters of loss of love and approval. These occurrences are very high among dialysis patients. We know from the social readjustment rating scale of Holmes and Rahe,[31] that the first three ranked events in terms of stressfulness were death of a spouse, divorce, and marital separation, and that these social readjustments received a very high correlation with onset of illness. We consider sexual dysfunction to be a significant illness which impairs the quality of most patients' lives.

4. They also fear economic deprivation due to loss of jobs and high medical expenses, and this fear all too often become a reality. Often these patients lose jobs which, in addition to providing financial stability, also contributed to their self-esteem, as they could feel pride in being hard-working, productive members of society. This important source of social gratification is totally, or at least partially, lost.

All of the psychologic and social aspects discussed lend credence to the theory that the sexual dysfunctions of uremic patients may also have a psychosocial basis. Certainly, sexual dysfunction has psychological and social consequences.

EVALUATION

Biopsychosocial sectors of inquiry in the evaluation of sexual dysfunction in ESRD should always be performed so that the treatment can address the major areas of difficulty in each sector.

Biological

The biological evaluation should include a thorough medical history with a detailed account of current medication and dose. Evidence which would suggest a purely psychosocial disorder is:

1. A negative medical history.
2. A negative drug history (prescribed and non-prescribed drugs).
3. A transient dysfunction (that is, less than 6 weeks duration).

4. A dysfunction that is present with spouse, absent with lover.
5. A patient's ability to masturbate to orgasm.
6. The presence of morning erections.

Actually in the seven uremic patients interviewed at the Bronx Dialysis Center, none of these six clinical aspects occurred. That is, they had a positive medical history, positive drug history (prescribed drugs), persistence with a lover (or partner other than spouse), could not masturbate to orgasm, and had an absence of morning erections.

A physical examination should be performed with special attention to the vasculature, musculature, and neurolgic status of the genitalia. Angiography and nerve conduction studies can be used for objective correlation.

Laboratory examination should include:

1. CBC.
2. SMAC 25.
3. Serum zinc.
4. Triiodothyrodine.
5. Parathyroid hormone.
6. Follicular-stimulating hormone (FSH), prolactin, luteinizing hormone, estrogen.
7. 24-hour hormone studies of adrenal androgens, if available.
8. Nocturnal penile tumescence (NPT) during REM sleep on two successive nights, if possible, for men,[35] and plethysmography for women,[36] if available.

These determinations can help differentiate whether the sexual dysfunction is primarily biological. If you find a patient has a primarily biologic dysfunction, for example, a hemotocrit of 17, your first treatment intervention would not be to send that patient for sex therapy, but to correct the low hematocrit.

Psychological

The psychological evaluation should include past psychiatric history and screening via structured questionnaire for depression, psychosis, hypochondriasis, anxiety, and organic brain syndrome. We recommend using the Beck Depression Inventory,[37,38] the Hamilton Anxiety Scale, [39],[40] and the Cognitive Capacity Screening Examination[41] for a more objective screen for depression, anxiety, and organic brain syndrome.

Social

The social evaluation should include:

1. Past social history, including relationship with spouse, living conditions, and economic situation with a work history.
2. Past sexual history and detailed information about the current problem. We find patients are often vague and have to be asked explicit questions.*
3. Evaluation of the spouse, including a psychosexual history. We sometimes get different or additional history. It is important to know if the spouse also has a sexual dysfunction which may require treatment, and how he/she feels about their partner's dysfunction and its treatment. It is also of utmost importance to know whether the partner understands and is willing to cooperate, particularly when treatment may involve them both, such as sex therapy or a penile implant.[42]

SUMMARY

An evaluation of sexual function in all three dimensions—biologic, psychologic, and social—is crucial to the development of the best possible treatment plan specific for the kind of disorder the patient has, a treatment with the greatest chance of success for both the patient and his/her mate.

REFERENCES

1. SCHMITT, G. W., SHEHADEH, I., and SAWIM, C. T. Transient gynecomastia in chronic renal failure during chronic intermittent hemodialysis. *Annals of Internal Medicine*, 1968, *69*, 73–79.
2. PHADKE, A. G., MACKINNON, K. J., and DOSSETOR, J. B. Male fertilty in uremia: Restoration by renal allografts. *Canadian Medical Association Journal*, 1970, *102*, 607–608.
3. BOMMER, J., RITZ, E., TSCHOPE, W., and ANDRASSY, K. Life on haemodialysis. *Lancet*, 1975, *2*, 511.
4. BOMMER, J., TSCHOPE, W., RITZ, E., and ANDRASSY, K. Sexual behavior of hemodialyzed patients. *Clinical Nephrology*, 1976, *6*, 315–318.
5. HARARI, A., MUNITZ, H., and WIJSENBEEK, H. Psychological aspects of chronic haemodialysis. *Psychiatrica Neurologica Neurochirurgica*, 1971, *74*, 219–223.
6. LEVY, N. B. Sexual adjustment to maintenance hemodialysis and renal transplantation: National survey by questionnaire: Preliminary report. *Transactions of American Society for Artificial Internal Organs*, 1973, *19*, 138–143.

*Available on request.

7. KARACAN, I., DERVENT, A., CUNNINGHAM, C., WEINMAN, E., CLEVELAND, S. E., SALIS, P., WILLIAMS, R. L., and KOPEL, K. Assessment of nocturnal penile tumescence as an objective method for evaluating sexual functioning in ESRD patients. *Dialysis and Transplantation*, 1978, *7*, 872–876.

8. GOLDEN, J. and MILNE, J. Somatopsychic sexual problems of renal failure. *Dialysis and Transplantation*, 1978, *7*, 879–890.

9. ZUMOFF, B., WALTER, L., ROSENFELD, R., DEGEN, K., STRAIN, J., STRAIN, G., LEVIN, J., and FUKUSHIMA, D. Subnormal plasma adrenal androgen levels in men with uremia. *Journal of Clinical Endocrinology and Metabolism*, 1980, *51*, 801.

10. SILVERBERG, D. S., ULAN, R. A., FAWCETT, D. M., DOSSETOR, J. B., GRACE, M., and BETTCHER, K. Effects of chronic hemodialysis on thyroid function in chronic renal failure. *Canadian Medical Association Journal*, 1973, *101*, 282–286.

11. RAMIREZ, G., O'NEILL, W., JUBIZ, W., and BLOOMER, H. A. Thyroid dysfunction in uremia: Evidence for thyroid and hypophysial abnormalities. *Annals of Internal Medicine*, 1976, *84*, 672–676.

12. GUPTA, D., and BUNDSCHU, H. D. Testosterone and its binding in the plasma of male subjects with chronic renal failure. *Cllinica Chimica Acta*, 1972, *36*, 479–484.

13. LIM, V. S. and FRANK, V. Restoration of plasma testosterone levels in uremic men with clomiphen citrate. *Journal of Clinical Endocrinology and Metabolism*, 1972, *43*, 1370–1377.

14. RAMIREZ, G., O'NEILL, W., BLOOMER, H. A., and JUBIZ, W. Abnormalities in the regulation of prolactin in patients with chronic renal failure. *Journal of Clinical Endocrinology and Metabolism*, 1977, *45*, 648–661.

15. HAGEN, C., OLGAARD, D., McNEILLY, A. S., and FISHER, R. Prolactin and the pituitary–gonadal axis in male uraemic patients on regular dialysis. *Acta Endocrinologica (KbH)*, 1976, *82*, 29–38.

16. BLAIR, A. J., MORGAN, R. D., and BECK, J. C. The plasma 17-hydroxy-corticosteroid levels in acute and chronic renal failure. *Canadian Journal of Biochemistry and Physiology*, 1961, *39*, 1617–1624.

17. McDONALD, W. J., GOLPER, T. A., MASS, R. D., KENDALL, J. W., PORTER, G. A., GIRARD, D. E., and FISCHER, M. D. Adrenocorticotropin–cortisol axis abnormalities in hemodialysis patients. *Journal of Clinical Endocrinology and Metabolism*, 1979, *48*, 92–95.

18. HALDSWORTH, S., ATKINS, R. C., and DE KRETSER, D. M. The pituitary testicular axis in men with chronic renal failure. *New England Journal of Medicine*, 1977, *296*, 1245–1249.

19. LIM, V. S., and FANG, V. S. Gonadal dysfunction in uremic men. A study of the hypothalamo-pituitary-testicular axis before and after renal transplantation. *American Journal of Medicine*, 1975, *58*, 655–662.

20. BENTLY, M. S., GANS, D., and HORTON, R. Regulation of gonadal function in uremia. *Metabolism*, 1974, *23*, 1065–1072.

21. ANTONIOU, R. D., SHALHOUB, R. J., SUDHAKAR, T., and SMITH, J. C. Reversal of uremic impotence by zinc. *Lancet*, 1977, *2*, 895–899.

22. MASSRY, S. G., GOLDSTEIN, D. A., PROCCI, W. R., and KLETZKY, O. A. Impotence in patients with uremia: A possible role for parathyroid hormone. *Nephron*, 1977, *19*, 305–310.

23. LOEW, H., SCHULTZ, H., and BUSCH G. Klinische aspekte der impotenz mannlichen dauerdia patienten. *Medizinische Welt*, 1975, *26*, 1651–1652.

24. FISCHER, C., GROSS, J., and ZUCH, J. Cycle of penile erection synchronous with dreaming (REM) sleep. *Archives of General Psychiatry*, 1965, *12*, 29–45.

25. KARACAN, I., GOODENOUGH, D. R., SHAPIRO, A., and STARKER, S. Erection cycle during sleep in relation to dream anxiety. *Archives of General Psychiatry*, 1966, *15*, 183–189.
26. JOVANOVIC, U., and NIPPERT, M. Erektionen im schlaf und sexualitat. *Journal of Nervo-Visceral Relations*, Supplement X, 1971, 580–590.
27. BAILEY, G. The sick kidney and sex. *New England Journal of Medicine* 1977, *276*, 1288–1289.
28. SALKIN, M. S. Uremic sex (letter). *New England Journal of Medicine*, 1977, *297*, 725–726.
29. KAPLAN DE-NOUR, A. Some notes on the psychological significance of urination. *Journal of Nervous and Mental Disease*, 1969, *148*, 615–623.
30. STRAIN, J. and GROSSMAN, S. Psychological reactions to medical illness and hospitalization. In J. Strain and S. Grossman (Eds.), *Psycholigical Care of the Medically Ill.* New York: Appleton-Century-Crofts, 1975.
31. DEGEN, K., and STRAIN, J. Unpublished data from research study 1977–79.
32. FINKELSTEIN, F., FINKELSTEIN, S., and STEELE, T. Assessment of marital relationships of hemodialysis patients. *American Journal of the Medical Sciences*, 1976, *271*, 21–28.
33. FRIEDMAN, E. A., GOODWIN, N. J., and CHANDHRY, L. Psychosocial adjustment of family to maintenance hemodialysis. Part II. *New York State Journal of Medicine*, 1970, *70*, 767.
34. HOLMES, T. H., and RAHE, R. H. The Social Readjustment Rating Scale. *Journal of Psychosomatic Research*, 1967, *11*, 213–218.
35. KARACAN, I., DERVENT, A., CUNNINGHAM, G., MOORE, C., WEINMAN, E., CLEVELAND, S. E., SALIS, P., WILLIAMS, R. L., and KOPEL, K. Assessment of nocturnal penile tumescence as an objective method for evaluating sexual functioning in ESRD patients. *Dialysis and Transplantation*, 1978, *7*, 872–922.
36. ABEL, G., MURPHY, W., BECKER, J., and BITAR, A. Womens' vaginal responses during REM sleep. *Journal of Sex and Marital Therapy*, 1979, *5*, 5–14.
37. BECK, A. T. *Depression: Clinical, experimental and theoretical aspects.* New York: Hober Medical Division, Harper and Row, 1967.
38. BECK, A. T., and BEAMESDERFER, A. *Assessment of depression: The depression inventory in psychological measurements of psychoparmacology.* Vol. 7. Basel: Pichot, 1974.
39. HAMILTON, M. The assessment of anxiety states by rating. *British Journal of Medical Psychology*, 1959, *32*, 50–55.
40. HAMILTON, M. Diagnosis and rating of anxiety. In M. H. Lader (Ed.), *Studies of anxiety. British Journal of Psychiatry*, Special Publication, 1969, *3*, 76–79.
41. JACOBS, J., BERNHARD, M., DELGADO, A., and STRAIN, J. J. Screening for organic mental syndromes in the medically ill. *Annals of Internal Medicine*, 1977, *86*, 40–46.
42. SCOTT, F., BYRD, G., KARACAN, I., OLSSON, P., BEUTLER, L. E., and ATTIA, S. Erectile impotence treated with an implantable, inflatable prosthesis. *Journal of the American Medical Association*, 1979, *241*, 2609–2612.

20

Impotence in Uremia
Preliminary Results of a Combined Medical and Psychiatric Investigation

WARREN R. PROCCI, DAVID A. GOLDSTEIN,
OSCAR A. KLETZKY, VITO M. CAMPESE, AND
SHAUL G. MASSRY

BACKGROUND OF THE PROBLEM

End-stage renal disease (ESRD) is a very stressful illness with many possible complications. One of the most disruptive of these potential complications for both males and females is sexual dysfunction. ESRD patients must make many sacrifices and they are required to give up many things. Assaults on their self-esteem are ubiquitous for these individuals. The loss of sexual functioning can deprive the patient of one of the key areas of gratification in his or her life. In this day and age, with so much emphasis on sexuality, the loss of the ability to perform sexually can be devastating to one's self-esteem. While sexual dysfunction had been sporadically mentioned over the course of many years and in numerous reports as a sequela of ESRD,[1,2] it wasn't until Levy's study that a large-scale, systematic analysis of this problem was presented.[3] Basically, Levy performed a national questionnaire survey of the membership of an organization of patients with ESRD of varying degrees. A total of over 500 patients on hemodialysis and with renal transplants were as-

WARREN R. PROCCI, M.D. • Director, Residency Education in Psychiatry, Harbor-UCLA Medical Center, Torrance, California; Visiting Professor of Psychiatry and the Biobehavioral Sciences, University of California at Los Angeles, School of Medicine, Los Angeles, California. DAVID A. GOLDSTEIN, M.D. • Associate Professor of Medicine, University of Southern California School of Medicine, Los Angeles, California. OSCAR A. KLETZKY, M.D. • Associate Professor of Obstetrics and Gynecology, University of Southern California School of Medicine, Los Angeles, California. VITO M. CAMPESE, M.D. • Associate Professor of Medicine, University of Southern California School of Medicine, Los Angeles, California. SHAUL G. MASSRY, M.D. • Professor of Medicine, University of Southern California School of Medicine, Los Angeles, California.

sessed. He found that a high percentage of male patients with ESRD suffered from erectile disturbances while a substantial number of women with ESRD complained of failure to experience arousal and achieve orgasm. A large number of both men and women reported declines in libido. The frequency of intercourse declined appreciably in most of these patients. Approximately 80% of both men and women on maintenance hemodialysis reported either no sexual activity or at most one episode of intercourse per month. Renal transplantation generally afforded some relief but it was in no way a panacea. Persistent deficits in sexual functioning were still noted in many patients. Approximately 60% of transplant recipients had intercourse no more than once a month. Levy speculated that emotional factors probably played a key role in these sexual disturbances. Since this work was reported, a large number of studies have investigated the effects of ESRD upon sexual functioning and, in general, they have provided strong support and confirmation of Levy's findings.[4-16]

Paralleling these psychological studies, there have been a number of studies which have examined the role of sex hormones in males with ESRD.[15,17-27] While there have been some discrepancies in the results of these studies, a general trend has been noted and several findings emerge as relatively constant. Serum testosterone levels are almost always observed to be low. The responsivity of testosterone to stimulatory hormones such as human chorionic gonadotropin or clomiphene has been variable. Follicle-stimulating hormone (FSH) levels in the sera of ESRD males are generally normal although some studies have reported elevations. Luteinizing hormone (LH) appears to be elevated in the sera of approximately 50% of ESRD males. Finally, serum prolactin levels have been observed to be elevated in many of these males although gynecomastia, which frequently coexists with hyperprolactinaemia, has not been noted as a regular occurrence. It has been suggested that the testosterone deficit combined with LH elevation is indicative of an unresponsive testicular end organ while the hypothalamic–pituitary portion of the endocrine axis remain intact. However, at this point in time our understanding of the nature of these hormonal abnormalities in uremic males is indeed incomplete. Similar lines of research have demonstrated menstrual and hormonal abnormalities in uremic women.[28]

SHORTCOMINGS OF PRIOR RESEARCH

Despite the impressive consistency which has been noted in both these lines of research, in truth little is known about the etiology of the sexual dysfunction of ESRD. That a problem exists both in sexual performance (in males and females) and in the hypothalamic–pituitary–gonadal axis (at least in men) is abundantly clear. There are a number of shortcomings of these studies which have precluded a more thorough understanding of these difficulties. First of all, with but few exceptions these psychiatric and hormonal studies exist strictly in parallel. There are scarcely any attempts to correlate and integrate these different lines of data. As a result, it is largely unclear whether or not any of the endocrine deficits are in anyway associated with the impairment of sexual performance. Similarly, there are a substantial number of unresolved questions concerning the role of depression in the sexual dysfunction of ESRD. Levy speculated that depression might play a major role in these sexual disturbances.[3] Despite the fact that depression has long been observed to be a frequent concomitant of ESRD[4,10,11,13] as well as having been recognized as an independent cause of sexual dysfunction,[29] surprisingly little information exists correlating the presence of depression in ESRD patients with sexual dysfunction. A further problem is that none of these studies have compared ESRD patients with a control group of patients suffering from other chronic illnesses. After all, it is possible that the sexual dysfunction noted in ESRD could be the result of the debilitating and depressing effects of severe chronic illness and not specifically related to renal disease *per se*. Also, none of the studies reported to date have attempted to control for the role of aging *per se* upon sexual functioning in ESRD. In general, of course, sexual functioning declines with the aging process. Since most ESRD patients are approaching middle age when maintenance hemodialysis is initiated (National Dialysis Registry statistics demonstrate that the average patient starting maintenance dialytic treatment is in his/her mid forties[30]), it may well be that the effects of the aging process play a significant role in uremic sexual dysfunction. Finally, nearly all of these studies rely exclusively upon interviews or questionnaires for gathering data concerning sexual performance. Few investigators to date have made use of objective mechanical techniques for evaluating sexual capability such as Nocturnal Penile Tumescence (NPT). NPT has been reported to be of enormous value in aiding in the differentiation of organic impotence from psychologically induced impotence.[31] Unfortunately, at the present time, there is no clinical instrument readily available for aiding in the objective evaluation of female sexual dysfunction although there is the promise of the development of such devices. Undoubtedly these shortcomings are a reflection of the fact that the systematic evaluation of sexual functioning in ESRD is still in its early stages. As is often the case for the beginning stages of investigation of a clinical problem, the available research methodology has not yet had the opportunity for the subtle refinements that come with the experience of performing many different studies over the course of many years and learning from the errors and shortcomings of one's predecessors. There simply hasn't been enough work done so far.

A COMBINED MEDICAL AND PSYCHIATRIC INVESTIGATION

At the USC School of Medicine we attempted to design a combined endocrinologic, nephrologic, and psychiatric investigation in order to help clarify some of these confusing questions. This study, conducted at the LAC/USC Medical Center in concert with several of our satellite dialysis units, has limited its focus to males with ESRD. Women were excluded only because there is at present no readily available objective mechanism for assessing their sexual arousability. We have utilized NPT, an objective measure of erectile capacity, in our assessment of the sexual functioning of uremic males. This study included both subjects currently being treated with maintenance hemodialysis and those recently diagnosed as having advanced chronic uremia who were not yet being treated with maintenance hemodialysis. We included subjects in the age range of 18–60. In addition to the NPT evaluation each subject received a detailed current and past sexual history utilizing a semistructured interview conducted by a psychiatrist (WRP). If the patient was married or had a regular sexual partner, an attempt was made to perform a conjoint interview. In order to examine the possible contributory role of depression in producing the sexual dysfunction of ESRD all subjects were carefully assessed for the presence of affective disorder by a thorough clinical interview and mental status examination complimented by three objective tests (Feighner[32], Beck[33], Raskin[34]). In order to examine the role of sexual hormones in these disturbances, we evaluated the hypothalamic–pituitary–testicular axis by obtaining sera for testosterone, FSH, LH, and prolactin levels. In addition, the responsivity of the endocrine axis was assessed by means of stimulation with gonadotropin releasing hormone (GNRH). The intactness of the autonomic nervous system was also studied and to pursue this we utilized a number of techniques including the Valsalva test.

All of the aforementioned studies were performed not only on the ESRD patients but also on two control groups. The first was a group of normal men and the second of these was a group of men with a variety of chronic illnesses but with normal renal functioning. In selecting these subjects with other chronic illnesses we specifically excluded any men with illnesses associated with major neurological or circulatory compromise of the genital region. Diseases such as rheumatoid arthritis, COPD, chronic asthma, chronic gout, and lymphoma or Hodgkin's Disease in remission provided the bulk of this patient sample. Patients with diabetes mellitus, either childhood or adult onset, were specifically excluded from any of the samples included in this study since sexual dysfunction is a common diabetic complication.[35] Similarly, any patient receiving the antihypertensive agents reserpine, methyldopa, or guanethedine was excluded. These drugs have all been reported to be associated with sexual dysfunction.

PRELIMINARY FINDINGS

Since research is still in progress, data analysis is not yet complete and our results must still be considered preliminary. To date we have studied 120 subjects. This includes 50 healthy individuals ("normals"), 22 patients with nonuremic chronic illnesses, 25 patients with ESRD who do not yet require maintenance hemodialysis, and 23 patients currently receiving maintenance hemodialysis.

At this early stage in our data collection and analysis, several findings are worthy of note. Table 1 represents data concerned with the frequency of intercourse and the occurrence of erectile failure. Patients with advanced uremia described a decline in frequency of intercourse from a mean of 10.8 times a month prior to the development of uremia to a frequency at present of 2.2 times per month ($p < 0.01$). Those patients currently receiving maintenance hemodialysis described a similar de-

TABLE 1

Summary of Data Concerning Frequency of Intercourse, Complaints of Erectile Failure, and NPT in Groups Studied

	N	Frequency of intercourse, times per month		Complaints of erectile failure		NPT change in circumference > 13mm (min)
		Prior to illness	Current	Prior to illness	Current	
Chronic illness controls						
Total	22	9.0	6.1	1 (5%)	4 (18%)	8.6 ± 7.3
18–39 y.o.	8	7.7	8.7	0 (0%)	1 (13%)	74.4 ± 11.9
40–60 y.o.	14	9.4	4.3	1 (7%)	3 (21%)	49.6 ± 8.6
Advanced uremia						
Total	25	10.8	2.2	1 (4%)	10 (40%)	28.5 ± 6.8
18–39 y.o.	16	12.1	2.9	1 (6%)	5 (31%)	36.0 ± 9.7
40–60 y.o.	9	8.8	1.1	0 (0%)	5 (56%)	15.2 ± 5.5
Maintenance hemodialysis						
Total	23	12.4	4.7	1 (4%)	11 (48%)	26.8 ± 5.9
18–39 y.o.	13	12.8	6.3	1 (8%)	5 (38%)	33.5 ± 9.3
40–60 y.o.	10	11.6	2.8	0 (0%)	6 (60%)	18.2 ± 5.7
Normal controls						
Total	50					78.8 ± 6.1
18–39 y.o.	37					84.8 ± 7.3
40–60 y.o.	13					59.8 ± 9.0

cline from 12.4 times per month prior to their illness to a current level of 4.7 times a month ($p < 0.01$). It is interesting to note that the maintenance hemodialysis patients have a greater frequency of intercourse than do the advanced uremics (4.7 versus 2.2 times per month). A previous study had described a progressive decline in sexual activity with the progress of uremia and further decrements after the institution of hemodialysis.[3] This was cited as evidence of a psychogenic etiology for uremic sexual dysfunction since a number of physical parameters improve during hemodialysis. Our data suggest that sexual functioning is not further compromised by the introduction of hemodialysis. Indeed, a slight amelioration of these problems may occur. Surprisingly, we found no such drastic decline in the frequency of intercourse for the nonuremic chronically ill. These patients describe a nonsignificant decline in the frequency of intercourse (9.0 times a month to 6.1 times a month, $p = NS$) with the onset of their illness as well as a higher frequency of current intercourse than either of the two uremic groups.

If we look at the numbers of patients who complain of serious problems in obtaining and/or maintaining an erection, an analogous pattern is observed. Few of the chronic illness controls describe such complaints as having existing prior to their illness and only a small number complain of such difficulties at present (from 5% before to 18% currently, $p = NS$). In both ESRD groups however, a substantial number of patients offer such complaints at present (40% of the advanced uremics, 48% of maintenance hemodialysis patients), while only a very small number described such problems as having existed prior to their illness (4% in both groups, $p < 0.01$ in both groups). In ESRD this complaint was somewhat more common in the older age group (56% and 60% for the advanced uremic and the maintenance hemodialysis patients, respectively) than in the younger group (31% and 38%, respectively).

It is very interesting to note the consistency of the finding that the older advanced uremic and maintenance hemodialysis patients seem to be more adversely affected than their younger counterparts. In both of these groups the decline in frequency of intercourse was more marked, the complaints of erectile failure were greater, and the current level of sexual activity was less for the 40- to 60-year-old men than it was for those 18–39 years old.

The predominant complaint in these ESRD males was the loss of ability to obtain and/or maintain an erection sufficient for intercourse. Only a very few patients complained of ejaculatory disturbances. We found a pronounced deficit in NPT values for both groups of ESRD patients but not for the patients with other chronic illnesses. For the NPT data, comparisons are most meaningful when the data is examined from the standpoint of the two different age groups. In the 18- to 39-year-old patients, normals had a mean NPT of 84.8 ± 7.3 (SE) minutes per night while the patients with nonuremic chronic illnesses had a mean of 74.4 ± 11.9 minutes (p = NS). However, both the advanced uremics (28.5 ± 6.8 minutes) and the maintenance hemodialysis patients (26.8 ± 5.9 minutes) had markedly reduced NPT compared to both the normals and the chronic illness controls ($p < 0.01$ for both comparisons). Furthermore, approximately one-half of these ESRD patients had NPT values lower than that of the normal control with the lowest value. The pattern was identical in the 40- to 60-year-old group with the normals (59.8 ± 9.0 minutes) and the chronic illness controls being very similar (49.6 ± 8.6 minutes, p = NS) but both the advanced uremics (15.2 ± 5.5 minutes) and the maintenance hemodialysis patients (18.2 ± 5.7 minutes) having significantly lower values than both of the control groups ($p < 0.01$). As in the younger age groups, approximately half of these ESRD patients had NPT values lower than that observed in the lowest normal subject. Again, it is of interest to note the similarity of NPT values, in both age groups, for the advanced uremics and the maintenance hemodialysis patients. This is further evidence against the hypothesis that maintenance hemodialysis produces even further deficits in sexual performance.

The NPT response criteria selected for analysis was the total duration of time throughout the evening during which penile circumference change of 13 mm or greater was maintained. This is a very conservative figure. It was suggested by previous research which had determined that organically impotent men were able to maintain a maximum penile circumference change of only 13 mm while the psychogenically impotent men, whose NPT is presumably normal, have a maximum change of over 20 mm.[36] Therefore the failure to maintain a penile circumference change of 13 mm for any length of time is almost certainly indicative of major deficit in erectile capacity.

To our surprise, we were unable to detect a strong relationship between depression and various complaints relating to impaired sexual performance. Also we did not see any relationship between depression and NPT, but we had not expected to see one. The ESRD patients did exhibit a reasonably high degree of depression. When compared to the nonuremic chronically ill controls, however, the number of ESRD patients meeting psychological test criteria for depression of at least a mild degree was not that much greater (6 of 22 chronically ill or 27%, 21 of 48 ESRD patients or 44%, p = NS). Without question this 44% figure indicates that the ESRD patients do indeed exhibit a marked degree of depression and it is a very serious problem in terms of their overall psychosocial functioning. However, it doesn't seem to have a consistent relationship to their sexual performance and it may not be that much more common in ESRD than it is in other chronic illnesses. Although we did not find a major role for depression in the sexual dysfunction of ESRD patients, there were a small number of patients with normal NPT, complaints of sexual dysfunction, and evidences of depression. All of these suggest that in an individual case depression does need to be considered as a possible cause of sexual dysfunction.

The results of hormonal studies, while similarly of a preliminary nature, are interesting. We observe a similar pattern to that seen with the sexual history and NPT data. The chronically ill patients have values similar to the normal controls while the ESRD patients have marked alterations. Specifically, in both groups of ESRD patients testosterone levels were low while FSH, LH, and prolactin levels were high. We have attempted to correlate the hormonal data with the results of NPT testing. We have found a strong direct correlation between NPT and serum testosterone levels. In addition, we have noted a trend suggesting that elevated prolactin levels are associated with diminished NPT while normal prolactin levels occur in congruity with normal NPT.

The results of autonomic nervous system testing, also very preliminary, suggest that ESRD patients have distinct deficits in autonomic nervous system functioning. We have observed a direct and significant relationship between impaired performance on Valsalva testing and reduction in NPT.

CONCLUSIONS

If we attempt to integrate all of this data several conclusions, albeit tentative, can be drawn. First, it appears clear that ESRD males have a definite organic deficit in their capacity to obtain and maintain erections. Approximately 50% of these men had NPT values lower than that of the lowest normal. Secondly, it does not appear to be the case that depression plays a major role in the genesis of sexual dysfunction in ESRD. Although a common occurrence, depression was not associated in a significant way with either the complaint of impotence or with reduced NPT. Males with ESRD appear to have major deficits in sexual hormone physiology. Testosterone is reduced while prolactin, FSH, and LH are elevated. Furthermore, the deficits in testosterone and the elevation of prolactin are apparently correlated with reduced NPT. Autonomic nervous system impairment, which occurs in ESRD, is also apparently correlated with reduced NPT. Aging seems to be associated with more pronounced sexual deficits in these ESRD patients. Finally, the state of being chronically ill does not play a major role in the sexual dysfunction observed in males with ESRD. Subjects with other chronic illnesses neither complain of sexual dysfunction to an appreciable degree nor do they have deficits in their NPT. Indeed, we think the evidence clearly supports the presence of a sexual dysfunction, erectile in nature and organic in etiology, which is specific for ESRD.

RECOMMENDATIONS

What then can we recommend at this time with regard to a therapeutic approach for these men? Probably the best recommendation we could offer for right now would be for a further clarification of the nature of this deficit. If there is indeed a physiological deficit, as suggested by this data, its exact nature needs to be further investigated. The possible relationship of elevated prolactin to the sexual deficits is very interesting. Several recent studies have found that hyperprolactinemia, from a variety of causes, is associated with erectile deficits.[37,38] Lowering of serum prolactin has, at least in some cases, restored erectile capacity.[39,40] Indeed there is one study which has suggested that the lowering of prolactin in impotent dialytic patients was associated with improved sexual performance.[41] This study relied solely on sexual history and did not include NPT evaluation. This matter obviously needs to be investigated more thoroughly in these patients and NPT assessment must be performed.

General guidelines for diagnostic and treatment approach to these patients should include first and foremost a thorough assessment with an accurate sexual history (with spouse if possible) as well as an assessment of: the nature of the relationship with the spouse, depression, NPT, hormonal studies, and autonomic nervous system studies. Where possible a specific therapy should be initiated based on the results of this assessment. For example, evidence for serious depression, coupled with complaints of impotence but normal or near-normal NPT would suggest a psychogenic impotence secondary to depression. Treatment of the depression in such cases should restore sexual performance. Individual and/or conjoint couples therapy perhaps with the use of antidepressant medication should be instituted. We could readily envisage another example in which complaints of sexual dysfunction were coupled with seriously reduced NPT and an elevated prolactin. This would suggest that a strategy for intervention should be directed towards lowering the elevated prolactin, perhaps with bromocriptine. Unfortunately, at this point in time, there are few specific therapies for organically based impotence. This is most likely due to the fact that precise etiological knowledge concerning organic causes of impotence in ESRD is, at present, nonexistent. Evidence of persistent, severe, and irreversible NPT deficits might raise consideration of the use of penile prostheses in certain cases. Finally, we should consider the institution of psychotherapeutic approaches even if impotence appears clearly organic in nature. The problem should be approached both from the point of view of the patient and from that of the dyadic unit. Specific sex therapy approaches can focus on teaching the couple to utilize as much as possible of the male's remaining capability for providing his spouse with warmth, closeness, and physical contact. Perhaps the male can still help bring his wife to arousal and orgasm. If this is not possible, due to personal preference or for some other reason, perhaps some other form of physical contact such as touching and caressing can be encouraged. Certainly emotional contact and closeness does not need to be lessened even with intractable impotence. Analogous considerations could be applied to females with ESRD although we have not specifically addressed their problems in this chapter.

Sexual behavior and performance is obviously complicated and involves an interplay of biological and psychological forces in an appropriate mix in order to occur satisfactorily. A deficit in any one area can impair optimal sexual functioning. The etiology of the sexual dysfunction in ESRD while becoming better understood remains unclear at this point in time.

REFERENCES

1. KAPLAN DE-NOUR, A. Some notes on the psychological significance of urination. *Journal of Nervous and Mental Disease*, 1969, *148*, 615–623.
2. FRIEDMAN, E. A., GOODWIN, N. J., and CHAUDHRY, L. Psychosocial adjustment of family to maintenance hemodialysis. Part II. *New York State Journal Medicine*, 1970, *70*, 767–774.
3. LEVY, N. B. Sexual adjustment of maintenance hemodialysis and renal transplantation: National survey by questionnaire: Preliminary report. *Transactions of the American Society of Artificial Internal Organs*, 1973, *19*, 138–143.
4. FOSTER, F. G., COHN, G. L., and McKEGNEY, F. P. Psychological factors and individual survival on chronic renal hemodialysis—a two year follow up: Part I. *Psychosomatic Medicine*, 1973, *35*, 64–82.
5. SALVATIERRA, O., FORTMANN, and J. L., BELZER, F. O. Sexual function in males before and after renal transplantation. *Urology*, 1975, *5*, 64–66.
6. ABRAM, H. S., HESTER, L. R., and SHERIDAN, W. F. Sexual functioning in patients with chronic renal failure. *Journal of Nervous and Mental diseases*, 1975, *160*, 220–226.
7. THURM, J. Sexual potency of patients on chronic hemodialysis. *Urology*, 1975, *5*, 60–62.
8. SHERMAN, F. P. Impotence in patients with chronic renal failure on dialysis: Its frequency and etiology. *Fertility and Sterility*, 1975, *26*, 221–223.
9. BOMMER, J., TSCHOPE, W., and RITZ, E. Sexual behavior of hemodialyzed patients. *Clinical Nephrology*, 1976, *6*, 315–318.
10. STEELE, T. E., FINKELSTEIN, S. M., and FINKELSTEIN, F. O. Hemodialysis patients and spouses: Marital discord, sexual problems and depression. *Journal of Nervous and Mental Disease*, 1976, *162*, 225–237.
11. BERGSTEIN, E., ASABA, H., and BERGSTROM, J. A study of patients on chronic hemodialysis. *Scandanavian Journal of Social Medicine*, 1977, *11*, 1–31.

12. MILNE, J. F., GOLDEN, J. S., and FIBUS, L. Sexual dysfunction in renal failure: A survey of chronic hemodialysis patients. *International Journal of Psychiatry in Medicine*, 1977/78, *8*, 335–345.

13. KAPLAN DE-NOUR, A. Hemodialysis: Sexual functioning. *Psychosomatics*, 1978, *19*, 229–235.

14. PROCCI, W. R., HOFFMAN, K. I., and CHATTERJEE, S. N. Sexual functioning of renal transplant recipients. *Journal of Nervous and Mental Disease*, 1978, *166*, 402–407.

15. HOLDSWORTH, S. R., DE KRETSER, D. M., and ATKINS, R. C. A comparison of hemodialysis and transplantation in reversing the uremic disturbance in male reproductive function. *Clinical Nephrology*, 1978, *10*, 146–150.

16. PROCCI, W. R., GOLDSTEIN, D. A., and ADELSTEIN, J. Sexual dysfunction in the male uremic patient: A reappraisal. *Kidney International*, 1982, *19*, 317–323.

17. GUEVARA, A., VIDT, D., and HALBERG, M. C. Serum gonadotropin and testosterone levels in uremic males undergoing intermittent dialysis. *Metabolism*, 1969, *12*, 1062–1066.

18. CHEN, J. C., VIDT, D. G., and ZORN, E. M. Pituitary–Leydig cell function in uremic males. *Journal of Clinical Endocrinology and Metabolism*, 1970, *31*, 14–17.

19. BAILEY, G. L., ROSEN, S., and WEINTRAUB, B. Serum testosterone and gonadotrophins in uremic males before and after hemodialysis. *Proceedings of the American Society of Nephrology*, 1970, *4*, 5.

20. FRANTZ, A. G., KLEINBERG, D. L., NOEL, G. L. Studies on prolactin in man. *Recent Progress in Hormonal Research*, 1972, *28*, 527–590.

21. NAGEL, T. C., FREINKEL, N., and BELL, R. H. Gynecomastia, prolactin, and other peptide hormones in patients undergoing chronic hemodialysis. *Journal of Clinical Endocrinology and Metabolism*, 1973, *36*, 428–432.

22. SAWIN, C. T., LONGSCOPE, C., and SCHMITT, G. W. Blood levels of gonadotropins and gonadal hormones in gynecomastia associated with chronic hemodialysis. *Journal of Clinical Endocrinology and Metabolism*, 1973, *36*, 988–990.

23. STEWART-BENTLY, M., GANS, D., and HORTON R. Regulation of gonadal function in uremia. *Metabolism*, 1974, *23*, 1065–1072.

24. DISTILLER, L. A., MORLEY, J. E., and SAGEL, J. Pituitary–gonadal function in chronic renal failure. The effect of luteinizing hormone-releasing hormone and the influence of dialysis. *Metabolism*, 1975, *24*, 711–720.

25. LIM, V. S., and FANG, V. S. Gonadal dysfunction in uremic men. A study of the hypothalamic–pituitary–testicular axis before and after transplantation. *American Journal of Medicine*, 1975, *58*, 655–662.

26. HAGEN, C., OLGAARD, K., and McNEILLY, A. S. Prolactin and the pituitary–gonadal axis in male uremic patients on regular dialysis. *Acta Endocrinologica Copenhagena*, 1976, *82*, 29–38.

27. HOLDSWORTH, S. R., ATKINS, R. C., and DE KRETSER, D. M. The pituitary–testicular axis in men with chronic renal failure. *New England Journal of Medicine*, 1977, *296*, 1245–1249.

28. PEREZ, R. J., LIPNER, M., and ABDULLA, N. Menstrual dysfunction of patients undergoing chronic hemodialysis. *Obstetrics and Gynecology*, 1978, *51*, 552–555.

29. BECK, A. T. *The diagnosis and management of depression.* Philadelphia: University of Pennsylvania Press, 1973.

30. BRYAN, F. A. The national dialysis registry. Development of a medical registry of patients on chronic dialysis. 7th Annual Progress Report, No. AK-7-7-1387, Artificial Kidney–Chronic Uremia Program, National Institute of Arthritis, Metabolism, and Digestive Diseases, National Institute of Health, October, 1975.

31. KARACAN, I. A simple and inexpensive transducer for quantitative measurements of penile erection during sleep. *Behavioral Research Methods and Instruments*, 1969, *1*, 251–252.

32. FEIGHNER, J. R., ROBBINS, E., and GUZE, S. B. Diagnostic criteria for use in psychiatric research. *Archives of General Psychiatry*, 1972, *26*, 57–63.
33. BECK, A. T., WARD, C. H., and MENDELSON, M. An inventory for measuring depression. *Archives of General Psychiatry*, 1961, *4*, 561–571.
34. RASKIN, A., SCHULTERBRAND, J., and REATIG, N. Factors of psychopathology in interview, ward behavior, and self-report ratings of hospitalized depressives. *Journal of Consultation Psychology*, 1967, *31*, 270–278.
35. KARACAN, I., SALIS, P. J., and WARE, J. C. Nocturnal penile tumescence and diagnosis in diabetic impotence. *American Journal of Psychiatry*, 1978, *135*, 191–198.
36. FISHER, C., SCHIAVI, R. C., and EDWARDS, A. Evaluation of nocturnal penile tumescence in the differential diagnosis of sexual impotence: A quantitative study. *Archives of General Psychiatry*, 1979, *36*, 431–437.
37. FRANKS, S., JACOBS, H. S., and MARTIN, N. Hyperprolactinaemia and impotence. *Clinical Endocrinology*, 1978, *8*, 277–287.
38. GLASSMAN, C. N., RIFE, C. C., and WILSON, C. B. Prolactin—Added dimension in male genitosexual disorders. *Urology*, 1980, *15*, 49–52.
39. SPARK, R. F., WHITE, R. A., and CONNOLLY, P. B. Impotence is not always psychogenic: Newer insights into hypothalamic–pituitary–gonadal dysfunction. *Journal of the American Medical Association*, 1980, *243*, 750–755.
40. NAGULESPAREN, M., ANG, V., and JENKINS, J. S. Bromocriptine treatment of males with pituitary tumors, hyperprolactinaemia, and hypogonadism. *Clinical Endocrinology*, 1978, *9*, 73–79.
41. BOMMER, J., DEL POZO, E., and RITZ, E. Improved sexual function in male hemodialysis patients on bromocriptine. *Lancet*, 1979, *2*, 496–497.

21

Uremia Therapy in the Twenty-First Century

ELI A. FRIEDMAN

INTRODUCTION

Planning for health care in the next century in a complex, computer-maintained society,[1] requires an inventory of current programs as well as a crystal ball. With less than 17 years remaining until the twenty-first century, it may be appropriate to assess the extraordinary progress of the past 20 years in treating renal failure. At the close of 1981, more than 145,000 persons around the world, who would formerly have died, are living because of a functioning kidney transplant or regular dialysis. In stark contrast, prior to Scribner's introduction of chronic hemodialysis by invention of the external plastic arteriovenous shunt in 1960, all that could be offered the dying uremic patient was early euthenasia. Addis's text illustrates this point:

> Paraldehyde gives a very natural and dreamless sleep. The dose can be repeated whenever the patient shows signs of restlessness, and the quantity given can be safely increased up to as much as 60 cc every 6 hr. or so, for here also uremia seems to carry with it a greatly increased tolerance, and there is a wide margin between the dose that makes the patient just drowsily unconscious and the amount required to induce a deep sleep. It is the quiet drowsiness we want. The disease itself will soon bring the deep sleep.[2]

Today, health planners must take into account great inequities in uremia therapy between nations and between social class within the same country. Once these evocative issues are faced squarely, a future strategy based on reality can be devised.

INEQUITIES IN DELIVERY OF UREMIA THERAPY

The study of any country-by-country listing of the number of patients sustained by dialysis or renal transplantation affords confirmation

---

ELI A. FRIEDMAN, M.D. • Professor of Medicine, Director of Renal Division, Downstate Medical Center, Brooklyn, New York.

TABLE 1
Uremia Therapy around the World[a]

Country	PD	HD	(% Home)	Transplant	Total
U.S.A.	5	205	(13%)	66	277
Japan	2	235	(1%)	14	251
Canada	29	92	(35%)	72	193
W. Germany	3	137	(21%)	14	161
U.K.	4	57	(64%)	48	111
E. Germany	1	37	(0)	16	56
S. Africa	2	15	(11%)	9	26
Poland	1	10	(0)	2	14
Egypt	0	1	(2%)	0	1

[a]Wing and Selwood for 1979–1980, per million, ISN 1981.

of the unavailability of modern uremia therapy to about four-fifths of the world. As shown in Table 1, a partial listing of a recent registry report,[3] underdeveloped countries like Egypt offer virtually no treatment for irreversible renal failure. Nigeria, for example, with a population of 70 million, has not a single hemodialysis unit or renal transplant facility. So-called third-world nations must place in perspective the need to cope with malaria (200 million cases annually, worldwide), trachoma (300 million cases), and malnutrition (undefined number of cases), before sophisticated, high-cost regimens like dialysis can be considered seriously. Political constraints also strongly influence availability of uremia therapy. Depending on which side of the Berlin Wall a citizen resides, his chances for acceptance into a hemodialysis program may vary by 400% (Table 1).

Class distinctions, mainly economic, determine which uremic patients will live in countries with some, but not sufficient uremia services. An extraordinary event at a recent international meeting made this clear. Greece, emerging from its former position as an underdeveloped nation, hosted a world congress of nephrology in 1981, and proudly issued a commemorative stamp (Figure 1). But as foreign guests entered the ancient amphitheatre on the acropolis to attend the opening ceremony, they were thrust into a Greek patient–government conflict. Leaflets protesting inadequate national programs for uremia therapy were handed out by chanting, picketing, angry patients. At the same time, representatives of a well-appointed proprietary dialysis unit distributed brochures soliciting vacationers for dialysis in a posh facility, at a cost of $300 (drugs extra) per dialysis (Figure 2). In the United States, debate over the morality of permitting profit-making dialysis units to continue their expansion is brisk and current.[4]

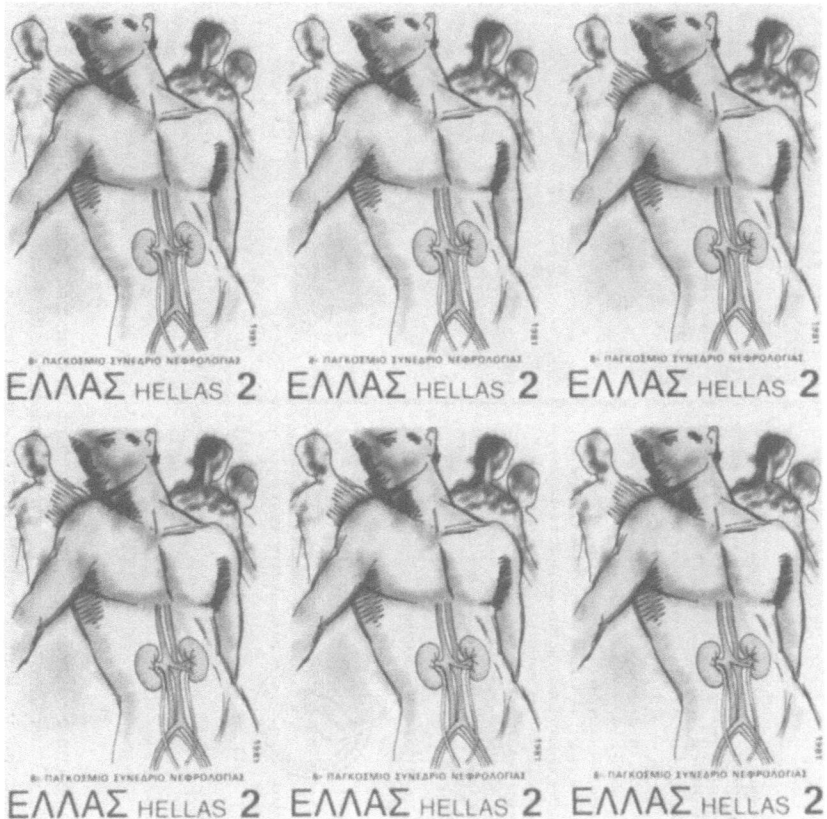

FIG. 1. Commemorative stamp issued by Greece in honor of 8th International Congress of Nephrology held in Athens in May, 1981.

PRESSURES IN PATIENT SELECTION

Assignment of a specific uremic patient to a designated treatment and facility represents a resultant vector in a parallelogram of forces, including the vested interests of physicians, surgeons, facilities, and governments. In Canada, for instance, dominance of one Toronto group has fostered a unique growth of peritoneal dialysis, to the extent that Canadian patients are six times more likely than their American neighbors to be initially treated by this option (Table 1). Physician bias in Japan has excluded home hemodialysis despite that country's position at the top of the list in rate per million receiving maintenance hemodialysis. Retention of patients by profit-making dialysis units in

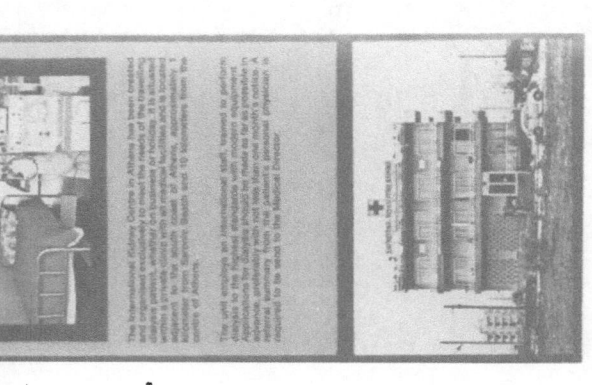

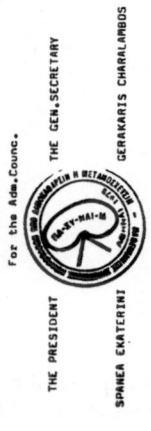

- 2 -

Request to see the de-ionization and the technical equipment. Request to see the places of transplantations and the surgical oper··i;r rooms for transplantations. Request them WHY the transplantations for dead bodies haven't been promoted in Greece, while since 3 years this Law has been passed. Request them for the Greeks'suffering from nephro- pathy recovery and for the social care of State for these patients. Request to know about the circumstances under which the most patients live and about their survival percentage. Request to know about the provincials who live obligatorily in Athens. Request to know all the above mentioned and then you'll understand WHY the Greek patients suf- fering from nephropathy complain. Only in this way,you'll have a console picture of this fascinating country which is called Greece and which has been the 10th member of ECC.

If the organizers of the Congress "omit" to let you know on the above mentioned or,perhaps they haven't the necessary informations than our Association will be in the position to give you these informations.

With friendly regards,

For the Adm.Counc.

THE PRESIDENT   THE GEN.SECRETARY

SPANEA EKATERINI   GERAKARIS CHARALAMBOS

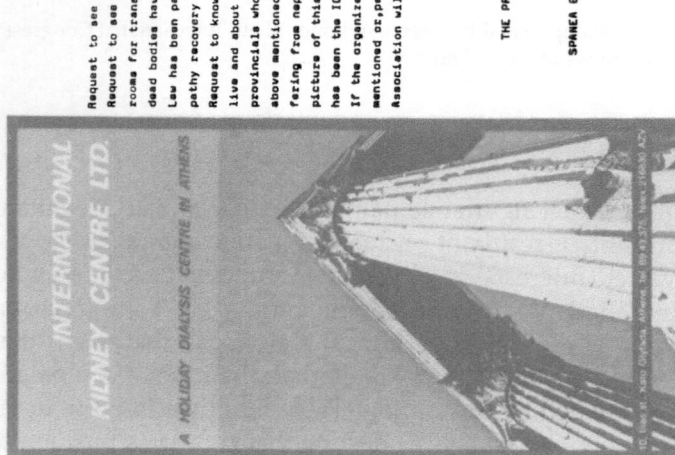

FIG. 2. Left and right are the front and back of a brochure advertising dialyses for tourists in an Athens suberb. Affluent guests are charged $300 per dialysis. Center shows a portion of a mimeographed leaflet handed out by a Greek patients' organization at the congress opening protesting inadequate renal therapy for Greek citizens.

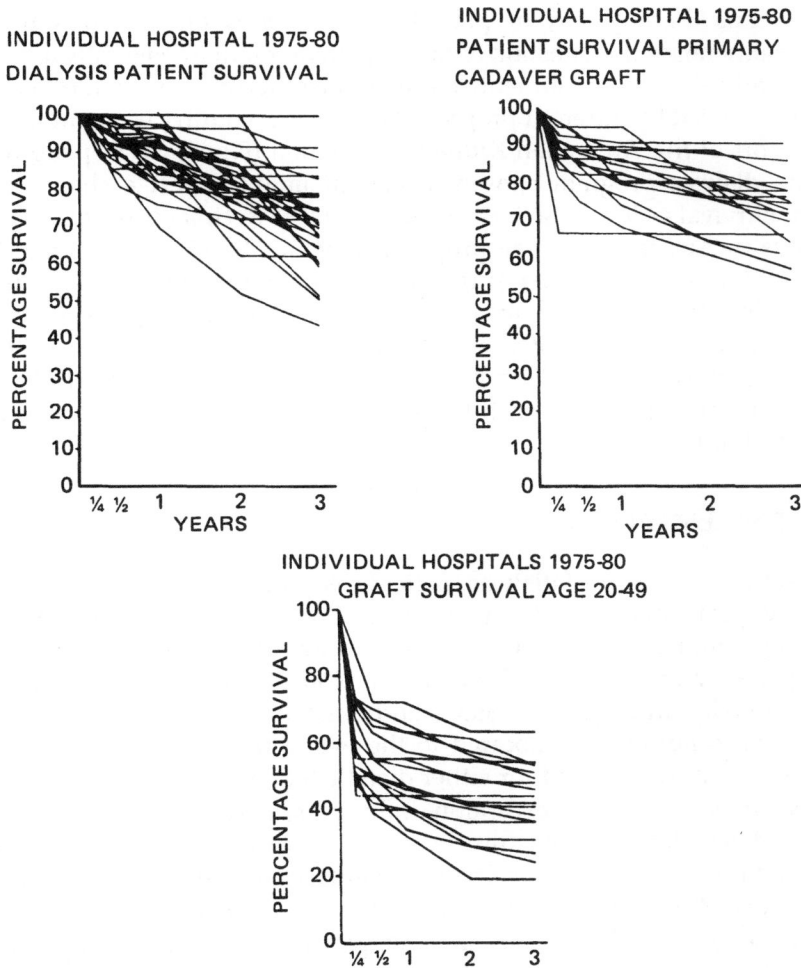

FIG. 3. A chart taken from the annual report of the Australian Kidney Foundation for 1980, issued in April 1981. There is a wide range from facility to facility in survival after renal transplantation or after beginning maintenance hemodialylsis.

the United States, retards their referral for either home hemodialysis or renal transplantation.[5] Great Britain, in a move to restrict health care costs, is attempting to impose an upper limit of age 50 years on reimbursement for uremia therapy,[6] an action which would have made Winston Churchill ineligible, though he later led that nation in its most desperate challenge.

Uremia therapy may be provided competently or incompetently. This reality raises the question of how a patient might intelligently avoid the added risk of bad treatment. The extreme range of survival rates currently achieved by different programs in the same country is apparent in the report of the Australian Kidney Foundation (Figure 3). Depending on the dialysis program chosen, a patient might expect a chance of 3-year survival as low as 46% or as high as 100%. Recipients of cadaveric kidneys in Australia in some programs have a 92% chance of living 3 years, while under another surgeon's care only 57% will live 3 years. Complaints about poor results in transplantation occasionally reach national attention in the United States.[7] Patients ought not to "belong" to any program or group. When properly informed as to the caliber of results to be anticipated by each therapy and program, patients will migrate to the best care.

PATIENT DESELECTION

In the early years of dialysis, patient selection committees struggled with the problem of deciding which few patients were deserving of life prolongation. Dialysis slots in the 1960s were allocated only after the patient passed a means test and satisfied dubious "worth to society" criteria. Gradually, in the United States and much of Western Europe, governmental funding was allocated to the extent that all clearly suitable patients are now accepted for either dialytic therapy or renal transplantation. Great Britain is an exception, inducing soul-searching and an understandably defensive posture by some program directors.[8,9] At the opposite pole of the patient selection quandary are equally vexing questions of: (1) Are there patients who ought to be denied dialysis? and (2) Should dialysis be discontinued in some patients who show no hope of rehabilitation?

Ethicists of the twenty-first century will continue the effort to define when an organism ceases to be a person even though some vital life processes continue. Fox[10] examined the dilemma of protracting a machine-dependent existence in a vegetative state, as in the Quinlan case. Quinlan has survived 5 years in an unresponsive state. Suppose Quinlan now develops uremia. Should she be started on dialysis, or given a kidney transplant? Should a 100-year-old patient be dialyzed? Is advanced malignancy, psychosis, or senility sufficient reason to preclude uremia therapy? What should be done to proprietary units who accept an inordinately high proportion of senile or other "inappropriate" patients? How does one actually discontinue dialysis? As noted by Shear, "I have become very humble about my own ability to decide for others whether to stop dialysis."[11]

TABLE 2
Choice of Uremia Therapy

Hemodialysis
    Home or center
    Acetate or bicarbonate
    Low or high osmolality
Peritoneal dialysis
    Intermittent (IPD)
    Continuous ambulatory (CAPD)
    Continuous cyclic (CCPD)
Renal Transplantation
    Living donor
    Cadaver donor
Hemofiltration
Hemoperfusion

BEST THERAPY

From a listing of currently utilized effective treatments for uremia (Table 2), it may be inferred that no one approach is universally "the" correct therapy. Peritoneal dialysis can be performed intermittently (IPD), continuously in ambulatory patients (CAPD), or as a combined nighttime-machine-cycled and daytime-long-dwell regimen (CCPD). Hemodialysis can be done at a facility or in the home. Dialysate may contain either bicarbonate or acetate as a buffer. Hemofiltration, a technique for extracting solutes from blood placed under pressure against a semipermeable membrane, may have either pre- or postfiltration infusion of buffered electrolyte solution into blood. Indicative of the unsettled status of the "best therapy" issue is the fact that hemofiltration is widely employed in Germany and France, but ignored in the United States where it was developed and in Canada. Hemoperfusion, a technique in which the patient's blood is directly exposed to a chemical sorbent such as activated charcoal, is still investigational. Completing the choices is the option for renal transplantation from either a living or cadaver donor. After pondering all of the selections in Table 2, the discerning reader might correctly surmise that as of late 1981 a single best choice cannot be identified. Nevertheless, it is possible to recognize a consensus of opinion as to which a certain type of patient reacts well to a particular treatment (Table 3).

FUTURE THERAPY

Throughout the 1980s, it is likely that health problems causing greater economic consequences than uremia will take precedence for

TABLE 3
Suiting Patient to Uremia Therapy

Strong indication
Renal transplantation
Infants
Diabetics
Well-matched siblings
CAPD
Solitary elderly resident
Individual factors most important
Hemodialysis
Nondiabetic
No intrafamilial donor
Toss-up
Choice between cadaveric transplant and home hemodialysis

most of the world. Egypt, for example, must be more concerned with its millions infectd with schistosomiasis than its thousands dying of uremia. Similarly, India requires a strategy to feed its 800 million population, before establishing a nationwide network of dialysis facilities. By the 1990s, however, advances in population control and enhanced food production may permit diversion of resources to less urgent medical problems. To gain a place on this secondary priority list, uremia therapy will have to come down in cost. There is little prospect, for instance, that China will be able to sustain patients at an annual cost of $25,000 per patient. Predicting how kidney failure will be handled a generation hence must therefore differentiate between rich and poor nations.

The industrialized West, at one extreme, will make smaller, more efficient dialysis devices (Figure 4), culminating in an implantable bionic kidney which might be mass-produced like a Japanese quartz watch. Enhanced immunosuppressive techniques, presaged by the synthesis of monoclonal antibodies, promise specific donor tolerance to organ transplants, avoiding the risk of sepsis. In less than a decade, renal allograft recipients should regularly have an annual graft survival in excess of 90%. As this century ends, xenografts should be readily tolerated, setting a value for best kidneys much above 69 per lb. There will thus continue to be a rivalry between medical and surgical approaches to uremia with the patient as beneficiary.

For the underdeveloped majority of the world however, uremia therapy must be made cheaper to become real. An equivalent to the Scribner shunt for the poor needs to be devised. Innovative therapies are in fact under laboratory test. Perhaps the most rational direction in uremia research is an effort to utilize the intestine as a substitute

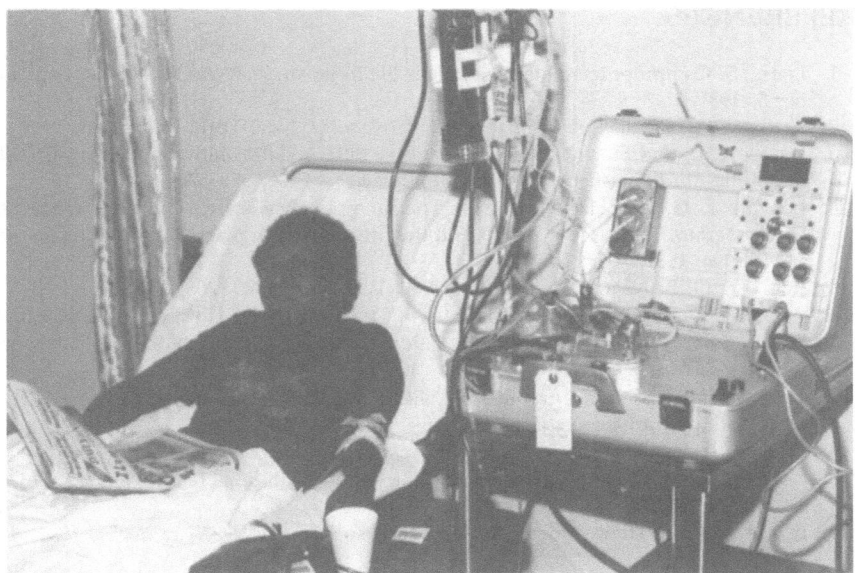

FIG. 4. An attache-case kidney. Developed by James Hutchisson and the author, this simplified dialysis system weighs 15 lb. and permits portable self-treatment. Dialysis equipment will get smaller as this century ends, culminating in an implantable bionic device.

nephron. Induction of controlled diarrhea and ingestion of oral sorbents are promising methods for extraction of nitrogenous solutes in feces. It may prove possible to program intestinal bacteria to convert nitrogenous wastes to essential amino acids. Alternatively, uremic patients might be fed bacterial enzymes synthesized *in vitro*, accomplishing the same end.

SUMMARY

Renal failure, once a universally fatal disease can be routinely treated today by several acceptable but imperfect therapies. Work in progress suggests that the lot of patients in renal failure will continue to improve. By the turn of the century it is anticipated that uremia will be treated by insertion of tiny bionic dialyzers and replacement kidneys obtained from animals. These therapies however, will be limited to rich nations until well into the twenty-first century. A search for a "poor man's" uremia therapy is now taking place. Reliance on the gut as a substitute nephron, seems the best hope, though an open mind may be rewarded by some other innovative approach.

REFERENCES

1. LOHR, S. Computer technology pervades life in Japan. *The New York Times*, September 5, 1981, 1.
2. ADDIS, T. *Glomerulonephritis diagnosis and treatment*. New York: Macmillan, 1949.
3. WING, A. J., and SELWOOD, N. H. Registry data-A collaborative exercises. *Proceedings of the 8th International Congress on Nephrology*, 1981, 575–576.
4. LOWRIE, E. G., and HAMPERS, C. L. The success of Medicare's end stage renal disease program: The case for profits and the private market place. *New England Journal of Medicine*, 1981, *305*, 434-438.
5. KOLATA, G. B. NMC thrives selling dialysis. *Science*, 1980, *208*, 379-382.
6. BERLYNE, G. M. Over 50 band Uremic = Death: The failure of the British National Health Service to provide adequate dialysis facilities. *Nephron* (Editorial), 1982, *31*, 189–190.
7. Time Magazine. Surgical trauma in California. Davis center suspends heart operations, kidney transplants. *Time Magazine*, July 20, 1981, 72.
8. Editorial. Ethics and the nephrologist. *Lancet*, 1981, *1*, 594–596.
9. PARSONS, V., and LOCK, P. Triage and the patient with renal failure. *Journal of Medical Ethics*, 1980, *6*, 173–176.
10. FOX, R. C. The sting of death in American society. *Social Service Review* 1981, *55*, 41–59.
11. COHEN, J. J., HARRINGTON, J. T., and KASSIRER, J. P. Exclusion from dialysis: A sociologic and legal perspective. *Kidney International*, 1981, *19*, 739–751.

III
Renal Transplantation

22

The Renal Transplant Patient
Three-Stage Model and Psychotherapeutic Strategies

HELLMUTH FREYBERGER

STAGE ONE: IMMEDIATE PRE- AND POSTOPERATIVE PERIOD

In the time period immediately preceding transplantation, patients have an awareness of the seriousness of their illness and tend to approach the transplant surgery with an air of expectation and optimism. In hospital units which include other patients anticipating similar surgery, patients also tend to feel secure. This security is further enhanced by the concentrated and competent care of trained transplant nurses.

In the immediate postoperative stage the patient becomes aware of the potential for transplant rejection, and awareness which will be ongoing. During this period patients are very appreciative of the many necessary contacts with medical personnel, particularly of staff who are willing to listen to fears, doubts, and questions about treatment progress. The strength of this early patient–medical team bond is of vital importance to the patient's emotional well-being should the transplant fail and the patient become more in need of a stable object relationship.[1]

STAGE TWO: THE EARLY STAGES FOLLOWING TRANSPLANTATION

If the immediate postoperative stage is free of medical complications, the patient begins to appreciate the freedom from the dependence on routine dialysis and its physical and psychological difficulties. Patients in this stage are characterized by feelings of thankfulness and elation. Other terms used to describe this phenomenon have been "born

HELLMUTH FREYBERGER, M.D. • Professor of Psychosomatics and Chairman, Center of Psychological Medicine, Department of Psychosomatics, Hannover Medical School, Hannover, German Federal Republic.

again" and "euphoric reaction."[2] Such terms have infrequently been applied to patients recovering from traditional surgery. This stage is also characterized by an increased awareness of the implications of transplant rejection resulting in patients' heightened interest in and attention to the details of their medical condition.

If the patient believes that the transplant has been successful he tends to become more relaxed and less self-absorbed. However, this tendency toward stability can be short-lived at the first sign of transplant rejection. Patients report the feeling of "sitting on a powder keg" at the first sign of possible transplant rejection. At this time patients present clinically as anxious and labile. They may be alternately agitated or depressed and pessimistic. Typically the patient uses massive denial and his outlook becomes very constricted.[2]

Individual patient situations can also have an impact on the psychological climate of the entire renal transplant unit. If most of the patients are doing well, the climate of the unit is usually cheerful and stimulating. If, however, many of the patients are experiencing symptoms of transplant rejection, the atmosphere in the unit can become constricted, anxious, and depressed. Fortunately, in our experience the majority of the transplant patients do well and the mood in the unit is usually more positive than negative.

Psychological Manifestations of the Unsuccessful Transplant

If the removal of the transplanted kidney is indicated, patients typically experience tremendous stress resulting in extremely labile moods and a return to the emotional reactions typical of dialysis patients in general. For patients who have effectively used the defense mechanism of denial and who are able to deal realistically with their situation, the difficulty in adjusting to the failed transplant is minimized. This is particularly true if the patient is able to communicate his feelings to others, especially to his family. In such circumstances, patients gradually regain emotional equilibrium and begin to look forward to the possibility of a second and hopefully more successful transplant.

In contrast, those patients who use denial in a maladaptive way and who have little capacity for introspection may be extremely unprepared to handle the crisis of transplant rejection. Such patients may internalize the stress at a deeper emotional level or may in fact be incapable of dealing with the crisis in a rational manner. These are often patients who have been uncooperative in the past and in our experience, continue to use massive denial in the renewed dialysis situation. Patients who do not fully process the loss of the transplanted kidney and who continue to use massive denial are considered at great risk for further psychosomatic complications.

STAGE THREE: THE LATER STAGE FOLLOWING TRANSPLANTATION

During this stage patients are usually receiving out-patient aftercare. Psychodynamic processes in this stage tend to parallel the experiences in the early stage following transplantation. Patients continue to ask themselves, "Will this success last or will I ultimately have to face rejection?" Patients who are progressing well also continue to appreciate the freedom from the rigors of dialysis and begin to make new life plans based upon the hope of continued success. In this stage, if any impairment of renal function is experienced, the patient will again report the precarious feeling of "sitting on a powder keg." This may lead to a further preoccupation with body functions and fears of transplant failure.

As transplant failure is generally recognized and dealt with in the early postoperative period, patients in the later stage of recovery are generally functioning satisfactorily. As a result the physician is usually dealing with patients who are for the most part continuing to appreciate a born-again feeling. The contrast between the emotional state of a successfully transplanted patient and that of a dialysis patient is marked. Only those who have worked with both groups of patients are in the position of truly appreciating these differences in psychological functioning. Indeed, without having been exposed to the differences between these groups of patients, an inexperienced physician may have a tendency to underestimate both the psychic difficulties of a dialysis patient and the degree of relief experienced by the transplant patient.

Psychotherapeutic Implications

Doctors and nurses working with in-patients as well as patients on follow-up care need to become aware of relevant clinical treatment strategies. One general principle underlies each of these strategies and that is the "emotional presence" of the nurse and the physician. Emotional presence implies the personal availability of the healer to be psychologically attuned to the patient at times of need. This principle is especially relevant given the following common patient characteristics in the postoperative period.

1. Patients' desire for details and discussion of their physical condition: The patient is greatly relieved if he has ample opportunity to dis-

cuss his doubts and fears about recovery. Such listening requires time and patience by the medical team. Following the patients' verbalizations, it is very important for the doctor or nurse to clearly express support and encouragement.

2. Patients' manifestations of passive–aggressiveness: Patients who are temporarily unable to express their negative emotions may express these emotions through passive yet visable means. Aggressive impulses may be increased if the patient perceives correctly or incorrectly that the medical team is not psychologically available. At the first sign of passive–aggressive patient behavior, the physician or nurse should approach the patient, recognize his frustration, and allow him to express himself in a more appropriate manner.

When the patient can count on the physical and psychological availability of the treatment team, the resulting emotional security predisposes the patient toward a more appropriate use of defense mechanisms and toward taking more personal responsibility for his physical and mental health. Furthermore, such stable object relationships promote outward-directed behavior which is more beneficial to the patient than constant introspection. Patients who are secure and well oriented to reality are in the best position to accept their condition and to follow therapeutic recommendations.

Special Psychotherapeutic Interventions

For the majority of patients, the emotional support of the doctors, nurses, and family members satisfactorily meets psychological needs in each of the three stages. In some cases more support is needed and more intensive psychotherapy is indicated. The technique which has been most successfully applied in transplant patients is supportive psychotherapy.

Supportive psychotherapy is characterized by the following three tasks[3]:

1. Establishing and maintaining a stable object relationship. This positive relationship is created and enhanced by the regular inpatient visits with the physician and by the out-patient contacts available during follow-up visits. Such contacts encourage positive transference when the physician answers questions, offers advice, and lets the patient know of his ongoing availability.
2. Allowing patients' expression of concerns and conflicts. Supportive psychotherapy also involves allowing patients to express their concerns, fears, and frustrations. Patients who are

able to describe their symptoms and emotions experience a significant reduction in stress.

3. Dealing with current conflict situations. When patients describe problematic situations, the physician can provide support through the use of gentle confrontation and simple interpretation.

When working with in-patients, there are several indications for the initiation of supportive psychotheraphy.

1. When the patient is in extreme distress as a result of transplant rejection and subsequent removal of the kidney, he may revert to earlier crisis patterns and may exhibit emotional lability and depression. In this situation psychotherapy is definitely indicated, although in our experience only two-thirds of these patients are amenable to treatment. Extreme psychopathology may be observed in this situation and patients may even refuse dialysis treatment if they are not well oriented to reality or are unable to mobilize defense mechanisms adequately. Under these circumstances it is not unusual to provide emergency psychotherapeutic intervention.[1,4]
2. Stress associated with the threat of rejection; this is later overcome.
3. Narcissistic personality disorders and inability to utilize denial appropriately, resulting in extremely poor patient cooperation.

Difficulties encountered in the out-patient treatment of transplant recipients include:

1. Noncompliance with diet resulting in excessive weight gain.
2. Conflicts between patients and their families.
3. Estrangement from the family and delayed resolution of problems.
4. Periodic discouragement of family members regarding treatment progress.
5. Problems inherent in the related-donor or live-donor situations both preoperatively and postoperatively.
6. Patients who are dealing with extreme neuroses and current life conflicts.

Consultation–Liaison Activities

Our consultation–liaison activities in the renal transplant unit may be summarized in the following five statements.[5]

1. It is understood that both surgeons and nurses are capable of engaging in problem solving with patients. However, the psychosomaticist is available for consultation in the event that intervention with the patient or his family is necessary.

2. In addition to being on call for consultations, the psychosomaticist initiates informal contacts with patients up to three times per week. During these visits the consultant assesses the degree to which patients are utilizing appropriate and adequate defense mechanisms. The consultant is then available to physicians and nurses to discuss details of case management for individual patients.

3. The psychosomaticist is available to the nurses for consultation about an individual patient's situation or about stress management in the work environment.

4. The consultant meets daily with student therapists placed in the unit.

5. The psychosomaticist meets with the surgeons weekly during their out-patient consultations. This participation includes the following two tasks: consultation and training with the surgeons and maintenance of ongoing contacts with the out-patients themselves.

The Role of Student Therapists

Therapist trainees provide consultation–liaison activities as long as they are involved in ongoing group supervision.[6] The Departments of Medicine and Surgery within our Medical School provide clinical services through three auxiliary therapist pools. There are 10 students in each of the three groups which are under the Department of Psychosomatics. These students are always on call to provide counseling services to patients and fill an important gap in traditional services to medical and surgical in-patients. These students are trained to provide psychotherapeutic services in the areas of denial and secondary hypochondria and are also able to consult with doctors and nurses about relevant patient issues.

The students also provide one-to-one psychotherapy if the transplant patients' psychopathology is not too severe.

We have observed several positive effects of the use of student therapists:

1. A significantly reduced work load for the professional therapists.

2. A cost-effective way to improve the level of patient care within the in-patient setting.
3. The possibility of forming more auxiliary therapist groups for the many available students provided that sufficient supervision is also available.

On the basis of our work with student auxiliary therapists, I predict that this way of providing psychological services will soon become the predominant form of psychotherapeutic intervention.

In summary, from the perspective of a psychosomatisist with 10 years of experience, 5 of which have been in a renal unit, I clearly affirm the thesis that renal transplantation is the best alternative for patients suffering from terminal renal failure. Indeed, from the perspective of the dialysis patient, a part of normal living is coming to an end while for the transplant patient a new life is beginning. This idea was stated by Eisendrath[7] as follows: "In most cases a successful kidney transplant is the best psychotherapy for anyone in renal failure, whatever their psychiatric problems."

REFERENCES

1. FREYBERGER, H. Renal transplant unit. In H. Freyberger (Ed.), *Psychotherapeutic interventions in life threatening illness. Advances in Psychosomatic Medicine*, Vol. 10. Basel: Karger, 1980, pp. 151–177.
2. CASTELNUOVO-TEDESCO, P. Transplantation: Psychological implications of changes in body image. In N. B. Levy (Ed.), *Psychonephrology I: Psychological factors in hemodialysis and transplantation*. New York: Plenum, 1981, pp. 219–226.
3. FREYBERGER, H. Six years experience as a psychosomaticist in a hemodialysis unit. In H. Freyberger (Ed.), *Topics of psychosomatic research*. Basel: Karger, 1973, pp. 108–113.
4. FREYBERGER, H. Psychosomatic aspects of an intensive care unit. In J. G. Howells (Ed.), *Modern perspectives in the psychiatric aspects of surgery*. New York: Brunner/Mazel, 1976, pp. 549–569.
5. FREYBERGER, H. Consultation liaison in a renal transplant unit. In N. B. Levy (Ed.), *Psychonephrology I: Psychological factors in hemodialysis and transplantation*. New York: Plenum, 1981, pp. 225–264.
6. FREYBERGER, H. Students working as auxiliary therapists with groups of psychosomatic and organically ill patients. In C. P. Kimball and A. J. Krakowski (Eds.), *The teaching of psychosomatic medicine and consultation–liaison psychiatry. Bibltheca psychiatrica, 159*. Basel: Karger, 1979, pp. 62–70.
7. EISENDRATH, R. M. Adaptation to renal transplantation. In J. G. Howells (Ed.), *Modern perspectives in the psychiatric aspects of surgery*. New York: Brunner/Mazel, 1976, pp. 549–569.

23

A Model for Social Work Intervention in Live–Related Kidney Transplantation

JUNE BURLEY

Live–related kidney transplantation has far-reaching implications for recipients, donors, their families, and the staff who care for them. The large body of psychosocial literature on this treatment modality focuses on the emotional reactions of donors and recipients before and after transplantation.[1] The purpose of this paper is to outline the psychosocial problems encountered in clinical practice with this patient population and to suggest a model of treatment intervention for the social worker in the transplant center. The role in orientation, assessment, individual, group and family counseling, and team consultation will be discussed. The material presented is experiential and is based on 4 years of experience as a nephrology social worker in a Canadian hospital, with involvement in 25 live–related transplants.

My first experience with a live–related transplant occurred in 1976 when I joined the renal team at University Hospital, London, Canada (the Southwestern Ontario transplant center). A 24-year-old diabetic male was receiving a kidney from his 26-year-old brother. While the surgery was in progress I received a referral from the team leader who was concerned about the behavior of the extended family in the waiting room. Crisis intervention with this family, which included the recipient's parents and two siblings and the donor's wife and her parents, revealed an uniformed, angry, overanxious group which was divided into two camps (donor and recipient), neither of which was speaking to the other. This situation made me acutely aware of the need for psychosocial intervention in live–related transplantation, intervention which would assist in preventing a situation such as the one described. Coincidentally, this incident occurred during the initial planning stages of a patient transplant orientation program on the unit and the role of the

JUNE BURLEY, A.I.M.S.W. • Social Worker, University Hospital, London, Ontario, Canada.

social worker in live–related transplantation was developed as an integral part of this program.

STRESSES IN LIVE–RELATED TRANSPLANTATION

In discussing the stresses associated with live–related transplantation we need to examine the specific problems which can be encountered by the donor, the recipient, and their families. Simmons has documented the internal stress of potential volunteer donors, the guilt experienced by the recipients, the conflict between potential donors and their spouses, the stress within the mutual family, and the feelings of anger which are directed at and reciprocated by less willing family members.[2] Although these problems would seem to be of a temporary nature, failure to identify the individual's ability to cope with them can lead to a perpetuation and a degree of stress within an individual or family which is so emotionally disabling as to threaten the final outcome of the transplant.[3] Social and economic consequences of donating a kidney, or in the case of the recipient, the results of several years of treatment on dialysis should also be recognized. The donor and recipient should be viewed in the context of their environment and the social worker is responsible for exploring, assessing, and treating the multiple factors which make up this environment. The following issues, therefore, need to be addressed in order to provide an effective social work service on a transplant unit:

1. Patient and family orientation
2. Identification of high-risk psychosocial factors
3. Treatment of psychosocial pretransplant problems
4. Posttransplant counseling
5. Team consultation

ORIENTATION

The pretransplant orientation of recipients, donors, and families is of major importance. Because most transplant units are regional centers, candidates for transplantation are referred from distant dialysis units. In our experience, patients usually have a strong allegiance to their own dialysis unit, fear separation from its support system, and view their new treatment center with apprehension. The Southwestern Ontario transplant orientation program attempts to deal with this problem, providing orientation sessions for patients and families with physician, surgeon, and other team members. The program includes a routine social work interview with the recipient for a psychosocial assessment and to establish a rapport and demonstrate a support system ready to take over from the recipient's own center when the transplant occurs.

The first social work contact with the donor is usually on admission for the medical work-up when he or she is referred routinely for a psychosocial assessment. This interview and subsequent short contacts during the admission will assist in establishing trust and rapport to form the basis of a sound professional relationship with the donor when the transplant takes place. The respective families too, may seek information and support and they are encouraged to do so through the recipient and donor.

IDENTIFICATION OF HIGH-RISK PSYCHOSOCIAL FACTORS

A psychosocial assessment of recipient and donor is a requirement of the unit's transplant protocol. The recipient is assessed in terms of reactions to illness thus far, adjustment to and compliance on dialysis, ego strengths and weaknesses, economic status, and family and social supports. The recipient's feelings as to acceptance of a relative's kidney are explored and inquiry made as to the responses within the extended family towards the potential transplant.

The donor is assessed in the context of family milieu and intrapsychic adjustment.[4] Significant factors affecting donation, such as motivation, spouse and family attitudes, employment, and economic status are explored. Previous psychiatric histories are of major importance and a recommendation for a psychiatric consultation will be made if there appears a possibility that kidney donation might exacerbate an already labile mental status. A routine MMPI is performed on every potential donor and collaboration with the psychologist and the psychiatrist can facilitate the social work role in working with the donor. The assessment interview serves a dual purpose. In addition to gathering psychosocial information, the donor is given the opportunity to share feelings and fantasies about the donation without fear of judgement. The social worker must achieve complete objectivity in this interview and be able to provide support without influencing the donor in any way.

By combining the findings of the recipient and donor assessments, much can be learned about the family dynamics surrounding the transplant. Ignorance, conflict, and anxiety can be identified. Meetings with families experiencing these problems to offer information and to provide opportunity for ventilation of feelings have proved very helpful in achieving a stable emotional background to the transplant.

All relevant information surrounding potential related transplants is communicated to the team via team meetings and written assessments. In cases where we anticipate specific psychosocial problems during the transplant process the social worker will meet with the nursing staff to discuss approaches to management, and ongoing consultation with the team is maintained.

Treatment of Psychosocial Pretransplant Problems

The need for pretransplant counseling resulting from assessment findings is agreed on as necessary by the recipient, donor, family members, and social worker. An example of pretransplant counseling is illustrated by the following case history.

> Mrs. D., a 29-year-old married woman, fourth in a line of eight siblings was referred to the transplant unit from a peripheral hospital after 3 years on hemodialysis. Her youngest sister was the only volunteer donor in the family and was found medically suitable. Mrs. D., the recipient, gave a history of emotional deprivation during childhood due to having been raised in a home where both parents drank heavily and where she was physically abused by her mother until her late teens. Ten years later the relationship with her mother was still poor. The recipient and donor assessments revealed serious family conflict regarding the potential transplant, including hostility on the mother's part towards her youngest daughter's wish to donate. Despite protestation from donor and recipient that the transplant was "their business" the conflict mainfested itself in telephone calls from the mother to other family members asking them to put pressure on the donor to change her mind. The recipient received abusive calls pressuring her to refuse the kidney. The recipient, already anxious about the transplant, became increasingly distressed, expressed guilt feelings, and questioned her original decision to accept her sister's kidney. Admission to the hospital provided a secure environment and she received daily individual counseling for 1 week. She was able to develop some insight into her mother's behavior and the reactions within the family. She was also introduced to a donor who had given a kidney to his brother 4 days earlier and who provided her with support and positive feedback which reduced Mrs. D.'s guilt feelings related to "donor suffering." The nephrologist and social worker invited the extended family to a meeting to discuss the transplant. The parents and one sister attended. All three were apprehensive and distrustful and required detailed explanations of the risks, procedure, and prognosis of the transplant. Following this meeting the phone calls ceased. The mother was seen once individually and the dynamics of her feelings explored. On the day of the transplant she expressed an appropriate concern and was supportive to both daughters postoperatively.

This case illustrates the importance of pretransplant counseling resulting from assessment findings. Failure to have dealt with this situation would have resulted in continuing disorganization with this family and traumatization of recipient and donor.

POSTTRANSPLANT COUNSELING

The posttransplant role of the social worker involves:

1. Provision of emotional support for family members.
2. Counseling with donor and recipient.
3. Team consultation.

Provision of Emotional Support for Family Members

On the day of the transplant the social worker is, whenever possible, available to the extended family for emotional support. One or two short meetings with them during the time that the donor and recipient are in the operating room provides opportunity for ventilation of anxiety. Even families who are normally self-sufficient experience a very high stress level at this time and reach out for support. The social worker needs to be flexible in intervention during the transplant process, leaving families to cope alone when able, but reinitiating contact when medical or social crises occur.

Counseling with the Donor and Recipient

Although most posttransplant counseling is done individually with recipient and donor they cannot be considered in isolation from one another. The first rejection episode will commonly occur on the sixth posttransplant day. The donor will still be in the hospital. At this point family and staff attention commonly shifts to the recipient who will require support. The donor often feels left out and forgotten[5] and it is important for the social worker to validate the donor's actions at this time and to help him or her deal with the anxiety about the future of the kidney. In the Southwestern Ontario transplant center, recipients and donors are nursed on the same floor and communication by bedside telephone and visiting is encouraged. This usually results in healthy and happy interaction and the strengthening of relationships between donor and recipient are frequently observed.

Group interaction can also provide effective support for transplant recipients. I am currently running a weekly group for recipients of cadaver and live–related kidneys. This group is open-ended and available to those recipients who are in the hospital recovering from transplant

surgery or who have been readmitted while experiencing kidney rejection or other medical complications. Each patient brings a different treatment experience to the group which can be led in a flexible way to provide an educational, problem-solving, or support focus—whichever is
the most appropriate for the members of the group in a particular week.

Team Consultation

Posttransplant counseling is approached holistically and involves
team consultation. The following case history of the unit's first transplant between two adolescents is of interest in the challenge it presented
to the team in postoperative management.

> Patricia B., a 14-year-old girl who had been on hemodialysis for 6 months,
> was referred from a peripheral hospital for a live–related transplant from her
> sister, Diane, aged 18. The recipient was an attractive, outgoing, well-
> adjusted teenager, as yet untouched emotionally by her disease and showing
> little outward signs of uremia. The potential donor was, in contrast, over-
> weight, sullen, and withdrawn. She had come to us for donor work-up with
> a documented history of alcoholism and drug abuse and had been dis-
> charged from an addiction treatment center 12 months previously. In the as-
> sessment interview Diane could not express any motivation for offering her
> sister a kidney. She did not feel close to her and denied coercion from her
> parents. She had "just heard about donating kidneys and thought it might be
> a good idea." There was complete denial of any risk and anxiety connected
> with the surgery. Diane was strongly critical of her parents, particularly her
> father, on whom she blamed her past difficulties. On the ward she was
> seductive in her behavior and attempted to avoid any situation (such as an
> appointment with the psychiatrist) which would involve confrontation. Fol-
> lowing my assessment, Diane was seen individually and with her family by
> the psychiatrist. The parents displayed strong denial of the seriousness of the
> situation,[6] felt that Diane might derive positive emotional gains from don-
> ating her kidney, and wished the transplant to take place. Diane was diag-
> nosed as a sociopathic personality and is an interesting example of "a black
> sheep donor." The sisters were HLA identical, the transplant was likely to
> succeed, and the psychiatrist would not say there was a psychiatric contrain-
> dication to using Diane as a donor. He did, however, recommend psycho-
> therapy to prepare this family for the transplant which went ahead.
>
> Postoperatively, the recipient regressed and became very demanding of
> staff attention. Diane, initially fussed over by her parents, was soon virtually
> ignored by them. She became depressed,[7] cried a great deal, and expressed
> her disappointment that Patricia had not thanked her for her kidney. In-
> stead, Patricia telephoned Diane numerous times during the day to complain
> of her various symptoms, symptoms which were promptly duplicated by
> Diane with unfailing regularity. One evening the sisters both pulled off their
> dressings 3 times in a few hours. The psychiatrist and social worker met with
> the nursing staff to interpret this behavior and to assist in formulating a care
> plan which would provide supportive structure and reduce the possibility of
> manipulation. The mother was asked to stay in a boarding home near the

hospital to facilitate daily visiting, but after years of being a housewife she had taken a full-time job. The father visited infrequently because of "pressures at work." Both denied the stress which their daughters were experiencing. The social worker met individually with the sisters on a daily basis and a joint session was held when the girls were encouraged to express their feelings about the transplant. Patricia could not express herself as an individual. She talked of "we" rather than "I" and referred to "our" kidney. She also expressed anxiety about her sister's impending discharge from hospital. Diane regretted having to separate from her but was pleased she would be leaving her kidney behind "to take care of Patricia." Patricia was carefully prepared for the separation from Diane. To alleviate her anxiety, the social worker arranged a tutor for the recipient and daily diversional therapy. She was counseled daily and the sisters talked on the telephone until Diane was well enough to visit, which she did, usually without her parents. This symbiotic relationship which developed between the sisters postoperatively proved to be of a temporary nature and Patricia remained in the hospital for another month with no further behavioral difficulties. A year later the donor had resumed full-time education and reported positive feelings about the donation.

Once out of hospital the goal for donor and recipient is "total" rehabilitation. For the donor this rarely proves a problem. All 25 donors with which I have been involved have returned to their previous occupations by 8 weeks postdonor nephrectomy. In the event of the rejection of a live–related kidney the unit philosophy is to offer emotional support to the donor, recipient, and family.

For the recipient, a successful transplant does not necessarily mean the end of physical, emotional, and economic difficulties. The patient's premorbid personality, the transition from the sick to the well role, and the expectations of family, society, and the health care team play a large part in the success or failure of rehabilitation.[8] The social worker will reassess counseling needs after the recipient is discharged from hospital and continue to work with high-risk patients on the psychosocial issues which are likely to affect reintegration into the family and society.

SUMMARY

Live–related transplantation is a stressful experience for recipients, donors, and families. Left untreated this stress can result in disorganization in families and trauma to recipients and donors. Communication should be opened up at all levels and orientation provided for the participants. The dynamics of this treatment modality require careful identification through psychosocial evaluation. Identified problems should be treated before and after transplantation and generous support provided for all concerned. In carrying out this role in collaboration with the team, the nephrology social worker makes a unique contribution to the total care of this patient population and is instrumental in the prevention and alleviation of psychosocial crises which can be seriously damaging to the transplant process.

REFERENCES

1. KEMPH, J. P. Psychotherapy with donors and recipients of kidney transplants. *Seminars in Psychiatry*, 1971, *3*(1), 145–158.
2. SIMMONS, R. G., KLEIN, S. D., and SIMMONS, R. L. *The gift of life*, New York: John Wiley and Sons, 1977.
3. HIRVAS, J. Psychological and social problems encountered in active treatment of chronic uremia, II. The living donor. *Acta Medical Scandanavia*, 1976, *200*, 17–20.
4. WHATLEY, L. W. Social work with potential donors for renal transplants. *Social Casework*, July 1972, *53*, 399–403.
5. SCHUMANN, D. The renal donor. *American Journal of Nursing*, 1974, *74*(1), 105–110.
6. CAIN, P. L. Casework with kidney transplant patients. *Social Work*, 1973, *18*, 76–83.
7. WENZL, J. E. Preparation of the patient and family for renal transplantation from a related donor. *Journal of Clinical Child Psychology*, 1975, *4*(3), 41–43.
8. SIMMONS, R. G. Social and psychological adjustment of adult post transplant patients. In E. A. Friedman (Ed.), *Strategy in renal failure*. New York: John Wiley and Sons, 1978, pp. 463–482.

24

Long-Term Reactions of Renal Recipients and Donors

ROBERTA G. SIMMONS

Questions of the quality of life of transplant *recipients* and the ethics of related *donation* remain important issues, even as these therapies become more routine.[1] Originally, when the federal HR-1 legislation to pay for transplantation and dialysis went into effect it was estimated that 70% of ESRD patients would be treated with kidney transplantation.[2] However, in 1979, only 8.6% of those treated have received a transplant; the vast majority of patients are receiving dialysis.[3] While there is much controversy as to the reasons for this low rate (perhaps it is simply that the new higher-risk patients being treated are too old or otherwise unsuitable for transplantation), many nephrologists have questioned whether the quality of life after transplantation is in fact as good as originally heralded.[1,4-8]

In addition, despite cadaver shortages and a history of higher success rates among recipients of kidneys from relatives, only 28% of transplants in the U.S. in 1979 had utilized the related donor.[3] Ethical questions remain—particularly questions as to the original willingness and long-term feelings of related donors.

Our earlier work[9,10] pointed to high levels of adjustment among successful transplant recipients 1 year after transplantation and to very positive reactions of living–related donors at the same time. However, it is possible that this positive level of adjustment is temporary. In fact Reichsman and Levy[11] have identified a "honeymoon period" among patients shortly after entering dialysis. Because these patients suddenly feel healthier, they experience relief. But this relief disappears with time as all the limitations of being on dialysis become more salient. The question is whether with time transplant patients also become disenchanted

ROBERTA G. SIMMONS, PH.D. • Professor of Sociology and Psychiatry, University of Minnesota, Minneapolis, Minnesota.
This work is supported in part by National Institute of Mental Health Grant 2K02-MH41688 and National Institute of Arthritis, Metabolism, and Digestive Diseases Grants 9R01-AM28618 and USPHS 5P01-AM13083 and NIMH 1R01-MH31249.

and whether their long-term adjustment deteriorates. Even up to a year after transplantation, patients used as a constant reference point the pretransplant period when many of them felt extremely ill and in danger of death. Against this comparison, their level of physical health at a year after the transplant is frequently cause for gratitude and even elation. With the further passage of time, does the pretransplant reference point fade along with feelings of physical and emotional well-being? Do long-term side effects become more important to the patient's self-evaluation? Similarly, once the recipient's new "health" can be taken for granted or once long-term side effects appear does the related donor react more negatively to his own loss of a body part?

It is the purpose of this research to begin to answer some of these questions. We have followed a cohort of patients transplanted between 1970 and 1973 to 1978–1980—that is, 5–9 years after transplantation.[12,13] Their live–related donors have also been studied.[14-16]

METHOD

Recipients

The total population of patients transplanted between 1970 and 1973 were followed (237 patients: 192 nondiabetics and 45 diabetics). Survey interviews were administered at 4 points in time: shortly before the transplant, 3 weeks after the transplant, 1 year after the transplant, and 5–9 years after the transplant. The data presented here focus on all the surviving adults (age 16 and older) who agreed to be interviewed 5–9 years after transplantation. This sample consisted of 148 patients: 123 nondiabetics and 25 diabetics. These last interviews were conducted in 1978–1980 at a time predetermined by the original month of the transplant. The small number of diabetic patients (due to their lesser likelihood of survival) renders our conclusions about this group more tentative.

The survey interview contained both (1) quantitative multiple-choice measures and scales and (2) open-ended in-depth segments. In terms of the quantitative information, self-esteem and depression scales were derived from well-known sources[17] and constructed from many multiple-choice items.

These same exact measures and scales were used at all four points in time and have been extensively described in prior publications.[9] It should be noted here, however, that score points on these scales have a relative rather than an absolute meaning. For example, there is no particular score on the depression scale that alerts us to pathological levels of depression in an individual; rather, groups of patients can be compared to one another to see in which group levels of depression are more unfavorable: diabetics can be compared to nondiabetics, pretransplant patients to themselves after transplantation. These scales then were not developed to be used as psychiatric diagnostic instruments on individuals, but rather as yardsticks with which to compare quality of life among subgroups. For the scales, reliability was satisfactory as measured by Cronbach's alpha, and the self-esteem scale has been extensively validated.[9] Where proportions are presented, tests of significance are based on chi-square analyses.

Donors

All 150 live–related donors used from 1970 to 1973 at the University of Minnesota constitute the population to be investigated. Of these, 135 were reachable and agreed to be interviewed 5–9 years after transplantation: 85 were "successful donors" in that their kidney was still functioning, and 50 were "unsuccessful" since the recipient had rejected the kidney and/or died. This same cohort of donors had been interviewed previously: before transplantation, 5 days after transplantation, and 1 year after transplantation. A control group of relatives ("nondonors") who did not volunteer to donate their kidneys, although they could have done so, were also interviewed at two points in time. Shortly after transplantation all such available relatives (186) were interviewed; at 5–9 years after transplantation, only one nondonor per family (randomly selected) was interviewed ($N=65$). The survey interview used, took from 45 minutes to approximately 1 hour and contained both (1) quantitative multiple-choice measures and scales and (2) open-ended segments.

FINDINGS

Recipients

Quality of life or rehabilitation are in themselves imprecise concepts and therefore have been conceptualized here into three major dimensions and multiple specific subdimensions (see Table 1). The three major dimensions are physical, emotional, and social well-being, and we focus on each in turn.

Physical Well-Being 5–9 Years after Transplantation

The vast majority of patients originally transplanted between 1970 and 1973 are still alive with high levels of graft survival. In our total co-

Table 1
Dimensions of Adjustment

Physical well-being
  Global feelings of well-being
  Symptoms of illness—frequency
  Ability to perform daily activities
Emotional well-being
  Happiness level
  Self-image level
    Self-esteem
    Stability of the self-picture
    Self-consciousness
    Feelings of independence
    Feelings of control over one's destiny
    Sense of distinctiveness
    Preoccupation with self
    Satisfaction with body image
    Perceived opinion of significant others (perceived popularity)
  Anxiety level (Gross psychopathology and suicidal behavior)
Social well-being in major life roles
  Social life
    Satisfaction
    Participation
  Vocation or school adjustment
    Satisfaction
    Participation
Adjustment of other family members
  Family disruption
  Individual adjustment

hort of 237 patients, 71% of those with related donors and 47% of those with cadaver donors have their first kidney still functioning 5–9 years after transplantation; 81% of those with related donors and 58% of those with cadaver donors are still alive. According to several measures, however, diabetic patients are doing substantially less well than nondiabetic patients physically. Whereas only 28% of nondiabetic patients have been hospitalized in the past year, 61% of diabetic patients have been hospitalized ($p < 0.01$).

According to two independent coders (with disagreements resolved by a third independent coder), 32% of nondiabetic patients with functioning kidneys are in excellent condition, 50% are in moderately good condition with some significant physical complaints, 8% are in poor condition, and 10% are chronically rejecting their kidneys. In contrast, no diabetic patients are in excellent condition, 56% are in moderately good condition, and 44% are in poor condition. Complications more common at 5–9 years after transplantation than earlier for nondiabetics appear to

TABLE 2
Percent of Patients Experiencing Difficulty with Daily Activities[a,b]

Activities	Nondiabetics			Diabetics		
	Pre-transplant (139)	1 year post-transplant (124)	5–9 years post-transplant (113)	Pre-transplant (38)	1 year post-transplant (32)	5–9 years post-transplant (25)
Getting out of bed	16%	7%	8%[d]	44%	6%	12%[c]
Walking[e]	41%	28%	31%	86%	52%	72%
Dressing	12%	5%	6%	56%	10%	12%[c]
Housework (women)	70%	27%	23%[c]	100%	31%	55%[c]
Lifting heavy objects	73%	44%	47%[c]	89%	81%	68%[d]
Eyesight	36%	41%	43%	83%	87%	96
Shopping	47%	12%	16%[c]	82%	52%	64%

[a]Patients 1-year after transplantation and 5–9 years after transplantation who have functioning kidney.
[b]Patients were asked "In which of the following activities do you have difficulty due to your health now? I will read you a list and you tell me if you have any difficulties with the activities due to your health."
[c]$p < 0.05$.
[d]$p < 0.10$.
[e]At 5–9 years after transplantation, there were no nondiabetics unable to walk, although three diabetics were confined to a wheelchair.

be arthritis, cataracts, fragile and easily broken bones, knee and hip replacements, hearing problems, skin cancer, skin bruising and tearing, steroid-induced diabetes, and heart problems. A person in "moderately good health" might suffer from one of these significant complications, but not to a debilitating extent.

For both diabetic and nondiabetic patients with functioning kidneys, all measured symptoms of kidney disease (nausea, weakness, headaches, tiredness, edema) have been dramatically and significantly reduced since the pretransplant period ($p < 0.05$ in all cases). Similarly, difficulties with daily activities (difficulty getting out of bed, with walking, dressing, housework, lifting heavy objects, shopping) have been substantially reduced for both diabetic and nondiabetic patients (Table 2). For example, 70% of nondiabetic women had difficulty with housework before transplantation compared to 23% 5–9 years after transplantation ($p < 0.05$); 73% of nondiabetic men and women had difficulty lifting heavy objects before transplantation compared to 47% 5–9 years after transplantation ($p < 0.05$). However, despite improvement, on almost all measures diabetic patients do substantially less well than nondiabetics and along some dimensions (walking, housework, eyesight, shopping) there is some loss from the 1-year posttransplant period.

One major problem with the diabetic patients transplanted in the period between 1970 and 1973 involves their eyesight. Almost all the diabetic patients have some eyesight problems with 15 out of 25 either totally blind, legally blind, or severely handicapped visually.

Emotional Well-Being

The same pattern of findings is reproduced for the several dimensions of emotional well-being, with both diabetics and nondiabetics showing improvement between the pretransplant and 5–9 years posttransplant period, and with nondiabetics doing better than diabetics. Before turning to the quantitative evidence for such assertions, we should look at the following quotations from nondiabetic patients as examples of the range of emotional and physical adjustment 5–9 years after transplantation. These examples also point to the interconnection of the emotional and physical realms. Two quotations from nondiabetic patients in excellent health and two others from nondiabetics in poor health illustrate the range of emotional and physical adjustment:

Excellent Health

CASE 1—I never realized I'd be able to return to full-time work as I have without any problems whatsoever. I've had no problems whatsoever since the day of the transplant.

CASE 2—I feel very grateful. I can't be thankful or grateful enough. I live and fulfill every day. I appreciate it and make it worthwhile.

Poor Health

CASE 3—I can't do things I did before. [I used to] always work . . . I was doing something all the time. Now I can't do nothing . . . I used to hunt and fish a lot and I can't do that anymore. I had to give up my ways. (This patient had a broken hip and a joint replacement, edema, pneumonia, and hearing difficulties.)

CASE 4—I can move around, there are some things I can do but everything is an effort, even taking a bath or washing my hair. (This patient had had a heart attack, mastectomy, cataracts, hypothyroidism, broken foot and ribs, shingles, edema, and suffered from fatigue.)

Table 3 shows the scores of the patients with functioning kidneys on the major sociopsychological scales of adjustment. The proportion scoring at the favorable end of the scale is presented. Both nondiabetic and diabetic patiens show considerable improvement from the pretransplant period in self-esteem, independence, and feelings of control over their own destiny. For example, 66% of nondiabetic patients score high in self-esteem 5–9 years after transplantation compared to only 35% who scored this high before transplantation ($p < 0.01$). In addition, both nondiabetic and diabetic patients show reductions in depression, in self-preoccupation, and in anxiety (that is, they are more likely

TABLE 3
Adjustment of Nondiabetic and Diabetic Patients on Social–Psychological Scales:
Proportion Scoring at Favorable End of Scales[a]

Psychological scales	Nondiabetics			Diabetics		
	Pre-transplant (139)	1 year post-transplant (124)	5–9 years post-transplant (113)	Pre-transplant (38)	1 year post-transplant (32)	5–9 years post-transplant (25)
High in self-esteem[e]	35%	59%	66%[b]	33%	55%	48%
High in independence	19%	80%	71%[b]	9%	50%	38%[c]
High in feeling of control over one's own destiny[e]	22%	68%	57%[b]	16%	46%	42%[d]
High in stability of self, sense of firm identity[e]	57%	61%	61%	37%	63%	50%
Low in preoccupation with oneself	22%	59%	68%[b]	24%	47%	54%
Low in depression	37%	81%	71%[b]	9%	72%	48%[b]
Low in anxiety	36%	58%	45%	32%	57%	40%

[a]Patients 1 year and 5–9 years after transplantation who have functioning kidney.
[b]$p < 0.01$.
[c]$p \leq .05$.
[d]$p \leq .10$.
[e]Nine item long-term recipient self-esteem scale (SERECS9), corrected independence, control-over-destiny, and stability scales.

to score at the low or favorable end of these scales now than they were before transplantation).

Once again, the diabetic patients are less likely than the nondiabetic patients to score at the favorable end of these scales. For example, 66% of the nondiabetics show high self-esteem 5–9 years after transplantation compared to only 48% of the diabetics. Finally, diabetics appear particularly likely to have had an unfavorable turn in depression since the 1-year posttransplant period (only 48% now score low in depression compared to fully 72% at 1 year), although they are still far better off than they were before transplantation (when only 9% scored low in depression).

Social Well-Being

The major dimension of rehabilitation used in most studies is vocational rehabilitation. As is obvious from this presentation, in our concep-

TABLE 4
Vocational Rehabilitation: Proportion Working or in School[a]

Time period	Male patients		Female patients	
	Nondiabetic	Diabetic	Nondiabetic	Diabetic
Before the disease	99%	100%	74%	76%
became serious	(71)	(21)	(66)	(17)
In the year prior	83%	67%	49%	47%
to the transplant	(71)	(21)	(63)	(17)
1 year after	88%	44%	44%	27%
the transplant	(56)	(18)	(64)	(15)
5–9 years after	82%	23%[b]	57%	33%
the transplant	(54)	(13)	(47)	(12)

[a]Patients 1 year after transplantation and 5–9 years after transplantation below age 62, with functioning kidneys.
[b]The difference between recipients the year prior to the transplant and 5–9 years after transplantation is significant; $p < 0.05$.

tion vocational rehabilitation is but one dimension of quality of life. Nevertheless, it is an important dimension. Table 4 shows that 82% of nondiabetic males, but only 23% of diabetic males, are working or in school at 5–9 years after transplantation. For the diabetic patients, these figures represent a major loss since the pretransplant period and a smaller loss since 1 year after transplantation. Most (76%) of the nondiabetic males are not only working or in school but are doing so full time. Also, 57% of the nondiabetic females are working or in school.

Patients were also asked about their satisfaction or dissatisfaction with their major life roles—their job situation, recreation, social life, relations with friends, and their role as a spouse and parent. Along all dimensions we see the same pattern we reported above for physical and emotional adjustment: Both diabetics and nondiabetics indicate much less dissatisfaction at 5–9 years after transplantation than during the pretransplant period ($p < 0.05$ in most cases for nondiabetics). Once again, diabetics usually indicate more dissatisfaction than do nondiabetics (for example, in terms of recreation: 48% versus 17%). Diabetics, but not nondiabetics, indicate a loss along these dimensions since the 1-year posttransplant period, although they still score more favorably than they did before transplantation.

Finally, impotence among male end-stage kidney patients has been noted as a major problem.[18] Table 5 indicates a steady improvement in sexual performance over time among married, nondiabetic male patients with functioning kidneys. At 5–9 years after transplantation 69% report no difficulty with sexual performance compared to only 19% before transplantation. Despite this substantial improvement, a sizeable minority (22%) of these 5–9 years posttransplant males are still reporting "a lot

TABLE 5
Impotence in Nondiabetic Married Male Patients

Difficulty with sexual performance	Pre- transplant	1 year posttransplant	5–9 years posttransplant
A lot	39%	28%	22%
Some	42%	16%	8%
No difficulty	19%	56%	69%
	100%	100%	100%
	(31)	(32)	(36)

[a]Patients were asked, "In the past couple of months, have you had a lot of difficulty with sexual performance, some difficulty, or no difficulty?"
[b]The difference between recipients the year prior to the transplant and 5–9 years after transplantation is significant; $p < 0.05$.

of difficulty." (There were not enough cases of male, married diabetics to examine them separately.)

Summary

The vast majority of patients originally transplanted between 1970 and 1973 at the University of Minnesota are still alive with high levels of graft survival. This study examined the quality of life of 123 nondiabetic and 25 diabetic patients 5–9 years after transplantation. Among nondiabetic patients, levels of physical, emotional, and social well-being have improved substantially and significantly since the pretransplant period and have remained about the same as at the 1-year posttransplant period although only one-third are rated in excellent health without a significant health complaint. Four-fifths of the nondiabetic males are working or in school (most of these full time); and males show considerably less sexual impotency 5–9 years after transplantation than before transplantation. The diabetic patients, despite considerable improvements since the pretransplant period, are less well-off than the nondiabetics along most dimensions and frequently show a loss since the 1-year posttransplant period. None of the diabetics are rated in excellent health, virtually all have eyesight problems, and only 23% of the males are working or in school.

Future analyses will focus on characteristics of the patients which affect their adjustment, other than those dealt with here.

Donors

The central ethical issue here is whether the psychological costs to the donor are too great to recommend related donation. The major theoretical question involves the effect extreme family altruism has upon individuals. In our original study of these donors,[9] we reported that family members were surprisingly willing to make this major sacrifice: 57% of all potential family donors in this population volunteered to donate and had their blood tested. How did they feel 5–9 years after transplantation?

First of all, to what extent were there negative feelings and regrets? Findings will be reported both for donors whose donated kidneys are still functioning in the recipient ("successful" donors) and for those whose kidneys were rejected or whose recipients died ("unsuccessful" donors).

At 5–9 years after transplantation the majority of long-term donors, both successful and unsuccessful, report positive attitudes and little regret, although regret is slightly more common among unsuccessful donors (12% versus 8%). Unsuccessful donors are also more likely than successful ones to report difficulty in their relationship with the recipient (18% versus 5%, $p < 0.01$) and less likely to indicate special closeness to the recipient (23% versus 40%, $p < 0.05$). Thus, negative reactions to donation are rare but not absent.

On the other hand, there is some evidence of psychological benefit from donation of a kidney. Table 6 shows that the mean self-esteem on the Rosenberg Self-Esteem Scale is significantly higher among donors after transplantation than before transplantation. Also, the donors score higher in self-esteem than the control group of nondonors at both points in time after transplantation. There is no significant difference in self-esteem 5–9 years after transplantation between successful and unsuccessful donors. However, in both successful and unsuccessful cases, donors show higher self-esteem than the control group of nondonors. The in-depth material from the donor is consistent with these indications of high donor self-esteem:

DONOR: It isn't a daily or a weekly thought. It's nonetheless kind of familiar. I'll remember it maybe when I'm having doubts about myself or analyzing myself in my introspective moods. It comes to mind . . . It's a tangible, quantifiable evidence of something I've done that I'm proud of. Sometimes if you've done a series of things wrong or for any reason you start to develop doubts about your own worth you say, "Wait a minute. I'm not all bad."

Clearly, relative to other family members, donation has not harmed the self-image and there is indication it may have helped.

In addition, after transplantation, donors are more likely to score favorably on a widely used measure of depressive-affect than are normal control groups. Approximately 30–37% of control groups from large-scale surveys ($N = 1460, 1501, 2460$) score favorably, that is, low in depression, on this measure.[19] Donors prior to the transplant score within this same range, as do normal controls from the Minneapolis region;

TABLE 6
Mean Self-Esteem[a] among Donors and Nondonors

	Donors	Nondonors
Pretransplant	4.34	
Shortly after transplantation	4.80[c]	3.58[b]
One year posttransplant successful	4.60	
Total 5–9 years post-transplant	5.08[d]	4.78

[a]9-item corrected scale, unrecoded.
[b]The difference between donors and nondonors is significant: $p < 0.001$.
[c]$p = 0.08$.
[d]$p = 0.01$.

nondonor controls also score close to this range at both times measured. However, at a year after transplantation donors are much more likely than all of these groups to score favorably, that is, low in depressive-affect: 60% of them do so, and 5–9 years after transplantation the proportion is 49%. The difference between donors and family nondonors is significant shortly after transplantation (60% versus 26%, $p < 0.001$) and at 5–9 years after transplantation (49% versus 34%, $p < 0.10$). Evidence of increased exhilaration among donors, *when the donation is made salient*, is further evidenced in the qualitative material:

FIRST DONOR (SON): Hey! I feel wonderful seeing Mom walk around and doing so much. I know I really did something for somebody and I feel good about it.
* * * *

SECOND DONOR (MOTHER): To me it was like I gave birth to him once and I gave birth to him a second time. It was like giving him life.
* * * *

INTERVIEWER TO THIRD DONOR: What words would you use to describe a living relative who donates a kidney?
DONOR(SISTER): It's a wonderful feeling, that's all.
* * * *

Finally, donors are significantly more likely than nondonors to report close relationships with recipients 5–9 years after transplantation (62% versus 37%, $p < 0.05$).

Summary

In summary most live-related donors maintain positive feelings about the donation and demonstrate greater closeness to the recipient than do nondonors. The majority of donors whose kidneys have not survived also maintain positive attitudes, although regret and lower levels of closeness to the recipient are somewhat more common in this group. Related donors show higher levels of self-esteem and lower levels of depressive-affect 5–9 years after transplantation (1) than they demonstrated themselves prior to the transplant and (2) than control groups of nondonors.

CONCLUSION

In conclusion, the reactions of both recipients and related donors remain relatively positive 5–9 years after transplantation. The live–related donors continue to report closer relations with the recipient than do other family members, and, at least when the transplant is made salient, levels of self-esteem seem relatively high overall and levels of depression low. Although there are differences among individuals, the evidence does not indicate that donors by and large are depressed and regretful over the loss of a body part. In fact, there are indications that for some donors, the fact of donation provides a boost for the self-image and an elation because of the increased health of a close family member. These findings are consistent with our earlier reports for these same donors[9] and with reports of other investigators.[20-22] For the majority of individuals studied here, altruism appears to have more psychological benefits than costs.

The recipients whose kidneys are still functioning show considerable improvement in quality of life since the pretransplant period. Nevertheless, the health of the majority is not equal to that of a normal population and certain complications are more frequent over the long term. Sexual potency for males, while markedly improved, still remains a considerable problem for a sizeable minority. Diabetic patients, despite improvement, remain a group whose quality of life is considerably compromised.

Comparison of the quality of life of transplant patients and patients undergoing alternate therapies (hemodialysis, CAPD) must await studies that compare them with the same social–psychological measurements. Such studies are badly needed.

REFERENCES

1. SIMMONS, R. G., and CROSNIER, J. (Co-Chair). Workshop—Ethical and social considerations in transplantation. *Proceedings of the VIII International Congress of the Transplantation Society*, 1981, 13, 1281–1283.
2. NATIONAL KIDNEY FOUNDATION. Position paper—Guidelines for the implication of public law 92-603, Title II, Section 2991 concerned with chronic kidney disease. April, 1973.
3. Health Care Financing Administration. Office of Special Programs End-Stage Renal Disease Second Annual Report to Congress FY 1980, Department of Health and Human Services, H. C. F. A., Figure 2, p. 2.
4. KEMPH, J. P. The kidney or the machine? *Journal of the American Medical Association*, June 6, 1977, 237, 2532.

5. KEMPH, J. P. Letters to the editor—Dialysis vs. transplant. *Journal of the American Medical Association*, Feb. 27, 1978, *239*, 830.

6. HOWARD, R. J., KJELLSTRAND, C. M., SUTHERLAND, D. E. R., and NAJARIAN, J. S. Letters to the editor—Dialysis vs. transplant. *Journal of the American Medical Association*, Feb. 27, 1978, *239*, 830.

7. HOWARD, R. J., and NAJARIAN, J. S. Letters to the editor—Dialysis vs. transplant. *Journal of the American Medical Association*, June 23, 1978, *239*, 2656.

8. JONASSON, O. Letters to the editor—Dialysis vs. Transplant. *Journal of the American Medical Association*, June 23, 1978, *239*, 2655–2657.

9. SIMMONS, R. G., KLEIN, S. D., and SIMMONS, R. L. *Gift of life: The social and psychological impact of organ transplantation.* New York: Wiley Interscience, 1977.

10. SIMMONS, R. G. Psychological reactions to giving a kidney. In N. B. Levy (Ed.), *Psychonephrology 1: Psychological factors in hemodialysis and transplantation.* New York: Plenum Publishing, 1981, pp. 227–245.

11. REICHSMAN, F., and LEVY, N. B. Problems in adaptation to maintenance hemodialysis. A four-year study of 25 patients. In N. B. Levy (Ed.), *Living or dying: Adaptation to hemodialysis.* Springfield, Ill.: Charles C. Thomas, 1974, pp. 30–49.

12. SIMMONS, R. G. Rehabilitation of renal patients: Issues of controversy. In G. E. Schreiner (Ed.), *Controversies in nephrology, 1979.* Washington, D.C.: Georgetown University, Nephrology Division, 1979, pp. 191–201.

13. SIMMONS, R. G., KAMSTRA-HENNEN, L., and THOMPSON, C. R. Psycho–social adjustment five to nine years post-transplant. *Proceedings of the VIII International Congress of the Transplantation Society*, 1981, *13*, 40–43.

14. SIMMONS, R. G., and KAMSTRA-HENNEN, L. The living related kidney donor: Psychological reactions when the kidney fails. *Dialysis and Transplantation*, 1979, *8*, 572–574.

15. KAMSTRA-HENNEN, L., and SIMMONS, R. G. Ethics of related donation: The unsuccessful case. *Proceedings of the Clinical Dialysis and Transplant Forum*, 1978, *8*, 25–29.

16. KAMSTRA-HENNEN, L., BEEBE, J. STUMM, S., and SIMMONS, R. G. Ethical evaluation of related donation: The donor after five years. *Proceedings of the VIII International Congress of the Transplantation Society*, 1981, *13*, 60–61.

17. ROSENBERG, M. *Society and the adolescent self-image.* Princeton, New Jersey: Princeton University Press, 1965.

18. LEVY, N. B. Sexual dysfunctions of hemodialysis patients: Psychological factors and treatment. In G. E. Schreiner (Ed.), *Controversies in nephrology, 1979.* Washington, D.C.: Georgetown University, Nephrology Division, 1979, pp. 141–149.

19. BRADBURN, N. M. *The structure of psychological well-being.* Chicago: Aldine, 1965.

20. FELLNER, C. J. and MARSHALL, J. R. Twelve kidney donors. *Journal of the American Medical Association*, 1968, *206*, 2703–2707.

21. EISENDRATH, R. M. The role of grief and fear in the death of kidney transplant patients. *American Journal of Psychiatry*, 1969, *126*, 381–387.

22. SAMPSON, T. F. Level of adjustment in one or more year post-transplant and in-center dialysis patients. Presented at the 81st Annual American Psychological Association Convention, Montreal, Quebec, Canada, August, 1973.

Index

This Index was prepared by June G. Rosenberg, Information Consultant, Brooklyn, New York.